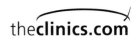

GASTROENTEROLOGY CLINICS OF NORTH AMERICA

Common Gastrointestinal and Hepatic Infections

GUEST EDITORS
Richard Goodgame, MD
David Y. Graham, MD

June 2006 • Volume 35 • Number 2

SAUNDERS
An Imprint of Elsevier, Inc.
PHILADELPHIA   LONDON   TORONTO   MONTREAL   SYDNEY   TOKYO

W.B. SAUNDERS COMPANY
A Division of Elsevier Inc.

Elsevier Inc. • 1600 John F. Kennedy Blvd., Suite 1800 • Philadelphia, Pennsylvania 19103-2899

http://www.theclinics.com

**GASTROENTEROLOGY CLINICS
OF NORTH AMERICA**
June 2006
Editor: Kerry Holland

Volume 35, Number 2
ISSN 0889-8553
ISBN 1-4160-3910-4

Reprints. For copies of 100 or more, of articles in this publication, please contact the Commercial Reprints Department, Elsevier Inc., 360 Part Avenue South, New York, New York 10010-1710. Tel. (212) 633-3813 Fax: (212) 462-1935 e-mail: reprints@elsevier.com.

The ideas and opinions expressed in *Gastroenterology Clinics of North America* do not necessarily reflect those of the Publisher. The Publisher does not assume any responsibility for any injury and/or damage to persons or property arising out of or related to any use of the material contained in this periodical. The reader is advised to check the appropriate medical literature and the product information currently provided by the manufacturer of each drug to be administered to verify the dosage, the method and duration of administration, or contraindications. It is the responsibility of the treating physician or other health care professional, relying on independent experience and knowledge of the patient, to determine drug dosages and the best treatment for the patient. Mention of any product in this issue should not be construed as endorsement by the contributors, editors, or the Publisher of the product or manufacturers' claims.

Gastroenterology Clinics of North America (ISSN 0889-8553) is published quarterly by W.B. Saunders, 360 Park Avenue South, New York, NY 10010-1710. Months of publication are March, June, September, and December. Business and Editorial Offices: 1600 John F. Kennedy Blvd., Suite 1800, Philadelphia, PA 19103-2899. Accounting and Circulation Offices: 6277 Sea Harbor Drive, Orlando, FL 32887-4800. Periodicals postage paid at New York, NY 10010, and additional mailing offices. Subscription prices are $195.00 per year (US individuals), $100.00 per year (US students), $290.00 per year (US institutions), $206.00 per year (Canadian individuals), $345.00 per year (Canadian institutions), $255.00 per year (international individuals), $130.00 per year (international students), and $345.00 per year (international institutions). Foreign air speed delivery is included in all *Clinics* subscription prices. All prices are subject to change without notice. POSTMASTER: Send address changes to *Gastroenterology Clinics of North America*, Elsevier Periodicals Customer Service 6277 Sea Harbor Drive, Orlando, FL 32887-4800. **Customer Service: 1-800-654-2452 (US). From outside of the US, call 1-407-345-4000. E-mail: hhspcs@harcourt.com**

Gastroenterology Clinics of North America is also published in Italian by Il Pensiero Scientifico Editore, Rome, Italy; and in Portuguese by Interlivros Edicoes Ltda., Rua Commandante Coelho 1085, 21250 Cordovil, Rio de Janeiro, Brazil.

Gastroenterology Clinics of North America is covered in *Index Medicus, Excerpta Medica, Current Contents/ Clinical Medicine, Science Citation Index, ISI/BIOMED,* and *BIOSIS*.

Printed in the United States of America.

GASTROENTEROLOGY CLINICS
OF NORTH AMERICA

Common Gastrointestinal and Hepatic Infections

GUEST EDITORS

RICHARD GOODGAME, MD, Professor, Department of Medicine, Baylor College of Medicine, Houston, Texas

DAVID Y. GRAHAM, MD, Professor, Department of Medicine, Baylor College of Medicine; Michael E. DeBakey Veterans Affairs Medical Center, Houston, Texas

CONTRIBUTORS

VICTOR ANKOMA-SEY, MD, Clinical Associate Professor, Department of Medicine, University of Texas Medical School, Houston, Texas

SAIMA ASLAM, MD, Medical Service (Infectious Disease Section), Michael E. DeBakey Veterans Affairs Medical Center; and Departments of Medicine, Molecular Virology and Microbiology, Baylor College of Medicine, Houston, Texas

ROBERT L. ATMAR, MD, Professor, Departments of Medicine, Molecular Virology & Microbiology, Baylor College of Medicine, Houston, Texas

PETER A. BANKS, MD, Professor, Department of Medicine, Harvard Medical School; and Director, Center for Pancreatic Disease, Division of Gastroenterology, Brigham and Women's Hospital, Boston, Massachusetts

TYLER M. BERZIN, MD, Clinical Fellow, Department of Medicine, Harvard Medical School; and Resident Physician, Department of Medicine, Brigham and Women's Hospital, Boston, Massachusetts

YONG U. CHOI, MD, Fellow, Minimally Invasive Surgery, Baylor College of Medicine, Houston, Texas

EDWARD P. DOMINGUEZ, MD, Fellow, Minimally Invasive Surgery, Baylor College of Medicine, Houston, Texas

HERBERT L. DUPONT, MD, FACP, Chief of Internal Medicine, St. Luke's Episcopal Hospital; Clinical Professor and Vice Chairman, Department of Medicine, Baylor College of Medicine; and Professor of Epidemiology and Director, Center for Infectious Diseases, University of Texas–Houston School of Public Health, Houston, Texas

MARY K. ESTES, PhD, Professor, Departments of Molecular Virology & Microbiology, Baylor College of Medicine, Houston, Texas

RICHARD GOODGAME, MD, Professor, Department of Medicine, Baylor College of Medicine, Houston, Texas

DAVID Y. GRAHAM, MD, Professor, Department of Medicine, Baylor College of Medicine; Michael E. DeBakey Veterans Affairs Medical Center, Houston, Texas

F. BLAINE HOLLINGER, MD, Professor of Medicine, Virology and Epidemiology, Departments of Medicine, Molecular Virology and Microbiology; and Director, Eugene B. Casey Hepatitis Research Center and Diagnostic Laboratory, Baylor College of Medicine, Houston, Texas

DAVID B. HUANG, MD, PhD, MPH, Assistant Professor, Division of Infectious Diseases, Department of Medicine, Baylor College of Medicine, Houston, Texas

ELIZABETH S. HUEBNER, MD, Fellow, Division of Gastroenterology, University of Washington School of Medicine, Seattle, Washington

DARYL T.-Y. LAU, MD, MSc, MPH, FRCP(C), Associate Professor of Medicine, Division of Gastroenterology and Hepatology, Department of Internal Medicine, The University of Texas Medical Branch at Galveston, Galveston, Texas; and Beth Israel Deaconess Medical Center, Harvard University, Boston, Massachusetts

VAROCHA MAHACHAI, MD, Associate Professor, Department of Medicine; and Chief, Division of Gastroenterology, Chulalongkorn University Hospital, Bangkok, Thailand

KOENRAAD J. MORTELE, MD, Associate Professor, Department of Radiology, Harvard Medical School; Associate Director, Division of Abdominal Imaging and Intervention; and Director, Division of Abdominal and Pelvic MRI, Department of Radiology, Brigham and Women's Hospital, Boston, Massachusetts

DANIEL M. MUSHER, MD, Medical Service (Infectious Disease Section), Michael E. DeBakey Veterans Affairs Medical Center; and Departments of Medicine, Molecular Virology and Microbiology, Baylor College of Medicine, Houston, Texas

WAQAR A. QURESHI, MD, FACG, FACP, Associate Professor, Department of Medicine; and Chief of Endoscopy, Department of Medicine, Baylor College of Medicine, Houston, Texas

HOMAYON SIDIQ, MD, Hepatology Fellow, St. Luke's Episcopal Hospital Center for Liver Disease, Houston, Texas

RISE STRIBLING, MD, Associate Professor, Departments of Medicine and Surgery; and Medical Director, Liver Transplantation, Baylor College of Medicine, Houston, Texas

CHRISTINA M. SURAWICZ, MD, Professor, Department of Medicine, University of Washington School of Medicine; and Section Chief, Gastroenterology, Harborview Medical Center, Seattle, Washington

NORMAN SUSSMAN, MD, Associate Professor, Departments of Medicine and Surgery; and Associate Medical Director, Liver Transplantatio, Baylor College of Medicine, Houston, Texas

JOHN F. SWEENEY, MD, Associate Professor, Department of Surgery, Baylor College of Medicine, Houston, Texas

JOHN M. VIERLING, MD, Chief of Hepatology; Director of Advanced Liver Therapies; and Director, Baylor Liver Health, Baylor College of Medicine, Houston, Texas

RATHA-KORN VILAICHONE, MD, PhD, Assistant Professor, Department of Medicine, Gastroenterology Unit, Thammasat University Hospital, Pathumthani, Thailand

A. CLINTON WHITE, MD, Professor, Division of Infectious Diseases, Department of Medicine, Baylor College of Medicine, Houston, Texas

GASTROENTEROLOGY CLINICS
OF NORTH AMERICA

Common Gastrointestinal and Hepatic Infections

CONTENTS

VOLUME 35 • NUMBER 2 • JUNE 2006

Helicobacter Pylori

Helicobacter pylori is a global human pathogen and the major cause of gastritis and the gastritis-associated diseases: gastric ulcer, duodenal ulcer, gastric cancer, and primary gastric B-cell lymphoma. Although several reliable diagnostic tests are widely available, the ideal regimen for treating the infection remains to be established. The current first-line or legacy triple therapy regimens fail in 20% to 40% of patients. Recent studies have confirmed older observations that the success rate of legacy triple regimens (proton pump inhibitor plus two antibiotics) can be improved if the duration is extended to 14 days or a third antibiotic is given. Confirmation of eradication using noninvasive diagnostic tests, such as a urea breath test or stool antigen assay, is now the standard of care.

Infectious Diarrhea

Acute infectious diarrhea is a yearly occurrence for most Americans. Up to 80% of cases of acute infectious diarrhea are caused by noroviruses, which produce a clinically mild illness with a predictable short course and good outcome. Most diarrhea-causing bacteria and protozoa can cause a clinical illness "like norovirus." The presence or absence of epidemiologic evidence (eg, travel, hospitalization, antibiotic use, other exposures) and clinical evidence (eg, diarrhea frequency and duration, severity of abdominal pain and fever, character of stool, presence of chronic illness or immune deficiency) can change the probability of "not norovirus" from as low as 8% to as high as 100%. Such probabilities guide the use of laboratory testing and antimicrobial therapy in patients who have acute infectious diarrhea.

Future approaches will be aimed at making host regions safer and providing more effective methods of treatment and prevention of enteric disease during short-term international travel.

Interest in the use of probiotics for the prevention and treatment of gastrointestinal infections has increased over the past few decades. Controlled trials support a role for probiotics in the prevention of antibiotic-associated diarrhea and in the treatment of recurrent *Clostridium difficile*–associated disease. In the pediatric population, controlled trials have shown efficacy in the prevention and treatment of acute diarrhea. Several studies have shown a suppressive effect of lactobacilli on *Helicobacter pylori*, and preliminary reports suggest that probiotics may decrease secondary infections in pancreatitis. Studies that evaluated their use for the prevention of traveler's diarrhea produced conflicting results. Additional trials are needed to define better the role of probiotics in the prevention and treatment of gastrointestinal diseases.

Diverticulitis and appendicitis are common infections of the gastrointestinal tract that require urgent medical and surgical attention. Successful management of these conditions requires a multidisciplinary approach among primary care providers, gastroenterologists, surgeons, and radiologists. The diagnosis of appendicitis, in particular, can be difficult. Advances in radiographic imaging have improved the diagnostic accuracy in these infections. Minimally invasive surgical techniques have improved the patient's postoperative recovery when surgery is necessary in the management of these conditions.

Pancreatic infection occurs most frequently in association with pancreatic necrosis, occasionally in extrapancreatic fluid collections and pancreatic pseudocysts, and rarely as a pancreatic abscess. It has been suggested that one half of deaths in acute pancreatitis are attributable to infected necrosis. The focus of this article is the recognition and management of pancreatic infections.

Acute bacterial cholangitis is a disease with substantial mortality. The two most important features are biliary obstruction and bacterial infection. It commonly presents with fever, jaundice, and right upper quadrant pain. Endoscopic decompression has become the cornerstone of management, although early diagnosis, prompt resuscitation, and antibiotics are required for successful treatment. Approaches to the successful management of this condition may vary but drainage is key to a positive outcome. Important decisions relating to the management of this condition include appropriate choice of antibiotics, imaging modalities before drainage, the timing and method of drainage, and the role of surgery.

Viral Infections of the Liver

Hepatitis B is a major public health problem in the world today. Since 1985, the number of reported cases has declined as a direct result of universal immunization of neonates, vaccination of at-risk populations, lifestyle or behavioral changes in high-risk groups, refinements in the screening of blood donors, and the use of virally inactivated or genetically engineered products in patients with bleeding disorders. New and potent antiviral agents being developed and evaluated provide hope and optimism for those who are chronically infected with hepatitis B virus. Prevention remains the most effective strategy in the global management of hepatitis B virus. Universal immunization programs prevent hepatitis B virus transmission and circumvent acute and chronic infection.

Approximately 175 million persons are infected chronically with the hepatitis C virus (HCV) worldwide, which causes chronic hepatitis, cirrhosis, liver failure, and hepatocellular carcinoma. The standard therapy for hepatitis C is a combination of pegylated interferon and ribavirin. The goal of therapy is a sustained virological response, defined as the absence of detectable HCV RNA at least 24 weeks after cessation of therapy. This article summarizes the treatment of chronic HCV infection, assesses the efficacy and safety of combination antiviral therapy for specific subsets of patients, and notes the new antiviral agents that are being introduced into clinical trials.

Homayon Sidiq and Victor Ankoma-Sey

Liver disease is an important cause of morbidity and mortality in persons who are infected with HIV-1. Myriad liver diseases occur in HIV-infected persons, including those that also affect non-HIV–infected counterparts (eg, hepatitis B and C, nonalcoholic steatohepatitis, alcoholic liver disease, drug-induced liver disease). Furthermore, rare opportunistic infections of the liver and biliary tree, including atypical mycobacterium, cryptosporidiosis, cytomegalovirus, and immunodeficiency-associated cancers with liver involvements (eg, lymphoma), can occur in HIV-infected individuals. This article focuses on HIV coinfections with hepatitis B and C and discusses antiretroviral-related liver toxicity, because these are common, but challenging, clinical issues.

GASTROENTEROLOGY CLINICS
OF NORTH AMERICA

GASTROENTEROLOGY CLINICS
OF NORTH AMERICA

ELSEVIER
SAUNDERS

PREFACE

Common Gastrointestinal and Hepatic Infections

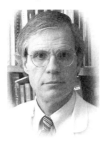 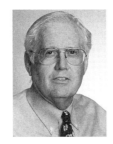

Richard Goodgame, MD
David Y. Graham, MD

Guest Editors

This issue is not about the rare, exotic, or seldom-visited gastrointestinal, hepatic, and pancreatic infections. It is about helping clinicians master some of most common and most significant "every day" infections of the gut, liver, and pancreas. Oliver Wendell Holmes said that we need education in the obvious more than investigation of the obscure. That has been our mantra. The goal of this issue is to present common gastrointestinal and hepatic infections with uncommon clarity, unusual practicality, and rare focus. Even familiar places are better understood with a set of carefully drawn maps and notes, and we thank each of the contributors for their outstanding efforts. We believe that many patients with these common infections will be well served.

For example, almost every American gets acute infectious diarrhea every year. Most cases are caused by norovirus which, although seldom lethal, wreaks havoc as our nation's number one cause of food-borne illness and epidemic diarrhea. Just ask cruise ship patrons and their hosts! The prevention and treatment of travel-related diarrhea is an issue with millions of traveling Americans, whether they travel by sea, air, or land. They are at risk for getting "not norovirus" traveler's diarrhea, which, along with other acute inflammatory bacterial infections of the intestine, are important and preventable causes of chronic irritable bowel syndrome.

0889-8553/06/$ – see front matter
doi:10.1016/j.gtc.2006.05.004

Questions about the diagnosis (ruling in and ruling out) of *Helicobacter pylori* infection and its evil twin, functional dyspepsia, are daily occurrences for many physicians. In the differential diagnosis of chronic gastrointestinal problems, whether dyspepsia, diarrhea, or chronic abdominal pain, some of the most common infections that must be considered are the frequently encountered protozoa: giardia, amoeba, and cryptosporidium. Unfortunately, our patients not only travel abroad but travel from their homes to the hospital, many because of acute severe infections. Acute appendicitis, diverticulitis, pancreatitis, and biliary sepsis are common reasons for hospital admission and involve common controversies about diagnostic imaging and medical, endoscopic, radiologic, laparoscopic, or standard surgical treatment. Surgeons were among the first in the United States to sound the alarm about the increasing frequency and lethality of *Clostridium difficile*. The approach to this common infection has included therapy with probiotics, which is attractive to many of our patients, if not many of our colleagues. Common liver infections, including hepatitis B and hepatitis C (with or without coinfection with immunodeficiency virus), have come to dominate inpatient and outpatient hepatology in recent years.

Each of these articles is an examination and elaboration of the ordinary. We hope that the whole endeavor makes us all extraordinary.

Richard Goodgame, MD
Baylor College of Medicine
1 Baylor Plaza, Room 525-D
Houston, TX 77030, USA

David Y. Graham, MD
Veterans Affairs Medical Center-111D
2002 Holcombe Boulevard, Room 3A-320
Houston, TX 77030, USA

E-mail addresses: goodgame@bcm.tmc.edu,
dgraham@bcm.tmc.edu

GASTROENTEROLOGY CLINICS
OF NORTH AMERICA

Helicobacter pylori Diagnosis and Management

Ratha-Korn Vilaichone, MD, PhD[a], Varocha Mahachai, MD[b],
David Y. Graham, MD[c,d],*

[a]Gastroenterology Unit, Department of Medicine, Thammasat University Hospital,
Pathumthani, 12120 Thailand
[b]Division of Gastroenterology, Department of Medicine, Chulalongkorn University Hospital,
Bangkok, 10330 Thailand
[c]Department of Medicine, Michael E. DeBakey Veterans Affairs Medical Center,
2002 Holcombe Boulevard, Houston, TX 77030, USA
[d]Baylor College of Medicine, 1 Baylor Plaza, Room 525-D, Houston, TX 77030, USA

In the early twentieth century, peptic ulcer disease was believed to be caused by stress and dietary factors. Basic remedies focused on hospitalization, bed rest, and prescription of special bland diets with antacids to neutralize gastric acid. Later, as gastric acid assumed more of a primary role in ulcer pathogenesis, antacids and medications that blocked acid production became standard therapy. The H_2-receptor antagonists were prominent in the mid-1970s but were replaced by the more potent proton pump inhibitors (PPIs) in the 1980s. Despite the high healing rates that were achieved with antisecretory agents, peptic ulcers typically recurred after cessation of therapy and necessitated long-term maintenance therapy [1].

Spiral-shaped microorganisms in the mucus layer overlying gastric mucosa were observed first at least 100 years ago. In the 1970s Steer and Colin-Jones [2–4] noted the association with gastritis and ulcer but failed in their attempt to culture the organism. In the late 1970s Warren also noted the bacteria, and in 1982 Barry Marshall and Robin Warren were able to culture the organism and

This material is based upon work supported, in part, by the Office of Research and Development Medical Research Service Department of Veterans Affairs and by Public Health Service grant DK56338, which funds the Texas Gulf Coast Digestive Diseases Center. Dr. Graham has received small amounts of grant support and/or free drugs or urea breath tests from Meretek, Janssen/Eisai, and TAP for investigator-initiated and completely investigator controlled research. In addition, Dr. Graham is a paid consultant for Otsuka Pharmaceuticals and is a member of the Board of Directors of Meretek Diagnostics, the manufacturer of the ^{13}C-urea breath test. Dr. Graham also receives royalties on the Baylor College of Medicine patent that covers the serologic test, HM-CAP.

*Corresponding author. Department of Medicine, Michael E. DeBakey Veterans Affairs Medical Center, 2002 Holcombe Boulevard, Houston, TX 77030. E-mail address: dgraham@bcm.tmc.edu (D.Y. Graham).

0889-8553/06/$ – see front matter
doi:10.1016/j.gtc.2006.03.004

Published by Elsevier Inc.
gastro.theclinics.com

proved the association with gastritis and peptic ulcer disease. For their discovery, they were awarded Nobel Prize in Medicine in 2005.

Helicobacter pylori is a gram-negative spiral bacterium and is estimated to infect more than half of the world's population, predominantly in developing countries. Furthermore, this organism is now well established as the cause of the gastritis-associated gastrointestinal diseases: gastric ulcer, duodenal ulcer, gastric cancer and gastric mucosal-associated lymphoid tissue (MALT) lymphoma (MALToma). Eradication of the organism from a population results in virtual disappearance of these diseases. Despite the fact that gastric cancer remains one of the most common preventable cancers, worldwide population-based eradication strategies have yet to be implemented. The focus on treating only symptomatic patients ensures a large pool of infected patients undergoing progressive damage to their stomachs and maintenance of a large pool for spreading the infection.

THE PREVALENCE OF *HELICOBACTER PYLORI* INFECTION

H pylori is one of the most common chronic bacterial infections among humans [5,6]. The prevalence of *H pylori* infection varies depending on age, socioeconomic status, and ethnic group. Typically, the infection is acquired in childhood and the rate of acquisition is related inversely to household hygiene and the general levels of sanitation; wherever sanitation and standards of living have improved, the incidence of transmission has declined. The low prevalence in middle and upper socioeconomic populations in Western Europe and North America reflect the different rates of improvements in sanitation and standards of living that have been achieved by different ethnic and racial groups. In the United States, the prevalence rate is approximately 50% in African Americans, 60% in Mexican Americans, and 26% in whites [7]. The prevalence in middle to upper income whites is now less than 20%. These differences are attributable to differences in socioeconomic status and household hygiene during childhood [8].

H pylori prevalence can be considered best in terms of birth cohorts, such that the prevalence of infection of the population of 20-year-olds defines the prevalence of that birth cohort throughout life. In developing countries, most children are infected before the age of 10, and the prevalence among persons who are older than 20 years of age typically is between 50% and 90% [5,9–13]. *H pylori* can be considered as a "situational opportunist," meaning that it will take advantage of any route available to gain access to the stomach. Infection is by person-to-person transmission, either directly or indirectly by fecal-oral or gastro-oral routes. Intrafamilial clustering of infection further supports person-to-person transmission and in most countries the primary caregivers (ie, mothers) are the reservoir that is responsible for spread of the infection to their children [14]. In areas with poor sanitation, contaminated water or food may be the primary reservoirs for transmission [15].

Helicobacter pylori–Associated Diseases

H pylori has a long latent period of subclinical infection during which it causes gastric mucosal inflammation and progressive mucosal damage. Although *H pylori* strains differ in their ability to provoke inflammation, no *H pylori* isolates have been identified that have not been associated with symptomatic *H pylori*–associated diseases (eg, gastric cancer or peptic ulcer) [16]. Clinical disease is believed to represent the outcome of interactions between the bacterium, the host, and the environment. The most virulent strains possess OipA, the outer inflammatory protein, and a functional *cag* pathogenicity island [17,18]. Strain virulence and the presence of polymorphisms in host genes that control the inflammatory response determine the severity of the inflammatory response that is modulated further (enhanced or reduced) by environmental factors, primarily diet [19].

One outcome of chronic gastritis is the development of mucosal atrophy with loss of function of the normal acid-secreting portion of the stomach. The degree and severity of gastritis is related directly to the risk of developing gastric cancer [20–23]. Before the discovery of *H pylori*, gastritis, particularly atrophic gastritis, was known to be associated tightly with gastric cancer. Discovery of *H pylori* also was the discovery of the cause of gastritis. Although the bacterium actually may not cause the cancer, it is a "necessary but not sufficient" factor in causation. The World Health Organization's International Agency for Research on Cancer has classified *H pylori* as a Group 1 or definite carcinogen. Eradication of *H pylori* worldwide essentially will eliminate gastric cancer and gastric MALT lymphoma. The lifetime risk for an *H pylori*–infected individual to develop peptic ulcer disease has been estimated at one in six. The risk for developing gastric cancer in countries with a high prevalence of *H pylori* infection ranges from 19.6% in Changle, China to 1.5% in the United Kingdom [24]. These differences reflect differences in *H pylori* prevalence and host and environmental factors [5].

Gastric MALT lymphomas were recognized recently. For decades these low-grade lymphomas were called pseudolymphoma, which reflected their indolent course and an association with gastric ulcers [25]. The association of gastric MALTomas with chronic gastritis was made at about the same time that *H pylori* was discovered [26]; many subsequent studies confirmed the association between *H pylori* infection and gastric MALToma [27,28]. The current understanding is that most gastric MALTomas are T-cell dependent B-cell lymphomas that respond to *H pylori* antigens. Most gastric MALTomas are low-grade lymphomas and approximately 75% undergo remission following eradication of *H pylori*, which removes the antigenic stimulus [29].

A consistent association among *H pylori* and functional dyspepsia has not been established. Approximately 10% of subjects who had documented non-ulcer dyspepsia and *H pylori* infection responded symptomatically to *H pylori* eradication therapy [30]. *H pylori* eradication is recommended for these patients (as it is for all patients in whom the infection is found) because it may result in resolution of symptoms, and largely prevents the subsequent development of peptic ulcer and gastric cancer as well as transmission of the infection to others [31]. Population-wide studies recently showed that eradication of *H pylori* resulted in a significant reduction in the number of people that consulted physicians for dyspepsia or had symptoms 2 years after treatment [32].

Studies on the effect of *H pylori* eradication and gastroesophageal reflux disease (GERD) have been conflicting. Overwhelming evidence shows that *H pylori* infection does not cause GERD nor does *H pylori* have a significant effect on the response of existing GERD to therapy; however, patients who have atrophy of the gastric corpus are "protected" from symptomatic GERD because they are unable to make sufficient acid to develop symptoms irrespective of the presence of a significant impairment of the gastroesophageal antireflux barrier [33]. Treatment of *H pylori* in persons who have severe corpus gastritis and asymptomatic reflux may result in improved acid secretion and development of symptomatic GERD (uncovering of GERD). Those who have severe corpus gastritis also are at increased risk for gastric cancer; therefore, development of mild, easy to treat GERD is a small price to pay for a reduction in cancer risk. Finally, *H pylori* eradication may improve vitamin B12 and iron absorption, and, thus, improve anemia [34].

DIAGNOSTIC TESTS FOR *HELICOBACTER PYLORI* INFECTION

The indications for testing for *H pylori* are shown in Box 1. All investigators agree that the diagnosis of an active *H pylori* infection should prompt treatment. Tests to diagnose whether a patient is infected with *H pylori* often are divided into those that require endoscopy or those that do not require endoscopy. The choice of test depends upon issues such as cost, availability, clinical situation, prevalence of infection, pretest probability of infection, and presence of factors (eg, the use of PPIs and antibiotics) that may influence test results.

Like syphilis and tuberculosis, long latent periods are the rule in *H pylori* infection. At least 20% of individuals who are infected with *H pylori* develop a symptomatic outcome, which is a higher percentage than latent syphilis or tuberculosis [35]. In contrast to syphilis and tuberculosis, latent *H pylori* is transmissible. Like previous campaigns to eradicate syphilis or tuberculosis, the questions of whom to test and when to test are public health issues. Despite its significance as a global pathogen and the high prevalence of *H pylori* and *H pylori*–related diseases in many countries, the focus is still on identifying and treating subjects who have symptomatic *H pylori* infections (eg, peptic ulcer disease, family history of gastric cancer, or uninvestigated dyspepsia) [16,36,37]. This approach results in *H pylori*–associated disease remaining an important cause of morbidity and mortality for decades to come. Simple approaches, such as testing (and treating when positive) at the time of application for a marriage license as was done for syphilis, would identify cases at an age when clinical outcomes can be prevented as well as prevent transmission of the infection within families. Such a strategy would result in complete elimination of *H pylori* and *H pylori*–related diseases within 30 or 40 years. Noninvasive tests include serologic tests, urea breath tests, and stool antigen tests [38,39]. IgM and IgA antibody testing have not proven to be useful clinically, whereas anti–*H pylori* IgG has a good track record. IgG anti–*H pylori* antibodies generally can be expected to be present by 4 weeks after infection. The three main

Box 1: Recommendations for testing for *Helicobacter pylori* infection

Definite

Duodenal or gastric ulcer (present or history of)

Gastric low-grade MALT lymphoma

Atrophic gastritis

Relatives of patients who have gastric cancer

After endoscopic resection of early cancer

Uninvestigated dyspepsia

Evaluate success of eradication therapy

Strongly recommended

Nonulcer dyspepsia

Chronic nonsteroidal anti-inflammatory drug/aspirin therapy[a]

Chronic antisecretory drug therapy (eg, gastroesophageal reflux disease)[b]

Relatives of patients who have duodenal ulcer

Relatives of patients who have *H pylori* infection

Patient desires to be tested

All patients who are proven to have an active *H pylori* infection should be treated

[a]When planning long-term therapy.
[b]When planning long-term antisecretory therapy.

formats for the serologic kits are ELISA, immunochromatography, and Western blotting. Urine and salivary testing for IgG antibody also are available. Urine testing has proven useful, whereas salivary testing has not. Most serologic tests have specificities and sensitivities of less than 90%, which makes their usefulness limited to cases with high (eg, peptic ulcer) and low (eg, GERD) pretest probabilities. For example, consider the interpretation of a serologic test with 85% sensitivity and specificity in two patients: a duodenal ulcer (DU) patient with a pretest probability of more than 90% and a patient who has GERD with a pretest probability of 20%. For 100 DU patients there would be 90 with *H pylori* and 10 without. The number of true positives would be 77 (90 × 85%). The number of false negatives would be 13. True negatives would be 9 (10 × 85%); there would be 1 false positive. Thus, a positive result definitely would be an indication for treatment (ie, 77 of 78 would be true positives). In contrast, more than 50% of the negatives (13 of 22) would be false negatives, such that retesting with a test for active infection would be indicated before deciding not to treat. The opposite conclusion would be the case for the patient who has GERD (low pretest probability) where the negative result would be highly reliable but the positive result would need confirmation

[16]. Antibody tests can remain positive for years after *H pylori* eradication and have limited value to confirm the cure of *H pylori* infection.

Urea breath testing provides a noninvasive method for the diagnosis of *H pylori* infections. Urea breath testing has the important advantage of being able to confirm *H pylori* eradication. Following ingestion of ^{13}C- or ^{14}C-urea, the urea is hydrolyzed by the *H pylori* urease enzyme to labeled ^{14}CO$_2$ or ^{13}CO$_2$, which can be detected in breath samples [39]. The nonradioactive ^{13}C test and the radioactive ^{14}C test have received US Food and Drug Administration approval for diagnosis of *H pylori* infection. Only the ^{13}C-urea test has been approved for posteradication testing. The dose of radiation in the ^{14}C-urea test is low but is cumulative and the test is not approved for use in children or pregnant women.

H pylori in the stomach eventually appears in the stool, which has led to the development of fecal assays, including *H pylori* culture, DNA detected by polymerase chain reaction, or *H pylori* antigen testing. Only stool antigen that uses enzyme immunoassay has proven to be useful clinically with reported sensitivities and specificities of more than 90% [39]. Stool antigen assay also is useful for documenting whether eradication has been successful.

To avoid false negative results, it is generally recommended that posttreatment testing with the urea breath test, histology, or culture be delayed for 4 weeks to ensure that any remaining organisms can repopulate the stomach. With stool antigen testing, the delay should be increased to 6 to 12 weeks [39].

Generally, invasive testing that requires endoscopy should be limited to patients who require endoscopy for therapy or as part of their diagnostic evaluation. Invasive tests include gastric biopsies for culture, histology, or rapid urease testing. *H pylori* culture is the absolute gold standard for detecting the bacterium; however, culture generally is not available. Experienced laboratories are able to culture *H pylori* from gastric biopsies with more than 95% success and also can offer susceptibility testing. Cultures also can be obtained using minimally invasive techniques, such as with an orogastric brush (Baylor brush) or string tests [40,41]. Histologic examination has potential advantages over other diagnostic tests because it also provides data regarding the severity of gastritis, the density of the organism, and the presence or absence of atrophy with or without intestinal metaplasia. The accuracy of histologic diagnosis of *H pylori* infection can be improved by adequate biopsies from antrum and corpus and by using special stains, such as a triple stain or the Diff-Quik stain [42]. Rapid urease tests contain a solution or gel with urea and a pH indicator color reagent. The presence of urease from *H pylori* results in hydrolysis of neutral urea to alkaline ammonia and is visualized by a change in color of the pH indicator. Most commercially available kits have similar diagnostic accuracy (eg, Hp*fast*, GI Supply, Camp Hill, Pennsylvania; CLOtest, TriMed Specialities, Inc., Lenexa, Kansas; PyloriTek, Serim Research Corp., Elkhart, Indiana) [43] with high sensitivity (90%–95%) and specificity (95%–100%) [31]. The high sensitivity and specificity of rapid urease test has led to its use by many physicians as their primary diagnostic test (ie, the samples for histology are discarded in those with positive rapid urease test results). Any maneuver that reduces bacterial load, such as the use of antibiotics or PPIs [44], may lead to false negative rapid urease tests such that a negative rapid urease test always must be confirmed by histology.

TREATMENT OF *HELICOBACTER PYLORI* INFECTION
The success rate for eradication of *H pylori* has decreased steadily. Worldwide, the most popular and highly promoted regimen is a triple therapy that consists of a PPI, amoxicillin (or metronidazole), and clarithromycin for 1 to 2 weeks. The average success rate for traditional triple therapy is approximately 70% (range, 60% to 85%). Success is best with at least 14 days of therapy (see later discussion) and the authors recommend that duration of therapy.

ANTISECRETORY AGENTS FOR *HELICOBACTER PYLORI* ERADICATION
H_2-receptor antagonists have no antimicrobial activity against *H pylori*, but they reduce gastric acidity and allow acid-sensitive drugs and those whose effectiveness as antimicrobial agents is reduced at acid pH (eg, amoxicillin and clarithromycin) to work more effectively. The H_2-receptor antagonist ranitidine also has been combined with bismuth in the form of ranitidine bismuth citrate (RBC), which produces a more soluble and possibly more effective form of bismuth. Comparative studies showed that the efficacy of RBC–triple therapy may be superior to PPI–triple therapy [45]. Unfortunately, RBC is not commercially available in many areas, including the United States. PPIs reduce acid secretion by blocking the hydrogen-potassium ATPase pump on the luminal border of gastric parietal cell, and are more effective antisecretory agents than are H_2-receptor antagonists. PPIs also have in vitro antimicrobial activity for *H pylori* [46]; however, the major activity of PPIs is believed to be on increasing intraluminal gastric pH (eg, head-to-head comparisons showed that H_2-receptor antagonist–containing triple therapy and PPI–containing triple therapies produce similar or equivalent results) [47].

ANTIMICROBIAL USE IN REGIMENS TO CURE *HELICOBACTER PYLORI*
There are probably few antimicrobial agents that have not been used in an attempt to treat *H pylori* infections. Amoxicillin is one of the most popular antibiotics that is used for the treatment of *H pylori* infection because it is inexpensive, well tolerated, and resistance is rare [48,49]. Amoxicillin inhibits the synthesis of the bacterial cell wall and can act topically and systemically after absorption into the bloodstream and delivery into the gastric mucosa and lumen. The antimicrobial effect of amoxicillin is pH dependent; the bactericidal activity increases as pH increases. Single agents have not provided sufficiently high cure rates to be used clinically, and thus, amoxicillin typically is combined with a second antibiotic, most often clarithromycin.

Clarithromycin is a 14-membered ring macrolide antibiotic. It is a derivative of erythromycin, with a similar spectrum of activity and clinical application; however, clarithromycin is the most acid-stable macrolide, has more consistent absorption, lower minimum inhibitory concentration (MIC) for H pylori, and has a longer elimination half-time than erythromycin. The antimicrobial effect results from its binding to bacterial ribosomes, which disrupts bacterial protein synthesis. Clarithromycin resistance is increasing and resistance predicts a marked reduction in treatment success. Increasing the dosage cannot overcome the problem of clarithromycin resistance. Clarithromycin commonly causes an alteration of taste sensation that can be sufficiently unpleasant to cause the cessation of treatment. Clarithromycin is one of the most expensive of the antimicrobial drugs that is used to treat H pylori infection and this increases the cost significantly.

Metronidazole is a nitroimidazole that is toxic to microarephillic organisms. Metronidazole is secreted actively into the gastric juice and saliva, and therefore, is active after absorption, with a half-life of 8 to 12 hours. Metronidazole is a prodrug and its activity is pH independent [50]. After entry into the bacterial cell, metronidazole undergoes transformation into a toxic form. Alteration in the bacterial enzymes that is required for this transformation results in metronidazole resistance that reduces the efficacy of treatment regimens that include this antimicrobial [51]. Unlike clarithromycin—because of the presence of alternate metabolic pathways in the cell and the high local levels of the drug—metronidazole resistance often can be overcome by increasing the dosage. The side effects of short-term use of metronidazole include interactions with alcohol and gastrointestinal symptoms.

Tetracycline is a close derivative of the polycyclic naphtacenecarboxamides and is an excellent anti–H pylori antimicrobial because it is inexpensive and pH independent. Tetracycline inhibits bacterial protein synthesis and seems to act luminally or topically [52]. The site of action of tetracycline is the bacterial ribosome, which results in the interruption of protein biosynthesis. In the United States, bacterial resistance to tetracycline is rare; however, the resistance is approximately 5% in Japan and South Korea [53]. This antibiotic should not be given to pregnant women or children because it causes permanent staining of developing teeth.

Fluoroquinolones have been used increasingly for H pylori eradication. These drugs block DNA gyrase and DNA synthesis in the organism. Resistance to fluoroquinolones develops rapidly, and previous use of these medications is associated with a high rate of resistance.

Furazolidone is a monoamine oxidase inhibitor with broad antibacterial activity that is based on interference with bacterial enzymes; it has proven to be an effective part of triple therapy [54]. H pylori resistance to furazolidone is rare, and furazolidone is an underused antimicrobial.

Rifabutin is a semisynthetic ansamycin antibiotic with low minimum inhibitory concentration (MIC) level for H pylori. Rifabutin use for H pylori treatment is becoming increasingly common and it is used primarily in combination with a PPI and amoxicillin as a rescue therapy.

Bismuth compounds are topically active pH-independent antimicrobial drugs that disrupt the integrity of bacterial cell walls. Bismuth was one of the first agents used against *H pylori* infection. There is evidence that bismuth is directly bactericidal, although its MIC is high for *H pylori*. In the United States, bismuth is available in the form of bismuth subsalicylate and bismuth subcitrate, both of which have equivalent effect as anti–*H pylori* therapy. *H pylori* resistance has not been reported for these medications.

THERAPEUTIC REGIMENS TO ERADICATE *HELICOBACTER PYLORI* INFECTION

Dual-therapy regimens that use a PPI plus one antibiotic (amoxicillin or clarithromycin) were the first therapies that were approved for *H pylori* eradication. They can no longer be recommended as primary therapy because their eradication rates are low [55] and they result in a high frequency of clarithromycin resistance among the treatment failures. The success of amoxicillin-PPI dual therapy seems to be enhanced if a higher or more frequent dose of PPI and amoxicillin [56].

The Maastricht Consensus Conference recommended that the initial therapy be a legacy therapy that consists of PPI-clarithromycin-amoxicillin (or metronidazole, if the primary resistance to clarithromycin in the area is <15%–20%). It also was agreed that there was a small advantage of using metronidazole in place of amoxicillin, and that this combination was preferred in areas where the prevalence of metronidazole resistance is less than 40%.

In clinical practice, the legacy regimen of a PPI, amoxicillin, and clarithromycin or a PPI plus clarithromycin and metronidazole/tinidazole standard triple therapies generally produce a lower than acceptable eradication rate that ranges from 60% to 80% [37,57,58]. For example, a recent study from the United States compared the efficacy of 3-, 7-, and 10-day triple therapies and found that they were equally poor with none achieving a cure rate as high as 80%. The rate of clarithromycin-resistant *H pylori* was 9% in that group [59]. A community-based study of 1161 patients resulted in an overall eradication rate of 61% (95% CI, 58%–64%) [60]. Another study of 1255 patients reported success in only 73% (95% CI, 58%–64%) [61]. These results are in line with a meta-analysis that compared the effectiveness of triple and quadruple regimens as first-line *H pylori* treatment [62,63]. The variability of treatment success with an individual regimen has been related to the presence of antimicrobial resistance, compliance with the drug regimen, and duration of therapy [37,51,57,58,64–66]. A 14-day course of therapy provides a higher eradication rate than does 7- or 10-day therapy (eg, by approximately 12%; 95% CI, 7%–17%) [37]. By definition, longer durations of therapy are more expensive than are shorter durations. Companies whose regimens are approved only for 7 days use "opinion leader" spokespersons to promote them as cost-effective. When one considers the serious consequences of *H pylori* infection and the cost of treatment failures, short-duration therapy cannot be considered to be cost-effective. The choice of the best initial therapy for individual regions can be made scientifically but requires knowledge of the rates of resistance in the local area; unfortunately, these data often are not available. Recommended treatment regimes are shown in Box 2.

TREATMENT SIDE EFFECTS

The main reasons for eradication failure include poor choice of regimen, inadequate duration of treatment, poor compliance with the regimen, and antibiotic resistance. Patient compliance can be improved by counseling the patient regarding the importance of completing the treatment regimen; however, compliance is reduced predictably when there are significant adverse effects of the medications. The adverse effects that are associated with *H pylori* therapy occur in up to 50% of patients; however, most usually are mild and less than 10% of patients stop treatment because of side effects [67]. Nausea is the most common and is present with most antibiotics. The short-term use of metronidazole can cause a disulfiram-like reaction when taken with alcohol, and the patient should be cautioned against using alcohol during the treatment period. Taste disturbance, such as metallic taste, can occur with metronidazole or clarithromycin use. Tetracycline can induce a photosensitivity reaction in some cases and should not be administered to pregnant women. Diarrhea is associated commonly with antibiotic therapy, especially amoxicillin. Pseudomembranous colitis and allergic reactions are rare but can occur. Patients who take bismuth salts

---

Box 2: Recommended antibiotic combinations for *Helicobacter pylori* infections

Legacy therapies

Triple therapy[a]: A PPI plus amoxicillin, 1 g, plus clarithromycin, 500 mg, or metronidazole/tinidazole, 500 mg, twice a day for 14 days

Quadruple therapy: Bismuth, metronidazole, 500 mg, tetracycline, 500 mg, three times a day plus a PPI twice a day for 14 days

Concomitant triple therapies

A PPI plus amoxicillin, 1 g, plus clarithromycin, 500 mg, and metronidazole/tinidazole, 500 mg, twice a day for 14 days

Sequential therapy[b]

A PPI plus 1 g amoxicillin, twice a day for 5 days. On day 6 stop amoxicillin and add clarithromycin, 250 or 500 mg and metronidazole/tinidazole, 500 mg, twice a day to complete the 10-day course.

Salvage therapy

Best if based on the results of susceptibility testing (see text for details)

[a]Should be replaced by concomitant triple therapies or sequential therapy.
[b]See text for details regarding doses, duration, and whether the sequential administration of drugs is needed. In general, the authors recommend 14 days of therapy until it can be shown that an acceptable success rate (>95%) can be achieved with a shorter duration.

have dark stools and should be warned so that it is not mistaken for gastrointestinal bleeding.

THERAPY AFTER INITIAL TREATMENT FAILURES

The initial eradication for *H pylori* fails in approximately 20% to 40% of patients. Retreatment with the same regimen (eg, PPI plus clarithromycin and amoxicillin) is not recommended because of a predictably low success rates. The rule of thumb is to change the antibiotics to ones that have not been used previously. This admonition does not include amoxicillin, which can be used repeatedly because resistance is rare. Thus, the second therapy might be a PPI plus amoxicillin plus a new antibiotic (eg, metronidazole).

Quadruple therapy (PPI twice a day plus 500 mg of metronidazole/tinidazole and 500 mg of tetracycline HCI plus bismuth given three times daily) is the most successful therapy that is available. It should be considered as initial anti–*H pylori* therapy in many areas with low success rates with traditional triple therapy [63]. Quadruple therapy is less convenient than is triple therapy because of the larger number of medications, the increased frequency of drug administration (ie, three times daily versus two times daily), and the possibility for increased frequency of side effects. The proportion that stops therapy because of side effects seems to be about the same as with the standard triple regimen.

Salvage therapies or therapies for those who have failed several courses, including quadruple therapy, are not standardized. One approach is to use quadruple therapy but to substitute a new drug for the metronidazole. Probably the most effective approach is to substitute furazolidone (eg, 100 mg three times a day) [68]. Another approach is to substitute a new drug for the clarithromycin/metronidazole in legacy triple therapy (eg, furazolidone, rifabutin, a fluoroquinolone) [37]. The authors prefer a sequential therapy using high-dose PPI and amoxicillin as the base (see later discussion). Outcome is predictably best if one chooses agents to which the organism is susceptible and where available, susceptibility testing is recommended.

ADJUVANTS TO TREATMENT

Alternative approaches and adjuvants include the use of probiotics, lactoferrin, or mucolytics. Some specific strains of lactic acid bacteria (probiotics) in dairy products adhere to human intestinal mucosa [69]. Lactic acid bacteria, including *Lactobacillus*, *Lactococcus*, *Pediococcus*, *Leuconostoc*, and *Bifidobacterium*, are found throughout the gastrointestinal tract. The predominant population of lactic acid–producing bacteria in the upper gastrointestinal tract are *Lactobacillus* spp. Recent studies reviewed the activities of other milk components, including lactoferrin [70,71]. Lactoferrin is a glycoprotein that is found in mammalian milk and is known to possess activity against a variety of gram-negative bacteria, including *H pylori*. The evidence is accumulating that lactic acid bacteria and lactoferrin may have roles in the management of *H pylori* infection. Moreover, such treatment counteracts the side effects of antimicrobial agents. In two studies, a 7-day triple regimen that included lactoferrin proved to be more effective in curing H pylori than did the same regimens without lactoferrin; this suggested a possible role for the agent in the eradication of the bacterium [70,71]. A third study that used a different 7-day triple therapy failed to confirm the results of the initial trials [72], which suggested that more work is needed. Lactoferrin, given as a single agent, does not effect H pylori eradication [73].

Oral administration of pronase is designed to remove gastric mucus and is used widely as a premedication for endoscopy [74]. Because H pylori colonize the mucus layer, pronase has been used with success and has improved the outcome with traditional triple therapy significantly [75]. Because N-acetylcysteine (NAC) is a mucolytic agent and a thiol-containing antioxidant, it may alter the establishment and maintenance of H pylori infection within the gastric mucus layer and mucosa. NAC also inhibited the growth of H pylori in agar and broth susceptibility tests. When NAC was used as an adjuvant to antibiotic therapy in clinical studies it resulted in an improvement in eradication rates [76,77].

Helicobacter pylori Eradication in the Twenty-First Century: Adjuvant and Sequential Therapy

Clearly, new approaches to therapy are needed. The use of probiotics, natural antimicrobial substances, or mucolytics as adjuvants showed promise; additional studies are warranted. Another approach has been to use current therapies in a sequential manner. Generally, sequential administration of antibiotics is not recommended because it is likely to promote drug resistance rather than result in increased eradication. The exceptions are the use of bismuth and amoxicillin because monotherapy with these drugs rarely promotes resistance. The underlying concept is to use initial therapy with drugs against which development of resistance is rare. This approach is designed to reduce the bacterial load markedly, which makes the presence of a preexisting small population of resistant organisms less likely. Then, another one or two drugs are added to kill the remaining organisms. A sequential treatment regimen using a PPI plus amoxicillin for 5 days followed the combination of a PPI plus clarithromycin (500 mg) and tinidazole (500 mg) for an additional 5 days has proven successful. Head-to-head comparisons have proven sequential quadruple therapy to be superior to the traditional triple therapy using a PPI plus two antibiotics (amoxicillin and clarithromycin) [78–80]. This concept has been extended to use a lower dose of clarithromycin (250 mg, twice a day) which, if confirmed, could reduce the cost of this therapy in areas where the cost of 250 and 500 mg of clarithromycin differ [81]. Sequential therapy also proved successful in children [80]. However, it is important to note that sequential therapy is the sequential administration of a dual therapy (PPI plus amoxicillin) followed by a triple therapy (a PPI, clarithromycin, and tinidazole/metronidazole). Four drug combinations (these three antibiotics and a PPI) given as a non-sequential therapy (concomitant therapy) for 5 days have been used previously with very good results (eg, per protocol cure rate of ranging from 89 to 96% with a PPI [82–84] or ranitidine bismuth citrate [85,86]. The comparisons of sequential therapy and traditional triple therapy have used different drug combinations (eg, clar-ithromycin–tinidazole versus clarithromycin amoxicillin) and have used a 7-day duration for the traditional therapy, which is no longer recommended. The differences would have likely been less if they had compared the same drug regimens and extended the duration of traditional therapy to the recommended 14 days. That said, the concept is very promising and studies evaluating doses, durations, formulation, the effect of pretreatment antibiotic resistance, and the administration of the drugs as concomitant therapy are clearly needed. Sequential therapy may be a reasonable alternate to standard triple therapy given for 14 days.

Another approach, and the one that the authors use, is to combine the "German" approach of high-dose PPI and high-dose amoxicillin into a sequential therapy. Studies from Germany showed that the combination of omeprazole, 40 mg, and amoxicillin, 750 mg, given three times daily for 14 days provided eradication rates that ranged from 67% to 91% [87–89]. Worldwide, this dual therapy provides variable eradication rates, but within a region the rates seem to be predictable. In the authors' experience, the cure rate has been approximately 75%. Their approach has been to use omeprazole or esomeprazole, 40 mg, and amoxicillin, 1 g, three times a day for 5 days. On day 6 a third antibiotic (eg, metronidazole or gatifloxacin) is added and continued as a triple therapy for a total of 12 to 14 days. This approach has proven highly successful in the presence of susceptible strains. The fact that resistant strains compromised the outcome suggests that pretreatment antibiotic susceptibility testing or the addition of a fourth antibiotic may have been useful. Clearly, variations on sequential therapy should be tested to search for a new and improved regimen. The authors believe that legacy PPI triple therapy generally should not be used, rather sequential quadruple therapy should be used if one wishes to use the traditional combinations.

CONFIRMATION OF CURE

The low eradication rates with current regimens and the availability of accurate, inexpensive noninvasive tests have made confirmation of cure the standard of care. The importance of confirming posttreatment eradication is related to recurrence of diseases and poor outcomes if the infection is not cured. Furthermore, the infected patients remain the source of infection to others, especially family members.

The primary reason for waiting before testing for cure is to allow regrowth of any remaining *H pylori* (ie, to reduce the false negative rate). Antibiotics and bismuth should be discontinued for at least 4 weeks before testing with urea breath test, histology, or culture. Stool antigen testing is a more widely available alternative but the waiting period is increased to approximately 6 to 12 weeks. If possible, PPIs should be stopped at least 1 week before testing is done to confirm *H pylori* cure. If testing is done earlier, a positive test is indicative of treatment failure, whereas a negative test could be a false negative result. Serology testing is not useful for confirming eradication because of the long-term elevation of antibody level.

SUMMARY

H pylori is a global human pathogen and is the major cause of gastritis and the gastritis-associated diseases: gastric ulcer, duodenal ulcer, gastric cancer, and primary gastric B-cell lymphoma (MALToma). Although several reliable diagnostic tests are widely available, the ideal regimen for treating the infection remains to be established. The current first-line or legacy triple therapy regimens fail in 20% to 40% of patients. Causes of treatment failure include antibiotic resistance, poor compliance, short (7–10 days) duration of therapy, and drug-related side effects. Fourteen-day triple therapy has an approximately 12% better cure rate than does 7-day therapy; therefore, shorter durations can no longer be recommended. Recent studies confirmed older observations that the success rate of legacy triple regimens (PPI plus two antibiotics) can be improved if the duration is extended to 14 days or if a third antibiotic is given. Sequential therapy (PPI plus amoxicillin followed by a PPI plus clarithromycin plus metronidazole) requires further evaluation although the concept appears very promising and therapy should probably replace the legacy triple therapies. More studies are needed to examine doses, durations, and the need for sequential administration of the drugs, which extends the duration to 14 days. Nonetheless, sequential quadruple therapy probably should replace the legacy triple therapies. Classic quadruple therapy contains bismuth, a PPI, 1500 mg of metronidazole, and 1500 mg of tetracycline. It provides the highest average eradication rates and in many regions should be considered as the initial approach. Confirmation of eradication using noninvasive diagnostic tests, such as a urea breath test or stool antigen assay, is now the standard of care. The diagnosis of latent or symptomatic *H pylori*, like the diagnosis of latent or symptomatic syphilis, always should prompt treatment. Because of decreasing cure rates, new and improved therapies are needed.

References

[1] Munnangi S, Sonnenberg A. Time trends of physician visits and treatment patterns of peptic ulcer disease in the United States. Arch Intern Med 1997;157(13):1489–94.

[2] Steer HW, Colin-Jones DG. Mucosal changes in gastric ulceration and their response to carbenoxolone sodium. Gut 1975;16(8):590–7.

[3] Steer HW. The gastro-duodenal epithelium in peptic ulceration. J Pathol 1985;146(4): 355–62.

[4] Steer HW. Ultrastructure of cell migration through the gastric epithelium and its relationship to bacteria. J Clin Pathol 1975;28(8):639–46.

[5] Breuer T, Malaty HM, Graham DY. The epidemiology of H. pylori-associated gastroduodenal diseases. In: Ernst P, Michetti P, Smith PD, editors. The immunobiology of H. pylori from pathogenesis to prevention. Philadelphia: Lippincott-Raven; 1997. p. 1–14.

[6] Graham DY, Adam E, Reddy GT, et al. Seroepidemiology of *Helicobacter pylori* infection in India. Comparison of developing and developed countries. Dig Dis Sci 1991;36(8): 1084–8.

[7] Everhart JE, Kruszon-Moran D, Perez-Perez GI, et al. Seroprevalence and ethnic differences in *Helicobacter pylori* infection among adults in the United States. J Infect Dis 2000;181(4): 1359–63.

[8] Malaty HM, Graham DY. Importance of childhood socioeconomic status on the current prevalence of *Helicobacter pylori* infection. Gut 1994;35(6):742–5.

[9] Hoang TT, Bengtsson C, Phung DC, et al. Seroprevalence of *Helicobacter pylori* infection in urban and rural Vietnam. Clin Diagn Lab Immunol 2005;12(1):81–5.

[10] Bodhidatta L, Hoge CW, Churnratanakul S, et al. Diagnosis of *Helicobacter pylori* infection in a developing country: comparison of two ELISAs and a seroprevalence study. J Infect Dis 1993;168(6):1549–53.

[11] Leal-Herrera Y, Torres J, Perez-Perez G, et al. Serologic IgG response to urease in *Helicobacter pylori*-infected persons from Mexico. Am J Trop Med Hyg 1999;60(4):587–92.

[12] Romero-Gallo J, Perez-Perez GI, Novick RP, et al. Responses of endoscopy patients in Ladakh, India, to *Helicobacter pylori* whole-cell and *cagA* antigens. Clin Diagn Lab Immunol 2002;9(6):1313–7.

[13] Youn HS. Baik SC, Cho YK, et al. Comparison of *Helicobacter pylori* infection between Fukuoka, Japan and Chinju, Korea. Helicobacter 1998;3(1):9–14.

[14] Mahachai V, Vilaichone RK. Intrafamilial transmission of *Helicobacter pylori* in Thailand. Am J Gastroenterol 2005;1006(9). Suppl:S133.

[15] Graham DY, Malaty HM. What remains to be done regarding transmission of *Helicobacter pylori*. Int J Epidemiol 2002;31(3):646–7.

[16] Shiotani A, Graham DY. Pathogenesis and therapy of gastric and duodenal ulcer disease. Med Clin North Am 2002;86(6):1447–66.

[17] Censini S, Lange C, Xiang Z, et al. *cagA* pathogenicity island of *Helicobacter pylori*, encodes type I-specific and disease-associated virulence factors. Proc Natl Acad Sci U S A 1996;93(25):14648–53.

[18] Yamaoka Y, Kwon DH, Graham DY. A M(r) 34,000 proinflammatory outer membrane protein (oipA) of *Helicobacter pylori*. Proc Natl Acad Sci U S A 2000;97(13): 7533–8.

[19] Vilaichone RK, Mahachai V, Tumwasorn S, et al. Gastric mucosal cytokine levels in relation to host interleukin-1 polymorphisms and *Helicobacter pylori cagA* genotype. Scand J Gastroenterol 2005;40(5):530–9.

[20] Correa P, Haenszel W, Cuello C, et al. A model for gastric cancer epidemiology. Lancet 1975;2(7924):58–60.

[21] Correa P. Precursors of gastric and esophageal cancer. Cancer 1982;50(11 Suppl): 2554–65.

[22] Correa P. The biological model of gastric carcinogenesis. IARC Sci Publ 2004;157: 301–10.

[23] Graham DY, Shiotani A. The time to eradicate gastric cancer is now. Gut 2005;54(6): 735–8.

[24] Parkin DM, Whelan SL, Ferlay J, et al, editors. Cancer incidence in five continents, vol. VIII. Lyon (France): IARC Scientific Publications No. 155; 2002.

[25] Perrillo RP, Tedesco FJ. Gastric pseudolymphoma. A spectrum of presenting features and diagnostic considerations. Am J Gastroenterol 1976;65(3):226–30.

[26] Vanden Heule B, Van Kerkem C, Heimann R. Benign and malignant lymphoid lesions of the stomach. A histological reappraisal in the light of the Kiel classification for non-Hodgkin's lymphomas. Histopathology 1979;3(4):309–20.

[27] Wotherspoon AC, Ortiz-Hidalgo C, Falzon MR, et al. *Helicobacter pylori*-associated gastritis and primary B-cell gastric lymphoma. Lancet 1991;338(8776):1175–6.

[28] Parsonnet J, Hansen S, Rodriguez L, et al. *Helicobacter pylori* infection and gastric lymphoma. N Engl J Med 1994;330(18):1267–71.

[29] Lee SK, Lee YC, Chung JB, et al. Low grade gastric mucosa associated lymphoid tissue lymphoma: treatment strategies based on 10 year follow-up. World J Gastroenterol 2004;10(2):223–6.

[30] Moayyedi P, Soo S, Deeks J, et al. Eradication of *Helicobacter pylori* for non-ulcer dyspepsia. Cochrane Database Syst Rev 2005;25(1):CD002096.

[31] Howden CW, Hunt RH. Guidelines for the management of *Helicobacter pylori* infection. Ad Hoc Committee on Practice Parameters of the American College of Gastroenterology. Am J Gastroenterol 1998;93(12):2330–8.

[32] Lane JA, Murray LJ, Noble S, et al. Impact of *Helicobacter pylori* eradication on dyspepsia, health resource use, and quality of life in the Bristol Helicobacter Project: randomized controlled trial. BMJ 2006;332(7535):199–204.

[33] Graham DY. The changing epidemiology of GERD: geography and *Helicobacter pylori*. Am J Gastroenterol 2003;98(7):1462–70.

[34] Kaptan K, Beyan C, Ural AU, et al. *Helicobacter pylori*–is it a novel causative agent in vitamin B12 deficiency? Arch Intern Med 2000;160(9):1349–53.

[35] Graham DY. Can therapy ever be denied for *Helicobacter pylori* infection? Gastroenterology 1997;113(6 Suppl):S113–7.

[36] Ofman JJ, Etchason J, Fullerton S, et al. Management strategies for *Helicobacter pylori*-seropositive patients with dyspepsia: clinical and economic consequences. Ann Intern Med 1997;126(4):280–91.

[37] Nakayama Y, Graham DY. *Helicobacter pylori* infection: diagnosis and treatment. Expert Rev Anti Infect Ther 2004;2(4):599–610.

[38] Graham DY, Qureshi WA. Markers of infection. Helicobacter pylori: Physiology and genetics. In: Mobley HLT, Mendz GL, Hazell SL, editors. Washington DC: ASM Press; 2001. p. 499–510.

[39] Vaira D, Malfertheiner P, Megraud F, et al. Diagnosis of *Helicobacter pylori* infection with a new non-invasive antigen-based assay. HpSA European study group. Lancet 1999;354(9172):30–3.

[40] Windsor HM, Abioye-Kuteyi EA, Marshall BJ. Methodology and transport medium for collection of *Helicobacter pylori* on a string test in remote locations. Helicobacter 2005;10(6):630–4.

[41] Graham DY, Kudo M, Reddy R, et al. Practical rapid, minimally invasive, reliable nonendoscopic method to obtain *Helicobacter pylori* for culture. Helicobacter 2005;10(1):1–3.

[42] El-Zimaity HM, Segura AM, Genta RM, et al. Histologic assessment of *Helicobacter pylori* status after therapy: comparison of Giemsa, Diff-Quik, and Genta stains. Mod Pathol 1998;11(3):288–91.

[43] Laine L, Lewin D, Naritoku W, et al. Prospective comparison of commercially available rapid urease tests for the diagnosis of *Helicobacter pylori*. Gastrointest Endosc 1996;44(5):523–6.

[44] Graham DY, Opekun AR, Hammoud F, et al. Studies regarding the mechanism of false negative urea breath tests with proton pump inhibitors. Am J Gastroenterol 2003;98(5):1005–9.

[45] Gisbert JP, Gonzalez L, Calvet X. Systematic review and meta-analysis: proton pump inhibitor vs. ranitidine bismuth citrate plus two antibiotics in *Helicobacter pylori* eradication. Helicobacter 2005;10(3):157–71.

[46] Figura N, Crabtree JE, Dattilo M. In-vitro activity of lansoprazole against *Helicobacter pylori*. J Antimicrob Chemother 1997;39(5):585–90.

[47] Graham DY, Hammoud F, El-Zimaity HM, et al. Meta-analysis: proton pump inhibitor or H2-receptor antagonist for *Helicobacter pylori* eradication. Aliment Pharmacol Ther 2003;17(10):1229–36.

[48] Duck WM, Sobel J, Pruckler JM, et al. Antimicrobial resistance incidence and risk factors among *Helicobacter pylori*-infected persons, United States. Emerg Infect Dis 2004;10(6): 1088–94.

[49] Watanabe K, Tanaka A, Imase K, et al. Amoxicillin resistance in *Helicobacter pylori*: studies from Tokyo, Japan from 1985 to 2003. Helicobacter 2005;10(1):4–11.

[50] van Zanten SJ, Goldie J, Hollingsworth J, et al. Secretion of intravenously administered antibiotics in gastric juice: implications for management of *Helicobacter pylori*. J Clin Pathol 1992;45(3):225–7.

[51] Dore MP, Leandro G, Realdi G, et al. Effect of pretreatment antibiotic resistance to metronidazole and clarithromycin on outcome of *Helicobacter pylori* therapy: a meta-analytical approach. Dig Dis Sci 2000;45(1):68–76.

[52] Tytgat GN. Treatments that impact favorably upon the eradication of *Helicobacter pylori* and ulcer recurrence. Aliment Pharmacol Ther 1994;8(4):359–68.

[53] Kwon DH, Kim JJ, Lee M, et al. Isolation and characterization of tetracycline-resistant clinical isolates of *Helicobacter pylori*. Antimicrob Agents Chemother 2000;44(11): 3203–5.

[54] Segura AM, Gutierrez O, Otero W, et al. Furazolidone, amoxycillin, bismuth triple therapy for *Helicobacter pylori* infection. Aliment Pharmacol Ther 1997;11(3):529–32.

[55] van der Hulst RW, Keller JJ, Rauws EA, et al. Treatment of *Helicobacter pylori* infection: a review of the world literature. Helicobacter 1996;1(1):6–19.

[56] Miehlke S, Mannes GA, Lehn N, et al. An increasing dose of omeprazole combined with amoxicillin cures *Helicobacter pylori* infection more effectively. Aliment Pharmacol Ther 1997;11(2):323–9.

[57] Fischbach LA, Goodman KJ, Feldman M, et al. Sources of variation of *Helicobacter pylori* treatment success in adults worldwide: a meta-analysis. Int J Epidemiol 2002;31(1): 128–39.

[58] Ford A, Moayyedi P. How can the current strategies for *Helicobacter pylori* eradication therapy be improved? Can J Gastroenterol 2003;17(Suppl B):36B–40B.

[59] Vakil N, Lanza F, Schwartz H, et al. Seven-day therapy for *Helicobacter pylori* in the United States. Aliment Pharmacol Ther 2004;20(1):99–107.

[60] Moayyedi P, Feltbower R, Crocombe W, et al. The effectiveness of omeprazole, clarithromycin and tinidazole in eradicating *Helicobacter pylori* in a community screen and treat programme. Leeds Help Study Group. Aliment Pharmacol Ther 2000;14(6):719–28.

[61] Della Monica P, Lavagna A, Masoero G, et al. Effectiveness of *Helicobacter pylori* eradication treatments in a primary care setting in Italy. Aliment Pharmacol Ther 2002;16(7): 1269–75.

[62] Gene E, Calvet X, Azagra R, et al. Triple vs. quadruple therapy for treating *Helicobacter pylori* infection: a meta-analysis. Aliment Pharmacol Ther 2003;17(9):1137–43.

[63] Fischbach LA, van Zanten S, Dickason J. Meta-analysis: the efficacy, adverse events, and adherence related to first-line anti-*Helicobacter pylori* quadruple therapies. Aliment Pharmacol Ther 2004;20(10):1071–82.

[64] Gisbert JP, Khorrami S, Calvet X, et al. Meta-analysis: proton pump inhibitors vs. H2-receptor antagonists–their efficacy with antibiotics in *Helicobacter pylori* eradication. Aliment Pharmacol Ther 2003;18(8):757–66.

[65] Laheij RJ, Rossum LG, Jansen JB, et al. Evaluation of treatment regimens to cure *Helicobacter pylori* infection—a meta-analysis. Aliment Pharmacol Ther 1999;13(7):857–64.

[66] Broutet N, Tchamgoue S, Pereira E, et al. Risk factors for failure of *Helicobacter pylori* therapy:–results of an individual data analysis of 2,751 patients. Aliment Pharmacol Ther 2003;17(1):99–109.

[67] de Boer WA, Tytgat GN. The best therapy for *Helicobacter pylori* infection: should efficacy or side-effect profile determine our choice? Scand J Gastroenterol 1995;30(5):401–7.

[68] Graham DY, Osato MS, Hoffman J, et al. Furazolidone combination therapies for Helicobacter pylori infection in the United States. Aliment Pharmacol Ther 2000;14(2): 211–5.
[69] Canducci F, Cremonini F, Armuzzi A, et al. Probiotics and Helicobacter pylori eradication. Dig Liver Dis 2002;34(Suppl 2):S81–3.
[70] Di Mario F, Aragona G, Dal Bo N, et al. Use of bovine lactoferrin for Helicobacter pylori eradication. Dig Liver Dis 2003;35(10):706–10.
[71] Di Mario F, Aragona G, Bo ND, et al. Use of lactoferrin for Helicobacter pylori eradication. Preliminary results. J Clin Gastroenterol 2003;36(5):396–8.
[72] Zullo A, De Francesco V, Scaccianoce G, et al. Quadruple therapy with lactoferrin for Helicobacter pylori eradication: a randomised, multicentre study. Dig Liver Dis 2005;37(7): 496–500.
[73] Guttner Y, Windsor HM, Viiala CH, et al. Human recombinant lactoferrin is ineffective in the treatment of human Helicobacter pylori infection. Aliment Pharmacol Ther 2003;17(1): 125–9.
[74] Fujii T, Iishi H, Tatsuta M, et al. Effectiveness of premedication with pronase for improving visibility during gastroendoscopy: a randomized controlled trial. Gastrointest Endosc 1998;47(5):382–7.
[75] Gotoh A, Akamatsu T, Shimizu T, et al. Additive effect of pronase on the efficacy of eradication therapy against Helicobacter pylori. Helicobacter 2002;7(3):183–91.
[76] Gurbuz AK, Ozel AM, Ozturk R, et al. Effect of N-acetyl cysteine on Helicobacter pylori. South Med J 2005;98(11):1095–7.
[77] Zala G, Flury R, Wust J, et al. Omeprazole/amoxicillin: improved eradication of Helicobacter pylori in smokers because of N-acetylcysteine. Schweiz Med Wochenschr 1994;124(31–32):1391–7.
[78] Zullo A, Vaira D, Vakil N, et al. High eradication rates of Helicobacter pylori with a new sequential treatment. Aliment Pharmacol Ther 2003;17(5):719–26.
[79] Zullo A, Gatta L, De Francesco V, et al. High rate of Helicobacter pylori eradication with sequential therapy in elderly patients with peptic ulcer: a prospective controlled study. Aliment Pharmacol Ther 2005;21(12):1419–24.
[80] Francavilla R, Lionetti E, Castellaneta SP, et al. Improved efficacy of 10-day sequential treatment for Helicobacter pylori eradication in children: a randomized trial. Gastroenterology 2005;129(5):1414–9.
[81] Hassan C, De Francesco V, Zullo A, et al. Sequential treatment for Helicobacter pylori eradication in duodenal ulcer patients: improving the cost of pharmacotherapy. Aliment Pharmacol Ther 2003;18(6):641–6.
[82] Nagahara A, Miwa H, Ogawa K, et al. Addition of metronidazole to rabeprazole-amoxicillin-clarithromycin regimen for Helicobacter pylori infection provides an excellent cure rate with five-day therapy. Helicobacter 2000;5(2):88–93.
[83] Treiber G, Ammon S, Schneider E, et al. Amoxicillin/metronidazole/omeprazole/clarithromycin: a new, short quadruple therapy for Helicobacter pylori eradication. Helicobacter 1998;3(1):54–8.
[84] Treiber G, Wittig J, Ammon S, et al. Clinical outcome and influencing factors of a new shortterm quadruple therapy for Helicobacter pylori eradication: a randomized controlled trial (MACLOR study). Arch Intern Med 2002;162(2):153–60.
[85] Gisbert JP, Marcos S, Gisbert JL, et al. High efficacy of ranitidine bismuth citrate, amoxicillin, clarithromycin and metronidazole twice daily for only five days in Helicobacter pylori eradication. Helicobacter 2001;6(2):157–62.
[86] Hopkins RJ. In search of the Holy Grail of Helicobacter pylori remedies. Helicobacter 2001;6(2):81–3.
[87] Bayerdorffer E, Miehlke S, Mannes GA, et al. Double-blind trial of omeprazole and amoxicillin to cure Helicobacter pylori infection in patients with duodenal ulcers. Gastroenterology 1995;108(5):1412–7.

[88] Miehlke S, Kirsch C, Schneider-Brachert W, et al. A prospective, randomized study of quadruple therapy and high-dose dual therapy for treatment of *Helicobacter pylori* resistant to both metronidazole and clarithromycin. Helicobacter 2003;8(4):310–9.

[89] Miehlke S, Mannes GA, Lehn N, et al. An increasing dose of omeprazole combined with amoxycillin cures *Helicobacter pylori* infection more effectively. Aliment Pharmacol Ther 1997;11(2):323–9.

Gastroenterol Clin N Am 35 (2006) 249–273

GASTROENTEROLOGY CLINICS
OF NORTH AMERICA

A Bayesian Approach to Acute Infectious Diarrhea in Adults

Richard Goodgame, MD

Department of Medicine, Baylor College of Medicine, 1 Baylor Plaza, Room 525-D, Houston, TX 77030, USA

A cute infectious diarrhea occurs when a microbial organism produces an illness that is characterized by at least three loose stools per day for less than 14 days. Although population-based data are sparse, such an illness probably occurs with an average frequency of a little less than once per year per person in the United States [1–4]. Out of these 250 million yearly episodes of acute infectious diarrhea, 1 million lead to hospitalization and 6000 lead to death [3]. Generally, mortality is seen only in infants, the elderly, and immunodeficient patients. About half of the episodes of acute infectious diarrhea occur in the setting of epidemics, usually from contaminated food or water [4]; the remainder occurs sporadically. More accurate estimates of the frequency and severity of acute infectious diarrhea are being generated by the Foodborne Diseases Active Surveillance Network [3,5,6], the principal foodborne disease component of the Centers for Disease Control and Prevention's (CDC) Emerging Infections Program. This program monitors 10 areas in the United States with a total population of 42 million people. Health care facilities that serve this monitored population are surveyed annually for the frequency, severity, and etiology of acute infectious diarrhea.

The diagnostic and management approach to acute infectious diarrhea requires constant mental shifting among three databases. Some of the numerous viruses, bacteria, and protozoa that cause acute infectious diarrhea are shown in Box 1. The Foodborne Diseases Active Surveillance Network (FoodNet) data give the probability of finding one of these pathogens in a given patient [3,5,6]; however, the probability of these pathogens changes dramatically in different epidemiologic settings. Some different epidemiologic settings of acute infectious diarrhea are shown in Box 2. The presence or absence of these settings can alter dramatically the probability that a certain pathogen is the cause of the diarrhea. The clinical and laboratory features that are associated with the diarrhea also influence the probability of each pathogen. These are shown in Box 3.

E-mail address: goodgame@bcm.tmc.edu

0889-8553/06/$ – see front matter
doi:10.1016/j.gtc.2006.03.003

Box 1: Infectious agents that cause diarrhea

Viruses

   Norovirus

   Rotavirus

   Astrovirus

   Adenovirus

Bacteria

   Clostridium difficile

   campylobacter

   Escherichia coli (enterotoxigenic; enterohemorrhagic [Shiga toxin producing or O157:H7]; enteroaggregative; enteropathogenic)

   salmonella

   shigella

   Yersinia

   vibrios

Protozoa

   giardia

   Entamoeba histolytica

   cryptosporidium

   Isospora belli

   Cyclospora

Different clinical features shift probabilities away from some pathogens and toward others. All of the items in Boxes 1 through 3 are relevant to the Bayesian logic by which the clinician constantly reassesses the probability of a specific pathogen being present. "Bayesian" refers to the process by which some bit of evidence (an epidemiologic setting or clinical feature) increases the probability of a specific pathogen relative to the probability without that bit of evidence. This probability governs the merits of specific diagnostic tests (or nontesting) and the use (or nonuse) of specific therapy. This is the logic behind the published practice guidelines on acute infectious diarrhea [2,7–9].

THE PATHOGENS

The FoodNet program by the CDC monitors only eight of the pathogens in Box 1; however, the monitored pathogens are the ones that are associated most commonly with mortality. The relative frequency of acute infectious diarrhea that is due to the monitored pathogens (in cases per 100,000 population) is as follows: salmonella, 14.4; campylobacter, 12.6; shigella, 7.3; *Escherichia coli* O157:H7, 1.1; cryptosporidium, 1.1; vibrio, less than 0.3; *Yersinia*, less than 0.4; and *Cyclospora*, less than 0.1 [10]. The same relative frequencies (but about

Box 2: Epidemiologic settings that change the likelihood of certain pathogens

Traveler

Hospital

Antibiotic exposure

Exposures (raw shellfish, farm animals, pet reptiles or amphibians, wilderness vacationer)

Epidemic (incubation a few hours, incubation 1 day, incubation longer)

Daycare center

Nursing home

Male homosexual

twice the rate) have been reported from Ontario, Canada [11]. If acute infectious diarrhea actually occurs one time per person per year, then these pathogens account for only 45 to 90 out of every 100,000 episodes of acute diarrhea. This means that the most common (probable) causes of diarrhea are not

Box 3: Clinical features that may change the probability of certain pathogens

Epigastric pain

Nausea and vomiting

Central abdominal pain

Watery stool

Bloody stool

Temperature greater than 101.3°F

Lower abdominal pain

Rectal pain and tenesmus

Diarrhea longer than 1 week

Diarrhea longer than 2 weeks

Hemolytic uremic syndrome

White cells in stool

Colonic ulceration

Proctitis

Pseudomembranes

Chronic disease (cirrhosis, diabetes mellitus)

Immunodeficiency (organ transplant, cancer chemotherapy, hypogammaglobulinemia)

HIV (CD4 greater than 200/mL, CD4 less than 200/mL, CD4 less than 75/mL)

included in the FoodNet data. The most common are the noroviruses, formally called "calicivirus," and "Norwalk-like virus" (see the article by Atmar and Estes elsewhere in this issue). True population-based surveys have not been done, but evaluation of epidemics and sporadic cases have shown that most acute infectious diarrhea in the United States is due to noroviruses [4,12–14]. Noroviruses account for 50,000 to 80,000 out of 100,000 episodes of acute infectious diarrhea. The next most common (probable) causes of acute infectious diarrhea are the diarrheagenic *E coli* (non-Shiga toxin producing) [15–17]. These organisms may cause up to 6000 per 100,000 cases of acute infectious diarrhea. Many of these episodes occur in travelers within the United States or internationally (see the article by DuPont elsewhere in this issue). Another unmonitored common cause of acute infectious diarrhea is *Clostridium difficile*. *Clostridium difficile* is increasing in frequency dramatically in outpatients and in-patients (see the article by Aslam and Musher elsewhere in this issue). Population-based data from Canada and the United States suggest that it may be the cause in up to 150 out of 100,000 episodes of acute infectious diarrhea [18–20], and up to 800 out of 100,000 episodes in the elderly [21,22]. Based on these frequency data, if all patients who had acute infectious diarrhea presented to a doctor after the first three loose stools, the probability of the infectious diarrhea being associated with a specific pathogen would be as follows: norovirus, 50% to 80%; diarrheagenic *E coli* (non-Shiga toxin producing), 6%; *Clostridium difficile*, 1.5%; invasive bacteria, 0.04%; Shiga toxin–producing *E coli* (STEC), 0.002%; and protozoa, 0.005%. Thus, norovirus is the starting point in the approach to acute infectious diarrhea.

The frequency of norovirus infection is related to its efficient transmission through multiple modalities (see the article by Atmar and Estes elsewhere in this issue). Two thirds of all foodborne illness is caused by norovirus [23]. Some contamination occurs at the food source, such as raw shellfish [24]. Most food contamination occurs through infected food handlers [25,26]. Waterborne epidemics also are well documented [27,28]. Swimming pools and recreational fountains also have been implicated [29]. Person-to-person transmission is important in home and institutional epidemics. Epidemics can last a long time because of environmental contamination coupled with person-to-person spread [30,31]. Airborne transmission also is well documented [32,33]. Norovirus infections are common in all age groups. Symptoms last for a median of 3 days but viral particles (perhaps infectious) can be detected in 26% of patients up to 3 weeks after the onset of illness.

Norovirus (and other viruses in Box 1) is suspected as the cause of acute infectious diarrhea when there are no epidemiologic clues from the history (eg, travel or antibiotic use) that suggest an alternate diagnosis and when the clinical features do not suggest bacterial infection (ie, high fever, bloody diarrhea, severe abdominal pain, more than six stools per 24 hours) or protozoa infection (ie, prolonged diarrhea). Clinicians (and most nonmedical personnel) recognize that "viral" (norovirus) gastroenteritis does not require specialized diagnostic testing or antimicrobial treatment. Therefore, diagnostic and management guidelines for adults who have acute infectious diarrhea recognize that most patients do not need extensive testing or specific treatment [2,7–9].

All of the pathogens in Box 1 can cause a clinical illness that is "like norovirus": nausea and vomiting, diarrhea with less than six stools per day, low-grade fever, mild abdominal pain, scant blood, and resolution in 3 to 5 days. Included in the definition of "like norovirus" is the absence of an epidemiologic setting (see Box 2) or clinical features (see Box 3) that increase the likelihood of "not norovirus" infection. To the extent that the bacteria (including salmonella, shigella, campylobacter, *E coli*, vibrios) and protozoa (including cryptosporidium, *Cyclospora*, giardia, and amoeba) cause an illness "like norovirus," diagnostic and treatment restraint are indicated.

EPIDEMIOLOGY

Acute diarrhea has a low (8%) probability of being "not norovirus." But there are epidemiologic settings that increase the probability of "not norovirus" well above this level. Most patients who have acute infectious diarrhea do not seek medical care. Up to 56% of adult patients who present to a health care facility because of acute nonepidemic diarrhea can have an enteropathogen identified through extensive testing: campylobacter, 13%; *Clostridium difficile*, 13%; enterotoxigenic *E coli*, 8%; salmonella, 7%; shigella, 4%; norovirus, 3%; rotavirus, 3%; giardia, 2%; and cryptosporidium, 2% [34]. Just coming to a health care facility alters the probability of "not norovirus" from about 8% in a population-based sample to about 50% in a clinic-based sample. Seeing a patient who has acute diarrhea at a health care facility is an epidemiologic fact. But the patient's decision to seek medical care likely is related to clinical features that are recognized by the patient as being more serious than "viral" gastroenteritis: more stools per day, more severe pain, higher fever, bloody stool, or prolonged diarrhea. The impact of these symptoms and signs is discussed in the next section.

Travel

When a patient who has acute infectious diarrhea gives a history of being a traveler or a returned traveler, the epidemiologic setting of travel changes the probability of "not norovirus" from between 8% and 17% to 80%. A history of travel, especially foreign travel, is associated with a high probability (80%) of bacterial diarrhea (see the article by DuPont elsewhere in this issue). Thirty to fifty percent of the 50 million Americans who travel annually to developing countries develop loose or liquid stools in the first few weeks of travel [35,36]; however, even travel within the United States is associated with a 4% rate of diarrhea. The major bacteria are the noninvasive diarrheagenic *E coli*: enterotoxigenic *E coli* [15] and enteroaggregative *E coli* [16,17]. These make up most identifiable cases in Mexico and South America. The invasive bacteria, such as *Campylobacter jejuni*, *Shigella* spp, and *Salmonella* spp, are seen much more commonly in travelers to southern Asia. Norovirus infection is the cause in up to 17% [37,38]. Protozoa (giardia, *Entamoeba histolytica*, cryptosporidium and the other spore-forming protozoa) are much less common causes of acute traveler's diarrhea but are important considerations when a traveler has persistent diarrhea (see "Clinical features") [39]. As the article by DuPont clearly states (elsewhere in this issue), presumptive antibiotic therapy combined with clinical observation is appropriate (Table 1). The clinical features (response to antibiotics and length of illness) may mandate stool examination and consideration of other pathogens (see "Clinical features").

Hospital Acquired and Antibiotic Associated

Although nosocomial diarrhea can have noninfectious causes, such as medication side effects, medication vehicles, and tube feedings, an infectious cause can be identified in about one third of cases [40,41]. Once the epidemiologic setting is "hospital-acquired acute diarrhea" the probability of "not norovirus" goes from 8% to 100%. The etiologic pathogen is almost always *Clostridium difficile* [40,41]. The article by Aslam and Musher (elsewhere in this issue) provides a comprehensive review of this important pathogen. *Clostridium difficile* is the only enteric infectious agent that merits serious initial consideration in a hospitalized patient who develops diarrhea after being in the hospital for 3 days or more [41]. Stool tests for other enteric pathogens (salmonella, shigella, campylobacter, protozoa) are almost never positive in patients who have hospital-acquired diarrhea [41]. Community-acquired *Clostridium difficile* infections also occur, especially in the elderly. These usually are associated with a history of antibiotic use or contact with health care personnel or institutions. When the epidemiology suggests increased risk (inpatient, recent hospitalization or antibiotic use, or contact with health personnel), stool should be sent for *Clostridium difficile* toxin assay (see the article by Aslam and Musher elsewhere in this issue for diagnostic test performance). A dramatic increase in the frequency and severity of *Clostridium difficile* infection is occurring [18–22]. The probability of *Clostridium difficile* being the cause of acute infectious diarrhea is so high in some epidemiologic settings that negative toxin assays by enzyme immunoassay (EIA) are likely to be false negatives. Negative tests in such settings must prompt further testing: repeat EIA, colonoscopy, or the bioassay for cytotoxin using tissue cell culture. Presumptive treatment while awaiting test results is appropriate in severely ill patients when the epidemiology makes *Clostridium difficile* highly probable.

Other Epidemiologic Features

In addition to the major epidemiologic associations with norovirus, diarrheagenic *E coli*, and *Clostridium difficile*, a few less common associations are listed in Table 2. It is difficult to quantify the exact change in the probability of encountering "not norovirus" that is associated with each of these epidemiologic details. But these epidemiologic clues should be used to direct diagnostic and treatment initiatives, especially in patients whose illness deviates clinically from that seen in typical viral gastroenteritis.

CLINICAL FEATURES

Some of the clinical features in Box 3 are those associated with norovirus infection or an illness "like norovirus": nausea, vomiting, watery diarrhea, mild to moderate epigastric and peri-umbilical abdominal pain, less than six stools per day, and less than 7 days of illness. But certain clinical features in Box 3 are associated with acute infectious diarrhea that has a high probability of being "not norovirus." Patients whose abdominal pain is severe, fever is high, or diarrhea is bloody are unlikely to have norovirus infection. Patients whose diarrhea persists for more than 7 days are likely to have "not norovirus." Published practice guidelines on the approach to acute infectious diarrhea [2,7–9] identify clinical features that require diagnostic testing and treatment that are appropriate for "not norovirus" illness.

Clinical Features of Potentially Lethal Bacterial or Amoebic Infection

Patients who have abdominal pain that is severe, temperature that is high (>101.3°F), and diarrhea that is voluminous or bloody have a subset of acute infectious diarrhea that is associated with the following probabilities of pathogens: salmonella, 7% to 20%; campylobacter, 10% to 30%; shigella, 4% to 10%; STEC, 2% to 4%; Yersinia or vibrios, 1% to 2%; and *Clostridium difficile*, 10% to 20% [5,11,34,42,43]. The clinical features of cholera—dehydrating, shock-producing, lethal watery diarrhea—are not included because clinical cholera that is due to *Vibrio cholera* O1 has disappeared from the United States mainland [44]. Other *Vibrio* spp cause mild gastroenteritis ("like norovirus") or severe disease that is indistinguishable from the other invasive bacterial pathogens [45].

The presence of severe clinical features mandates stool tests to look for bacterial or amoebic infection (see Table 1). In ambiguous cases the stool can be assessed for polymorphonuclear white blood cells (neutrophils) by microscopy or by immunoassay for the neutrophil protein lactoferrin [46,47]. If these tests are positive there is an increased probability of finding an invasive pathogen. Bloody stool without white blood cells is a common feature of STEC (eg, *E coli* O157:H7) and colitis that is due to *Entamoeba histolytica*. Definitive stool tests for specific pathogens include culture for salmonella, shigella, campylobacter, and *E coli* O157:H7; assay for Shiga toxin; and microscopy or antigen assay for *Entamoeba histolytica* (see Table 1). Flexible sigmoidoscopy that shows endoscopic evidence of acute colitis increases the probability of one of these pathogens. Pseudomembranes make *Clostridium difficile* infection highly probable. Biopsy can confirm amoebic colitis. If the symptoms and signs are severe, presumptive antibiotic therapy is recommended (unless *E coli* O157:H7 is likely, see later discussion) because of the high probability of campylobacter, shigella, and severe salmonella infection and the efficacy of antibiotics for these conditions (see Table 1) [2]. Precise diagnosis depends on the results of stool culture and microscopy, but almost half of the cases that fulfill the above criteria for bacterial colitis are culture negative on extensive testing. Probabilities that are based on published series are weighed heavier than stool culture results in individual patients.

Salmonella *species*

Salmonellae are widespread bacterial pathogens that are important causes of sporadic and epidemic acute infectious diarrhea. Most outbreaks are related

Table 1
Approach to acute infectious diarrhea in adults

	Epidemiology and clinical features	Probability of "not norovirus"	Prominent pathogens	Diagnosis	Treatment	Comments
Acute infectious diarrhea "like norovirus" epidemiologically and clinically	Epidemic or sporadic community acquired, nonbloody diarrhea, less than six stools per day, temperature less than 101.3°F, mild abdominal pain, less than 5 days in duration	8%	Norovirus (≤80%) Rotavirus Adenovirus Astrovirus The mild cases of bacteria and protozoa	No specific diagnostic tests indicated. Ask about drugs, unusual foods, shellfish, pets, animals, travel, immune disorder, chronic illnesses.	Avoid milk products. Oral hydration. Eat small, frequent, easily digested meals. Loperamide 4 mg once and 2 mg with each liquid stool (evidence reviewed in Ref [2]).	Most diarrhea-causing pathogens can cause mild self-limited illness, "like norovirus," not requiring laboratory testing or antimicrobial treatment
Epidemiologic setting suggesting "not norovirus"	Seen in acute care setting	50%	campylobacter 13% salmonella 7% shigella 4% non-STEC E coli 8% C difficile 13% giardia 2% cryptosporidium 2%	Diagnostic studies based on epidemiologic and clinical features below	Treatment based on epidemiologic and clinical features below	Salmonella, shigella, and STEC should be reported to public health authorities

Travel	80%	Non-STEC 50%–80% Invasive bacteria 5%–30%	Treatment for bacteria without diagnosis recommended [DuPont]. Diagnostic studies if unresponsive or prolonged [DuPont].	Suspected travel-related bacterial diarrhea: rifaximin, 200 mg three times daily for 3 d; if poor response, azithromycin, 1000 mg once [DuPont].	The efficacy of rifaximin in established dysentery is not certain
Hospital acquired or antibiotic use	Up to 100% if infectious	C difficile unless immunosuppressed or hospital epidemic of another pathogen	C difficile toxin assay by EIA or tissue culture assay [Aslam]. Consider colonoscopy.	Suspected C difficile: metronidazole, 500 mg three times daily [Aslam]. Consider oral nitazoxanide or vancomycin [Aslam].	

(continued on next page)

Table 1
(continued)

Clinical features suggesting "not norovirus"	Epidemiology and clinical features	Probability of "not norovirus"	Prominent pathogens	Diagnosis	Treatment	Comments
Severe bacterial or amebic disease	Bloody diarrhea More than six stools per day Temperature greater than 101°F Severe abdominal pain	Up to 100%	salmonella 7%–20% campylobacter 10%–30% shigella 4%–10% STEC 2%–4% yersinia 1%–2% vibrios 1%–2% C difficile 10%–20% Amoeba <1%	Culture for salmonella, shigella, campylobacter, and E coli O157:H7 [2] EIA for Shiga toxin, E histolytica, and C difficile toxin [Aslam]. Stool stain for white blood cells (evidence reviewed in Ref [2]). Stool assay for lactoferrin (evidence reviewed in Ref [2]).	Suspected Shiga toxin producing E. coli: no antibiotics or antidiarrhea agents Suspected severe bacterial enteritis: levofloxacin, 500 mg daily for 3 d [evidence reviewed in ref 2] and azithromycin 1000 mg once	Salmonella, shigella, and shiga toxin producing E. coli should be reported to public health authorities

Hemolytic-uremic syndrome	Hemolysis Thrombocytopenia Uremia	Up to 100%	STEC, either O157:H7 (63%) or non-O157 (uncommon)	EIA for Shiga toxin Culture of E coli O157:H7	Hydration Avoid nephrotoxic drugs Dialysis Intravenous immunoglobulin Plasmapheresis	Notify public health authorities. Assess family members and close contacts.
Prolonged diarrhea	Diarrhea longer than 7–14 d	Up to 100%	No reliable probabilities Protozoa and microsporidia C difficile campylobacter Shiga-producing E coli	Stool cultures for bacteria EIA for C difficile, Shiga toxin, E histolytica, giardia [Huang]. Immunofluorescent microscopy for giardia and cryptosporidium [Huang]. Stool microscopy for other spore-forming protozoa and microsporidia.	Suspected giardia: metronidazole, 250 mg three times daily for 5–7 d, or tinidazole, 2 g [Huang]. Suspected E histolytica: metronidazole, 750 mg three times daily for 10 d, followed by iodoquinol, 650 mg three times per day for 20 d	Giardia and cryptosporidium should be reported to public health authorities

(continued on next page)

Table 1
(*continued*)

Epidemiology and clinical features	Probability of "not norovirus"	Prominent pathogens	Diagnosis	Treatment	Comments
d. Immunocopromised Host					
Organ transplant	Increased, and bad outcome more likely	Abnormally severe illness from rotavirus and adenovirus. Increased frequency of cytomegalovirus. Severe illness from bacteria. Spore-forming protozoa and microsporidia.	Most common cause is noninfectious: drugs and graft-versus-host disease. Stool cultures for bacteria and viruses. EIA for *C difficile* [Aslam], cryptosporidium, and giardia [Huang]. Stool microscopy for protozoa and microsporidia. Endoscopy for cytomegalovirus and graft-versus-host disease.	Suspected cryptosporidium or giardia: nitazoxanide, 500 mg twice daily for 3 d [Huang]. Suspected cytomegalovirus: ganciclovir, 5 mg/kg twice daily IV, or valganciclovir, 900 mg twice daily.	

HIV/AIDS	Increased, and bad outcome more likely	Severe illness from bacteria. Spore-forming protozoa and microsporidia. Increased frequency of cytomegalovirus and Mycobacterium avium complex.	Most common cause is drug, especially protease inhibitors. Stool cultures for bacteria. EIA for C difficile [Aslam], cryptosporidium [Huang], and giardia [Huang]. Stool microscopy for spore-forming protozoa and microsporidia. Endoscopy for cytomegalovirus and Mycobacterium avium complex.	Suspected Isospora or Cyclospora: trimethoprim-sulfamethoxazole, 160–800 mg twice daily for 7–10 d. Suspected microsporidia: albendazole, 400 mg twice daily for 2–4 wk	Treatment with antiretrovirals to increase CD4 count is associated with reduced opportunistic infections
Chronic disease Age older than 60 y	Increased, and bad outcome more likely	Severe illness from bacteria and viruses	Stool cultures for salmonella, shigella, campylobacter. EIA for Shiga toxin and C difficile toxin.	Low threshold for presumptive treatment for suspected pathogens while waiting for test results	

Abbreviations: C difficile, Clostridium difficile; E histolytica, Entamoeba histolytica; EIA, enzyme immunoassay; IV, intravenously.

Table 2
Association between some epidemiologic features and specific pathogens

Epidemiologic feature	Specific pathogen
Epidemic gastroenteritis in institutions, hospitals, nursing homes, cruise ships, vacation-recreation-cultural venues	Norovirus; less commonly, *Campylobacter jejuni, Salmonella* species, cryptosporidium.
Hospital-acquired diarrhea or history of antibiotic use or contact with health care personnel or institutions	*Clostridium difficile*
Traveler's diarrhea or recent history of travel	Diarrheagenic *E coli;* less commonly other bacteria and protozoa.
Epidemic of severe gastroenteritis traced to eggs, poultry, meat, or dairy products	*Campylobacter jejuni, Salmonella* species
Pets, especially reptiles (turtles, lizards, and snakes) and amphibians (frogs, toads, newts, and salamanders)	*Salmonella* species
Animal contact at agricultural fairs, petting zoos, and county fairs	*E coli* O157:H7 and non-O157 Shiga toxin–producing *E coli*
Daycare client or worker	Rotavirus, Norovirus, shigella, giardia
Bloody diarrhea in an immigrant or traveler	*Entamoeba histolytica*
Shellfish ingestion	Norovirus or *Vibrio* spp
Hiker or vacationer drinking untreated water	Giardia or cryptosporidium

to contacts with animals [48]. Virtually all mammals, birds, reptiles, and many insects can be infected [49–51]. Contact with animal products, especially milk, beef, chicken, and eggs, is a common mode of transmission [52]. Salmonella is the leading cause of food-related deaths in the United States [53]. As with other invasive bacteria, gastrointestinal disease shows the full spectrum, from mild watery diarrhea ("like norovirus") to severe colitis that lasts for several weeks. Bacteremia predisposes to complications. Metastatic infection and abscesses occur in such organs as the heart, bones, or meninges [54,55]. Sometimes the clinical features of bacteremia (fever, malaise, inanition, delirium) can exist with few gastrointestinal symptoms (typhoidal salmonellosis). A mild case of salmonella enteritis ("like norovirus") does not need specific diagnosis or treatment in most patients. Antibiotics do not shorten the length of illness in salmonella enteritis and they may prolong the excretion of organisms. Antibiotics are indicated for salmonella infection in patients at extremes of age [53] and those with underlying diseases, such as cancer, cirrhosis, immunodeficiency, and abnormal heart valves and prostheses [55–58]. Antibiotics also are given for severe enteritis, bacteremia, and localized extraintestinal infection [54]. Therapy is guided by sensitivity testing but usually is initiated with fluoroquinolones because of widespread resistance to ampicillin, sulfonamides, tetracycline, and chloramphenicol and emerging resistance to ciprofloxacin and ceftriaxone [59–61]. Fluoroquinolone resistance is recognized increasingly, especially in foreign-acquired infections [62,63].

Campylobacter jejuni

Campylobacter jejuni is one of the most commonly recognized causes of bacterial gastroenteritis in the world [64]. American cases generally result from contact with untreated water, animals, and contaminated food products, especially chickens and poultry [65]. Most cases are sporadic, but food (poultry) and waterborne epidemics have been identified [66,67]. Most cases are mild and are "like norovirus." Diarrhea usually resolves in 1 week but persistent diarrhea for more than 2 to 3 weeks is not rare. Local (hemorrhage, megacolon) [68] and bacteremic (cellulitis, arthritis, meningitis) complications occur [69], mainly in the elderly and immunocompromised patients. Antimicrobials (quinolones and macrolides) shorten the duration of illness and reduce infectious complications [64]. Recent studies showed that 10% of *Campylobacter jejuni* infections are now resistant to fluoroquinolones because of the use of these medicines in poultry farming [64,70,71]. Infection with this organism is the most common identifiable cause of Guillain-Barré syndrome, especially the axonal subtypes [72]. There is molecular mimicry between the lipo-oligosaccharide of *Campylobacter jejuni* and gangliosides, components of the peripheral nerves. About one fourth of patients who have Guillain-Barré syndrome have evidence of preceding *Campylobacter jejuni* infection, but this complication occurs in less than 1 out of 1000 episodes of campylobacter enteritis. An abnormal host response to *Campylobacter jejuni* also may be important in the pathogenesis of immunoproliferative small intestinal disease [73].

Shigella *species*

Shigella infections are less frequent in the United States than are the other bacterial pathogens. Because there are no nonhuman hosts for these organisms, transmission requires close personal contact [74] or a major breakdown in sanitation [75]. High-risk groups include clients and workers in daycare centers [76,77] and nursing homes, and male homosexuals [74]. Mild infections ("like norovirus") resolve in 1 week and usually are not diagnosed. In severe cases, lower abdominal pain, fever, and diarrhea evolve into severe colitic symptoms with blood, pus, urgency, tenesmus, and systemic toxicity. Severe infections benefit from antibiotic therapy (see Table 1). In the appropriate setting, a fecal smear that shows numerous white blood cells makes shigellosis a likely diagnosis. Stool culture provides definitive etiologic diagnosis and antibiotic-sensitivity testing.

Shiga toxin–producing Escherichia coli

E coli O157:H7 (also called STEC or verotoxin-producing *E coli*) gained prominence 20 years ago as a consequence of numerous infections that were caused by fast-food restaurants serving contaminated, poorly cooked beef [78]. Now STEC is a frequently recognized cause of sporadic and epidemic acute infectious diarrhea in the United States [79], and a serious worldwide public health threat. Beef and milk products have been implicated in most outbreaks [80], but contamination of fruits, vegetables, and water also has been reported [79]. A wide variety of healthy animals (importantly cattle, sheep, goats, deer) harbor the organism. Agricultural fairs, county fairs, and petting zoos are well-known sites of infection [81,82]. A small inoculum of organisms can cause clinical disease. *E coli* O157:H7 initially causes watery diarrhea and cramps ("like norovirus"). A study from The Netherlands indicated that only 20% of community-acquired cases become severe enough to cause the patient to seek medical attention [83]. The FoodNet data are laboratory based, and so they may underestimate the frequency of infections drastically [79]. Among cases that are identified clinically, nonbloody diarrhea predominates [84]. The more severe cases evolve into a hemorrhagic colitis. Fever is much less prominent than in other bacterial diarrhea. In some patients, right lower quadrant pain, which mimics acute appendicitis, predominates. About 5% to 15% of severely symptomatic infections lead to the development of the hemolytic uremic syndrome (HUS), a potentially lethal (5%) multisystem disease that is characterized by microangiopathic hemolytic anemia, renal failure (50% need dialysis), and thrombocytopenia [85]. The pathogenesis is not well known. Five percent of survivors have major complications, such as chronic renal failure and stroke [83]. Local colitis and systemic disease (HUS) are related to the production of Shiga toxins, which are potent inhibitors of protein synthesis. Factors that may predict the occurrence of HUS in patients who present with diarrhea are a young (<15 years) or old (>65 years) age, short incubation period, high white blood cell count, high C-reactive protein, and low albumin [78,85].

A reliable method to screen for *E coli* O157:H7 is the culture of stool on sorbitol-MacConkey agar. Positive colonies are tested for Shiga toxin antigens to confirm diagnosis; however, there are STEC that are non-O157. These are not detected well on the sorbitol-MacConkey agar. Sensitive and specific stool-based EIAs for Shiga toxins 1 and 2 are available [86]. Patients who have frankly bloody stool are the ones who are most likely to have a positive culture or toxin assay. Clinical laboratories should screen bloody stool specimens ("not norovirus") routinely with the Shiga toxin assays. Accurate diagnosis is important for public health purposes. Product recall early in an epidemic can save many lives. All positive cases should be reported to public health authorities immediately [85]. The current recommendation is not to use antibiotics for suspected *E coli* O157:H7. This can be confusing because the decision to withhold antibiotics is supposed to be made based on epidemiologic and clinical features that are associated with STEC: a known recent or nearby epidemic, bloody diarrhea without high fever, blood much greater than diarrhea, and few white blood cells in the stool [2]. These features are of unknown sensitivity and specificity. Antibiotic use has been associated with the increasing risk for HUS [87]. These studies may be flawed because patients who received antibiotics were the most severely ill [88]. Nevertheless, the conclusive benefit of antibiotics has not been demonstrated and at least one animal model showed that antibiotics may worsen outcome [89].

Entamoeba histolytica

Bloody diarrhea, especially in an immigrant or traveler, always should raise the possibility of amoebic infection [90]. *Entamoeba histolytica* is the only intestinal protozoal disease that commonly causes death. Transmission occurs through contaminated food or water or by sexual practices. Trophozoites invade the colonic mucosa and cause discrete punched-out ulcers, most commonly in the right colon. The ulcers can enlarge to greater than 2 cm and can cause perforation. Diarrhea can be mild and intermittent ("like norovirus"). In endemic areas, new infections and reinfections with *Entamoeba histolytica* come and go without symptoms [91]. Diarrhea can be severe and persistent ("not norovirus"). Complications include severe bleeding, toxic megacolon, and mass lesions that lead to intussusception, stricture and obstruction, and perforation.

Microscopic examination cannot distinguish between the two most common strains: *Entamoeba histolytica* (10% of all infections) and the more common, but nonpathogenic *Entamoeba dispar* (90% of all infections). Almost all asymptomatic patients have *Entamoeba dispar* infection. In patients who present with an illness that is compatible with invasive amebiasis, a stool that is positive for amoeba by microscopy is assumed to be the pathogenic strain, but correlation between clinical symptoms and stool test results is poor. Microscopy on a single stool can miss almost half of infections. Colonoscopy may demonstrate ulcerations or, less commonly, mass lesions. Biopsy shows trophozoites in about 50% of cases; multiple scrapings of ulcers that are placed on a slide immediately usually yield the diagnosis. Because of poor sensitivity and specificity of microscopy, the new monoclonal antibody-based EIA for *Entamoeba histolytica* antigen (95% sensitive and specific for *Entamoeba histolytica*) should be used [92]. This test should reduce the need to perform multiple stool examinations, colonoscopy, and serology in an effort to diagnose *Entamoeba histolytica* infection accurately.

Asymptomatic infections that are identified by stool microscopy should not be treated. Asymptomatic *Entamoeba histolytica* infection (identified by the newer EIA tests) in nonendemic areas can be treated to eliminate the risk of developing invasive disease and to prevent its spread to others. The treatment of choice remains metronidazole, 750 mg three times per day for 10 days (for trophozoites), plus iodoquinol, 650 mg three times per day for 20 days (for cysts). A follow-up stool examination 2 to 4 weeks after treatment is recommended.

Hemolytic Uremic Syndrome

HUS—hemolysis, thrombocytopenia, and decreased renal function [78,85]—is the leading cause of renal failure in childhood and it also occurs in healthy adults [93]. Most cases are due to STEC. Stool samples from patients who have HUS are positive for *E coli* O157:H7 63% of the time [94]. In the setting of acute infectious diarrhea, early detection of this severe complication prompts confirmation of STEC infection and notification of public health officials. Early public health intervention can limit exposure and save lives [80]. In the affected individual, antibiotic treatment should be withheld, but efforts to maximize renal function (hydration, avoidance of nephrotoxic drugs, dialysis) can be implemented. Specific treatment (intravenous immunoglobulin or plasma exchange) can be considered. Family members and close contacts should be assessed.

Prolonged Acute Diarrhea

Most cases of acute infectious diarrhea are resolved by 5 days. The pathogen is norovirus or a bacteria or protozoa that produces an illness "like norovirus." The longer the diarrhea lasts, the higher is the probability that another pathogen is the cause ("not norovirus"). *Campylobacter jejuni* infections frequently last longer than 1 week. Some STEC have been associated with prolonged diarrhea [95]. The major clinical feature of protozoa infection is prolonged diarrhea. Patients who have persistent diarrhea should have stools tested for *Entamoeba histolytica* antigen, *Giardia intestinalis* antigen, and *Cryptosporidium parvum* antigen by EIA (see the article by Huang and White elsewhere in this issue). The other protozoa (*Isospora belli* and *Cyclospora cayatenensis*) and microsporidia (*Enterocytozoon bieneusi* and *Encephalitozoon intestinalis*) are uncommon causes of prolonged diarrhea in immunologically normal adults and children [39,96]. Stool tests for these pathogens are indicated when acute diarrhea fails to resolve in 1 to 2 weeks. Chronic infection can be difficult to distinguish from postinfectious irritable bowel syndrome (see the article by DuPont elsewhere in this issue) [42,97].

Immunocompromised Host

Diagnostic and treatment restraint is a guiding feature of the approach to acute infectious diarrhea because "like norovirus" is overwhelmingly probable and is associated with a good outcome is most cases. Patients who have the following clinical features require a more aggressive approach: extremes of age, chronic disease (hemoglobinopathy, lymphoproliferative disease, cirrhosis, diabetes, prosthetic valves or other hardware), immune suppression (organ transplant, cancer chemotherapy, steroid therapy), and acquired or inherited immune deficiency syndromes. Acute diarrhea in these settings requires a lower threshold for performing diagnostic testing, expanded diagnostic testing for unusual pathogens, and earlier presumptive treatment while awaiting test results.

The increased frequency and severity of invasive bacterial infections in immunocompromised hosts is well documented. Hospitalization, bacteremia, metastatic infections, and death due to salmonella infections correlate strongly with age and serious underlying conditions [49,53,55–57]. For example, almost all of the Spanish patients who were involved in a nosocomial outbreak of *Salmonella enteriditis* were immunocompromised [58]. Rare cases of disseminated infection from *Campylobacter jejuni* usually are related to immune compromised states [69]. Patients who have more severe underlying illnesses are more likely to develop *Clostridium difficile* colitis [98].

Organ transplantation

When acute infectious diarrhea occurs in a patient who has undergone organ transplant, early identification of an infectious cause is important [99]. This begins with testing for "not norovirus" pathogens that are common in patients with normal immunity, such as *Clostridium difficile* [100] and invasive bacteria. Viruses that cause self-limited mild viral gastroenteritis in a normal host (adenovirus and rotavirus [101]) may cause severe and prolonged enteric infections in patients with transplants. The use of prophylactic antiviral therapy (valganciclovir) has reduced the frequency of enteric infections with cytomegalovirus (CMV) dramatically; however, in a high-risk setting (donor CMV positive and recipient CMV negative) early endoscopy is indicated to investigate for CMV enteritis as a cause of acute infectious diarrhea [102,103]. The spore-forming protozoa and microsporidia also are more frequent pathogens in this setting [96]. A major diagnostic challenge is differentiating noninfectious diarrhea that is due to drugs [104] or graft-versus-host disease [105] from infectious causes.

Acquired immunodeficiency syndrome

Chronic, rather than acute, infectious diarrhea is a major problem in AIDS, but its frequency has been reduced by the ability of combination antiretroviral therapy to keep immunity (CD4 lymphocyte count) above 300 cells/mL [106]. Some acute gastrointestinal infections occur with a frequency and severity that are unrelated to the severity of immune deficiency. These include *Clostridium difficile*, *Giardia intestinalis*, and *Entamoeba histolytica*. At CD4 counts around 200 cells/mL, bacterial infections (salmonella, shigella, campylobacter) can be severe and prolonged if antibiotic therapy is delayed. At CD4 counts that are less than 200 cells/mL, more frequent and prolonged infection with spore-forming protozoa and microsporidia occurs [97]. When the CD4 count is less than 75 cells/mL, infections with CMV [103] and *Mycobacterium avium* complex become more frequent. The wide range of unusual gastrointestinal infections in AIDS, such as toxoplasma, histoplasma, bartonella, and pneumocystis, usually occurs in patients who have very low CD4 counts.

Evaluation of patients who have AIDS and acute infectious diarrhea should begin with stool tests (tailored to the clinical setting), including *Clostridium difficile* toxin assay; culture for invasive bacteria; microscopy for cryptosporidium, microsporidia, *Isospora*, and *Cyclospora*; and EIA for giardia antigen (see Table 1). Alternatively, the fluorescent, monoclonal antibody–based test for cryptosporidium and giardia can be used. A single stool in highly symptomatic patients has adequate sensitivity for most pathogens; however, three stools have been recommended for complete evaluation. Specific treatment is available for most pathogens. But the best treatment and prevention for acute and chronic infectious diarrhea is maintenance of high CD4 counts with highly active antiretroviral therapy [106].

Since the advent of combination antiretroviral therapy, most acute and chronic diarrhea has a noninfectious cause. Major causes of diarrhea include the protease inhibitors, especially nelfinavir (≤49% with diarrhea [107]) and the combination lopinavir/ritonavir (≤17% with diarrhea [107,108]). Diarrhea is one of the most common reasons for stopping or switching antiretroviral therapy when these agents are used [108]. The relationship between antiretro-virals and diarrhea is complex because infectious diarrhea can lead to low levels or poor compliance and high levels can be associated with symptoms [109].

SUMMARY

Acute infectious diarrhea is a yearly occurrence for most Americans, and is associated with 1 million hospitalizations and about 6000 deaths in the United States annually. Up to 80% of acute infectious diarrhea is caused by norovi-ruses, which produce a clinically mild illness with a predictable short course and good outcome that make laboratory testing and antimicrobial treatment unnecessary. Most diarrhea-causing bacteria and protozoa can cause a clinical illness "like norovirus"; when they do so in healthy adults neither specialized testing nor antimicrobials is required. The presence or absence of epidemio-logic evidence (such as travel, hospitalization, antibiotic use, other exposures) and clinical evidence (such as diarrhea frequency and duration, severity of ab-dominal pain and fever, character of stool, presence of chronic illness or im-mune deficiency) can change the probability of "not norovirus" from as low as 8% to as high as 100%. Such probabilities guide the use of laboratory testing and antimicrobial therapy in patients who have acute infectious diarrhea.

References

[1] Flint JA, Van Duynhoven YT, Angulo FJ, et al. Estimating the burden of acute gastroenteritis, foodborne disease, and pathogens commonly transmitted by food: an international review. Clin Infect Dis 2005;41:698–704.

[2] Thielman MN, Guerrant RL. Acute infectious diarrhea. N Engl J Med 2004;350: 38–47.

[3] Imhoff B, Morse D, Shiferaw B, et al. Burden of self-reported acute diarrheal illness in Food-Net surveillance areas, 1998–1999. Clin Infect Dis 2004;38(Suppl 3):S219–26.

[4] Musher DM, Musher BL. Contagious acute gastrointestinal infections. N Engl J Med 2004;351:2417–27.

[5] Allos BM, Moore MR, Griffin PM, et al. Surveillance for sporadic foodborne disease in the 21st century: the FoodNet perspective. Clin Infect Dis 2004;38(Suppl 3):S115–20.

[6] FoodNet. Available at: http://www.cdc.gov/foodnet/. Accessed May 8, 2006.

[7] DuPont HL. Guidelines on acute infectious diarrhea in adults. Am J Gastroenterol 1997;92: 1962–75.

[8] Manatsathit S, Dupont HL, Farthing M, et al. Guideline for the management of acute diar-rhea in adults. J Gastroenterol Hepatol 2002;17(Suppl 17):S54–71.

[9] Guerrant RL, Van Gilder T, Steiner TS, et al. Practice guidelines for the management of infectious diarrhea. Clin Infect Dis 2001;32:331–51.

[10] FoodNet Report 2003. Available at: http://www.cdc.gov/foodnet/pub.htm. Accessed on February 10, 2006.

[11] Lee MB, Middleton D. Enteric illness in Ontario, Canada, from 1997 to 2001. J Food Prot 2003;66:953–61.

[12] Fankhauser R, Noel J, Monroe S, et al. Molecular epidemiology of "Norwalk-like viruses" in outbreaks of gastroenteritis in the United States. J Infect Dis 1998;178:1571–8.

[13] Fankhauser R, Monroe S, Noel J, et al. Epidemiologic and molecular trends of "Norwalk-like viruses" associated with outbreaks of gastroenteritis in the United States. J Infect Dis 2002;186:1–7.

[14] CaliciNet. Available at: http://www.cdc.gov/mmwr/preview/mmwrhtml/mm5203a1. htm. Accessed on August 31, 2005.

[15] Jiang ZD, Mathewson JJ, Ericsson CD, et al. Characterization of enterotoxigenic *Escherichia coli* strains in patients with travelers' diarrhea acquired in Guadalajara, Mexico, 1992–1997. J Infect Dis 2000;181:779–82.

[16] Adachi JA, Jiang ZD, Mathewson JJ, et al. Enteroaggregative *Escherichia coli* as a major etiologic agent in traveler's diarrhea in 3 regions of the world. Clin Infect Dis 2001;32: 1706–9.

[17] Huang DB, Okhuysen PC, Jiang ZD, et al. Enteroaggregative *Escherichia coli*: an emerging enteric pathogen. Am J Gastroenterol 2004;99:383–9.

[18] Pépin J, Valiquette L, Alary M-E. *Clostridium difficile*–associated diarrhea in a region of Quebec from 1991 to 2003: a changing pattern of disease severity. CMAJ 2004;171: 466–72.

[19] Archibald LK, Banerjee SN, Jarvis WR. Secular trends in hospital acquired *Clostridium difficile* disease in the United States, 1987–2001. J Infect Dis 2004;189:1585–9.

[20] National Clostridium difficile Standards Group. Report to the Department of Health. J Hosp Infect 2004;56(Suppl 1):1–38.

[21] Public Health. *Clostridium difficile* infection in hospitals: A brewing storm. CMAJ 2004;171:27–9.

[22] Noren T. Outbreak from a high-toxin intruder: *Clostridium difficile* [editorial]. Lancet 2005;366:1053–4.

[23] Bresee J, Widdowson M, Monroe S, et al. Foodborne viral gastroenteritis: challenges and opportunities. Clin Infect Dis 2002;35:748–53.

[24] Le Guyader F, Neill F, Estes MM, et al. Detection and analysis of a small round-structured virus strain in oysters implicated in an outbreak of acute gastroenteritis. Appl Environ Microbiol 1996;62:4268–72.

[25] Daniels NA, Bergmire-Sweat DA, Schwab KJ, et al. Foodborne outbreak of gastroenteritis associated with Norwalk-like viruses: first molecular traceback to deli sandwiches contaminated during preparation. J Infect Dis 2000;181:1467–70.

[26] Hirakata Y, Arisawa K, Nishio O, et al. Multiprefectural spread of gastroenteritis outbreaks attributable to a single genogroup II norovirus strain from a tourist restaurant in Nagasaki, Japan. J Clin Microbiol 2005;43:1093–8.

[27] Nygard K, Vold L, Bringeland E, et al. Waterborne outbreak of gastroenteritis in a religious summer camp in Norway, 2002. Epidemiol Infect 2004;132:223–9.

[28] Carrique-Mas J, Andersson Y, Peterson B, et al. A norwalk-like virus waterborne community outbreak in a Swedish village during peak holiday season. Epidemiol Infect 2003;131: 737–44.

[29] Hoebe CJ, Vennema H, Husman AM, et al. Norovirus outbreak among primary schoolchildren who had played in a recreational water fountain. J Infect Dis 2004;189:699–705.

[30] Cheesbrough J, Green J, Gallimore CI, et al. Widespread environmental contamination with Norwalk-like viruses (NLV) detected in a prolonged hotel outbreak of gastroenteritis. Epidemiol Infect 2000;125:93–8.

[31] Kuusi M, Nuorti JP, Maunula L. A prolonged outbreak of Norwalk-like calicivirus (NLV) gastroenteritis in a rehabilitation centre due to environmental contamination. Epidemiol Infect 2002;129:133–8.

[32] Evans M, Meldrum R, Lane W, et al. An outbreak of viral gastroenteritis following environmental contamination at a concert hall. Epidemiol Infect 2002;129:355–60.

[33] Marks PJ, Vipond IB, Regan FM, et al. A school outbreak of Norwalk-like virus: evidence for airborne transmission. Epidemiol Infect 2003;131:727–36.

[34] Svenungsson B, Lagergren A, Ekwall E, et al. Enteropathogens in adult patients with diarrhea and healthy control subjects: a 1-year prospective study in a Swedish clinic for infectious diseases. Clin Infect Dis 2000;30:770–8.

[35] World Health Organization. The state of world health. In: The World Health Report 1996—fighting disease, fostering development. Geneva (Switzerland): World Health Organization; 1997. p. 1–62.

[36] Ramzan NN. Traveler's diarrhea. Gastroenterol Clin North Am 2001;30:665–78.

[37] Chapin AR, Carpenter CM, Dudley WC, et al. Prevalence of norovirus among visitors from the United States to Mexico and Guatemala who experience traveler's diarrhea. J Clin Microbiol 2005;43:112–7.

[38] Ko G, Garcia C, Jiang ZD, et al. Noroviruses as a cause of traveler's diarrhea among students from the United States visiting Mexico. J Clin Microbiol 2005;43(12): 6126–9.

[39] Goodgame RW. Emerging causes of travelers diarrhea: cryptosporidium, cyclospora, isospora, and microsporidia. Curr Infect Dis Rep 2003;5:66–73.

[40] Poutanen SM, Simor AE. Clostridium difficile–associated diarrhea in adults. CMAJ 2004;171:51–8.

[41] Gopal R, Ozerek A, Jeanes A. Rational protocols for testing faeces in the investigation of sporadic hospital-acquired diarrhoea. J Hosp Infect 2001;47:79–83.

[42] Rees JR, Pannier MA, McNees A, et al. Persistent diarrhea, arthritis, and other complications of enteric infections: a pilot survey based on California FoodNet surveillance, 1998–1999. Clin Infect Dis 2004;38(Suppl 3):S311–7.

[43] Dryden MS, Gabb RJ, Wright SK. Empirical treatment of severe acute community-acquired gastroenteritis with ciprofloxacin. Clin Infect Dis 1996;22:1019–25.

[44] 150 years of cholera epidemiology. Lancet 2005;366:957.

[45] McLaughlin JB, DePaola A, Bopp CA, et al. Outbreak of Vibrio parahaemolyticus gastroenteritis associated with Alaskan oysters. N Engl J Med 2005;353:1463–70.

[46] Choi SW, Park CH, Silva TM, et al. To culture or not to culture: fecal lactoferrin screening for inflammatory bacterial diarrhea. J Clin Microbiol 1996;34:928–32.

[47] Savola KL, Baron EJ, Tompkins LS, et al. Fecal leukocyte stain has diagnostic value for outpatients but not inpatients. J Clin Microbiol 2001;39:266–9.

[48] Cherry B, Burns A, Johnson GS, et al. Salmonella typhimurium outbreak associated with veterinary clinic. Emerg Infect Dis 2004;10:2249–51.

[49] Hoag JB, Sessler CN. A comprehensive review of disseminated Salmonella arizona infection with an illustrative case presentation. South Med J 2005;98:1123–9.

[50] Centers for Disease Control and Prevention (CDC). Salmonellosis associated with pet turtles–Wisconsin and Wyoming, 2004. MMWR Morb Mortal Wkly Rep 2005;54:223–6.

[51] Centers for Disease Control and Prevention (CDC). Reptile-associated salmonellosis–selected states, 1998–2002. MMWR Morb Mortal Wkly Rep 2003;52(49):1206–9.

[52] Olsen SJ, Ying M, Davis MF, et al. Multidrug-resistant Salmonella typhimurium infection from milk contaminated after pasteurization. Emerg Infect Dis 2004;10:932–5.

[53] Kennedy M, Villar R, Vugia DJ, et al. Emerging Infections Program FoodNet Working Group. Hospitalizations and deaths due to Salmonella infections, FoodNet, 1996–1999. Clin Infect Dis 2004;38(Suppl 3):S142–8.

[54] Fisker N, Vinding K, Molbak K, et al. Clinical review of nontyphoid Salmonella infections from 1991 to 1999 in a Danish county. Clin Infect Dis 2003;37(4):e47–52.

[55] Hsu RB, Tsay YG, Chen RJ, et al. Risk factors for primary bacteremia and endovascular infection in patients without acquired immunodeficiency syndrome who have nontyphoid salmonellosis. Clin Infect Dis 2003;36(7):829–34.

[56] Santos-Juanes J, Lopez-Escobar M, Galache C, et al. Haemorrhagic cellulitis caused by Salmonella enteritidis. Scand J Infect Dis 2005;37:309–10.

[57] Hsu RB, Chen RJ, Chu SH. Nontyphoid Salmonella bacteremia in patients with liver cirrhosis. Am J Med Sci 2005;329:234–7.

[58] Guallar C, Ariza J, Dominguez MA, et al. An insidious nosocomial outbreak due to Salmonella enteritidis. Infect Control Hosp Epidemiol 2004;25(1):10–5.

[59] Chiu CH, Su LH, Chu C, et al. Isolation of *Salmonella enterica* serotype *choleraesuis* resistant to ceftriaxone and ciprofloxacin. Lancet 2004;363:1285–6.

[60] Thaver D, Zaidi AK, Critchley J, et al. Fluoroquinolones for treating typhoid and paratyphoid fever (enteric fever). Cochrane Database Syst Rev 2005;2:CD004530.

[61] Pitout JD, Reisbig MD, Mulvey M, et al. Association between handling of pet treats and infection with *Salmonella enterica* serotype *newport* expressing the AmpC beta-lactamase, CMY-2. J Clin Microbiol 2003;41:4578–82.

[62] Kristiansen MA, Sandvang D, Rasmussen TB. In vivo development of quinolone resistance in *Salmonella enterica* serotype *typhimurium* DT104. J Clin Microbiol 2003;41(9): 4462–4.

[63] Walia M, Gaind R, Mehta R, et al. Current perspectives of enteric fever: a hospital-based study from India. Ann Trop Paediatr 2005;25:161–74.

[64] Butzler JP. Campylobacter, from obscurity to celebrity. Clin Microbiol Infect 2004;10: 868–76.

[65] Potter RC, Kaneene JB, Hall WN. Risk factors for sporadic *Campylobacter jejuni* infections in rural Michigan: a prospective case-control study. Am J Public Health 2003;93(12): 2118–23.

[66] Heryford AG, Seys SA. Outbreak of occupational campylobacteriosis associated with a pheasant farm. J Agric Saf Health 2004;10:127–32.

[67] Gillespie IA, O'Brien SJ, Adak GK, et al. Campylobacter Sentinel Surveillance Scheme Collaborators. Point source outbreaks of *Campylobacter jejuni* infection–are they more common than we think and what might cause them? Epidemiol Infect 2003;130(3): 367–75.

[68] Tracz DM, Keelan M, Ahmed-Bentley J, et al. pVir and bloody diarrhea in *Campylobacter jejuni* enteritis. Emerg Infect Dis 2005;11:838–43.

[69] Monselise A, Blickstein D, Ostfeld I, et al. A case of cellulitis complicating *Campylobacter jejuni* subspecies *jejuni* bacteremia and review of the literature. Eur J Clin Microbiol Infect Dis 2004;23(9):718–21.

[70] Engberg J, Neimann J, Nielsen EM, et al. Quinolone-resistant *Campylobacter* infections: risk factors and clinical consequences. Emerg Infect Dis 2004;10:1056–63.

[71] Allos BM. *Campylobacter jejuni* infections: update on emerging issues and trends. Clin Infect Dis 2001;32:1201–6.

[72] Hughes RA, Cornblath DR. Guillain-Barre syndrome. Lancet 2005;366:1653–66.

[73] Lecuit M, Abachin E, Martin A, et al. Immunoproliferative small intestinal disease associated with *Campylobacter jejuni*. N Engl J Med 2004;350(3):239–48.

[74] Centers for Disease Control and Prevention (CDC). *Shigella flexneri* serotype 3 infections among men who have sex with men–Chicago, Illinois, 2003–2004. MMWR Morb Mortal Wkly Rep 2005;54:820–2.

[75] Kimura AC, Johnson K, Palumbo MS, et al. Multistate shigellosis outbreak and commercially prepared food, United States. Emerg Infect Dis 2004;10:1147–9.

[76] Centers for Disease Control and Prevention (CDC). Day care-related outbreaks of rhamnose-negative *Shigella sonnei*–six states, June 2001–March 2003. MMWR Morb Mortal Wkly Rep 2004;53(3):60–3.

[77] Genobile D, Gaston J, Tallis GF, et al. An outbreak of shigellosis in a child care centre. Commun Dis Intell 2004;28:225–9.

[78] Mead PS, Griffin PM. *Escherichia coli* O157:H7. Lancet 1998;352:1207–12.

[79] Bender JB, Smith KE, McNees AA, et al. Emerging Infections Program FoodNet Working Group. Factors affecting surveillance data on *Escherichia coli* O157 infections collected from FoodNet sites, 1996–1999. Clin Infect Dis 2004;38(Suppl 3):S157–64.

[80] Jay MT, Garrett V, Mohle-Boetani JC, et al. A multistate outbreak of *Escherichia coli* O157:H7 infection linked to consumption of beef tacos at a fast-food restaurant chain. Clin Infect Dis 2004;39(1):1–7.

[81] Centers for Disease Control and Prevention (CDC). Outbreaks of *Escherichia coli* O157:H7 associated with petting zoos–North Carolina, Florida, and Arizona, 2004 and 2005. MMWR Morb Mortal Wkly Rep 2005;54:1277–80.

[82] Varma JK, Greene KD, Reller ME, et al. An outbreak of *Escherichia coli* O157 infection following exposure to a contaminated building. JAMA 2003;290:2709–12.

[83] Havelaar AH, Van Duynhoven YT, Nauta MJ, et al. Disease burden in The Netherlands due to infections with Shiga toxin-producing *Escherichia coli* O157. Epidemiol Infect 2004;132:467–84.

[84] Beutin L, Krause G, Zimmermann S, et al K. Characterization of Shiga toxin-producing *Escherichia coli* strains isolated from human patients in Germany over a 3-year period. J Clin Microbiol 2004;42:1099–108.

[85] Ochoa TJ, Cleary TG. Epidemiology and spectrum of disease of *Escherichia coli* O157. Curr Opin Infect Dis 2003;16:259–63.

[86] Gavin PJ, Peterson LR, Pasquariello AC, et al. Evaluation of performance and potential clinical impact of ProSpecT Shiga toxin *Escherichia coli* microplate assay for detection of Shiga toxin-producing *E. coli* in stool samples. J Clin Microbiol 2004;42:1652–6.

[87] Wong CS, Jelacic S, Habeeb RL, et al. The risk of the hemolytic–uremic syndrome after antibiotic treatment of *Escherichia coli* O157:H7 infections. N Engl J Med 2000;342: 1930–6.

[88] Safdar N, Said A, Gangnon RE, et al. Risk of hemolytic uremic syndrome after antibiotic treatment of *Escherichia coli* O157:H7 enteritis: a meta-analysis. JAMA 2002;288: 996–1001.

[89] Zhang X, McDaniel AD, Wolf LE, et al. Quinolone antibiotics induce Shiga toxin-encoding bacteriophages, toxin production, and death in mice. J Infect Dis 2000;181:664–70.

[90] Stanley SL Jr. Amoebiasis. Lancet 2003;361:1025–34.

[91] Blessmann J, Ali IK, Nu PA, et al. Longitudinal study of intestinal *Entamoeba histolytica* infections in asymptomatic adult carriers. J Clin Microbiol 2003;41(10):4745–50.

[92] Tanyuksel M, Yilmaz H, Ulukanligil M, et al. Comparison of two methods (microscopy and enzyme-linked immunosorbent assay) for the diagnosis of amebiasis. Exp Parasitol 2005;110(3):322–6.

[93] Teel LD, Steinberg BR, Aronson NE, et al. Shiga toxin-producing *Escherichia coli*-associated kidney failure in a 40-year-old patient and late diagnosis by novel bacteriologic and toxin detection methods. J Clin Microbiol 2003;41:3438–40.

[94] Chang HG, Tserenpuntsag B, Kacica M, et al. Hemolytic uremic syndrome incidence in New York. Emerg Infect Dis 2004;10:928–31.

[95] Spacek LA, Hurley BP, Acheson DW, et al. Shiga toxin-producing *Escherichia coli* as a possible etiological agent of chronic diarrhea. Clin Infect Dis 2004;39:e46–8.

[96] Goodgame R. Understanding intestinal spore-forming protozoa: cryptosporidia, microsporidia, isospora, and cyclospora. Ann Intern Med 1996;124:429–41.

[97] Wang LH, Fang XC, Pan GZ. Bacillary dysentery as a causative factor of irritable bowel syndrome and its pathogenesis. Gut 2004;53:1096–101.

[98] Kyne L, Sougioultzis S, McFarland LV, et al. Underlying disease severity as a major risk factor for nosocomial *Clostridium difficile* diarrhea. Infect Control Hosp Epidemiol 2002;23(11):653–9.

[99] Fishman JA, Rubin RH. Infection in organ-transplant recipients. N Engl J Med 1998;24: 1741–51.

[100] Niemczyk M, Leszczyniski P, Wyzgal J, et al. Infections caused by clostridium difficile in kidney or liver graft recipients. Ann Transplant 2005;10(2):70–4.

[101] Stelzmueller I, Dunst KM, Hengster P, et al. A cluster of rotavirus enteritis in adult transplant recipients. Transpl Int 2005;18:470–4.

[102] Korkmaz M, Kunefeci G, Selcuk H, et al. The role of early colonoscopy in CMV colitis of transplant recipients. Transplant Proc 2005;37:3059–60.

[103] Goodgame R. Gastrointestinal cytomegalovirus disease. Ann Intern Med 1993;119: 924–35.

[104] Kamar N, Faure P, Dupuis E, et al. Villous atrophy induced by mycophenolate mofetil in renal-transplant patients. Transpl Int 2004;17:463–7.

[105] Iqbal N, Salzman D, Lazenby AJ, et al. Diagnosis of gastrointestinal graft-versus-host disease. Am J Gastroenterol 2000;95:3034–8.

[106] Palella FJJ, Delaney KM, Moorman AC, et al. Declining morbidity and mortality among patients with advanced human immunodeficiency virus infection. N Engl J Med 1998;338:853–60.

[107] Guest JL, Ruffin C, Tschampa JM, et al. Differences in rates of diarrhea in patients with human immunodeficiency virus receiving lopinavir-ritonavir or nelfinavir. Pharmacotherapy 2004;24:727–35.

[108] Bongiovanni M, Cicconi P, Landonio S, et al. Predictive factors of lopinavir/ritonavir discontinuation for drug-related toxicity: results from a cohort of 416 multi-experienced HIV-infected individuals. Int J Antimicrob Agents 2005;26:88–91.

[109] Bushen OY, Davenport JA, Lima AB, et al. Diarrhea and reduced levels of antiretroviral drugs: improvement with glutamine or alanyl-glutamine in a randomized controlled trial in northeast Brazil. Clin Infect Dis 2004;38:1764–70.

GASTROENTEROLOGY CLINICS
OF NORTH AMERICA

The Epidemiologic and Clinical Importance of Norovirus Infection

Robert L. Atmar, MD*, Mary K. Estes, PhD

Departments of Medicine, Molecular Virology & Microbiology, Baylor College of Medicine,
1 Baylor Plaza, MS BCM280, Houston, TX 77030, USA

Viruses have been suspected as the cause of outbreaks of nonbacterial gastroenteritis for more than 75 years. In 1929, Zahorsky [1] proposed the name "winter vomiting disease" to describe such outbreaks because of their increase in incidence during the winter months. In the 1940s, Gordon and colleagues [2] collected stool samples from patients in an institutional outbreak of nonbacterial gastroenteritis and pooled the stool filtrates to infect volunteers experimentally. The inoculated volunteers developed gastroenteritis within 1 to 5 days of inoculation, and the infecting agent could be passed serially through humans. The ability of the inoculum to induce gastroenteritis was lost following heat inactivation by autoclaving. Attempts to identify a viral pathogen by culture in embryonated chicken eggs failed.

The Centers for Disease Control and Prevention investigated an outbreak of winter vomiting disease that occurred in an elementary school in Norwalk, Ohio in October–November of 1968 [3]. Fifty percent of the students and teachers developed gastroenteritis, and approximately one third of family contacts of ill individuals also became sick. Initial attempts to identify a causative agent failed, but stools that were collected from ill persons were used to make new challenge inocula for experimental studies at the National Institutes of Health [4]. Subsequently, Kapikian and colleagues [5] used immune electron microscopy to identify viral particles in the stools of volunteers who were infected with a passage of the Norwalk virus inoculum. These viruses initially were classified by their appearance in electron micrographs (Fig. 1) as small round structured viruses (SRSVs) or small round viruses, but they were reclassified as caliciviruses when the genome was cloned [6]. Later studies demonstrated that almost all of the SRSVs were related genetically to Norwalk virus.

THE VIRUS

Caliciviruses (family *Caliciviridae*) are a group of nonenveloped, icosahedral viruses with a single-stranded, positive sense RNA genome [7]. Four genera

*Corresponding author. *E-mail address*: ratmar@bcm.edu (R.L. Atmar).

0889-8553/06/$ – see front matter
doi:10.1016/j.gtc.2006.03.001

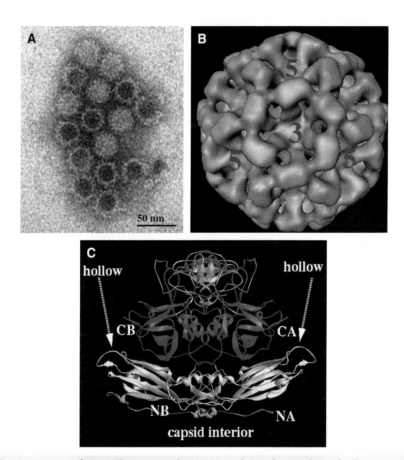

Fig. 1. Structure of Norwalk virus particles. (A) Virus detected in stool samples by negative-stain electron microscopy. (B) Surface representation of a Norwalk virus-like particle that consists of 90 dimeric arches that emanate from the surface of the particles. (C) A dimer of the VP1 protein that makes up the structure of the capsid. CA and CB show the carboxy and amino termini, respectively, of the A protein (right side of the dimer) and CB and NB show the carboxy and amino termini, respectively, of the B (left side of the dimer). (*Adapted from* Hutson AM, Atmar RL, Estes MK. Norovirus disease: changing epidemiology and host susceptibility factors. Trends Microbiol 2004;12(6):279–87; with permission; and Estes MK, Atmar RL. Viral pathogens of the intestine. In: Hecht G, editor. Microbial pathogenesis and the intestinal epithelial cell. Washington DC: ASM Press; 2003. p. 525–45; with permission.)

are recognized in the *Caliciviridae* family: *Norovirus, Sapovirus, Lagovirus,* and *Vesivirus.* Viruses in the latter two genera infect only animals. The *Norovirus* and *Sapovirus* genera contain human and animal virus strains, but cross-species transmission of strains within these genera has not been recognized to occur. Human noroviruses cannot be grown in vitro, but a recently described mouse norovirus strain grows in mouse dendritic cells and macrophages [8,9].

The norovirus genome is 7.5 to 7.7 kilobase in length and it has three open reading frames (ORFs). The first ORF encodes a large polyprotein that is cleaved after synthesis into several nonstructural proteins that are important for replicating the virus but are not found in virus particles, including a nucleotide triphosphatase, genome-linked viral protein (VPg), viral protease, and polymerase [10]. The second ORF encodes the major structural protein VP1; the third ORF encodes VP2, a basic protein that also is a minor structural protein. The viral capsid contains 180 copies of the VP1 protein, and in vitro expression of VP1 leads to the spontaneous assembly of the protein into virus-like particles (VLPs) [11]. The VLPs are antigenically and morphologically similar to native virions (see Fig. 1). VLPs are useful reagents to produce antiserum for diagnostic assays and are a candidate vaccine.

Noroviruses are genetically and antigenically diverse. The lack of an in vitro culture system or animal model prevents classification into serotypes, so the primary means of classification is through genetic analysis. Genetic characterization is used in molecular epidemiology analyses of outbreaks to try and identify the source and patterns of spread and evolution of these viruses. Five genetic groups (called genogroups) of noroviruses exist based on phylogenetic analysis of the complete capsid (VP1) gene [12]. Three of these genogroups (I, II, and IV) contain human strains, whereas genogroup III contains bovine strains and genogroup V contains mouse strains. Genogroups I, II, and III are divided further into genetic clusters, or genotypes, and contain 8, 17, and 2 clusters, respectively [12]. Norwalk virus is the prototype norovirus strain; it belongs to genogroup I, cluster 1 (I.1).

EPIDEMIOLOGY

Noroviruses infect persons of all ages. Previously, these viruses were believed to infect only school-aged children and adults, but recent studies indicate that they also infect young children and are second to rotaviruses in causing infants to be hospitalized. Noroviruses cause infection throughout the year, although there is a peak incidence during the cold-weather months [13]. Mead and colleagues [14] estimated that there are 23 million norovirus infections per year in the United States, which constitutes 60% of the illness burden that is caused by known enteric pathogens. Noroviruses are the major cause of epidemic nonbacterial gastroenteritis worldwide, and have been identified as the cause of 73% to more than 95% of outbreaks and approximately half of all gastroenteritis outbreaks (Table 1) [15–25]. Noroviruses also are a common cause of sporadic cases of gastroenteritis and are the most common viral cause of gastroenteritis identified in recent community-based studies (Table 2) [26–35]. In developed countries, seroprevalence increases during the first several years of life and reaches 80% to 90% by young adulthood [36].

Genogroup I and II strains cause infection in the community, although recent studies have shown a predominance of genogroup II strains. During the mid-1990s, a GII.4 strain emerged as the principal genotype that causes outbreaks of infection worldwide [37]. Since that time, this strain has evolved,

Table 1
Frequency of norovirus infections in outbreaks of acute gastroenteritis

Country [reference]	Years of study	Number of outbreaks of gastroenteritis	Frequency of norovirus infection	Genogroup distribution of noroviruses
The Netherlands [15]	1996	69	87%	7% GI; 91% GII; 2% GI and GII
United Kingdom [16]	1996–1997	94	68%	1% GI; 52% GII; 47% unknown
United States [17]	1996–1997	90[a]	96%	6% GI; 94% GII
Japan [18]	1996–1999	64[a]	73%	21% GI; 66% GII; 13% GI & GII
United States [19]	1997–2002	233[a]	93%	26% GI; 73% GII; 1% GIV
Japan [20]	1997–2004	60[a]	77%	11% GI; 72% GII; 17% GI & GII
Finland [21]	1998–2002	416	61%	13% GI; 86% GII; 1% GI & GII
Spain [22]	2000–2001	30	47%	21% GI; 79% GII
United States [23]	2000–2004	226[a]	81%	~20% GI; ~74% GII; 6% GI & GII
Australia [24]	2001	59	51%	3% GI; 90% GII; 7% unknown
The Netherlands [25]	2002	281	54%	Not reported

[a]Nonbacterial outbreaks only.

but it continues to be the major cause of outbreaks in many parts of the world [38,39]. Most infections and outbreaks are caused by a single strain of norovirus, but coinfections occur, especially after exposure to shellfish or sewage-contaminated water [40]. Recombination (exchange of genetic material) can occur following coinfection and lead to the generation of new virus strains [41].

Norovirus infections cause notable problems in several special populations. They are a significant cause of outbreaks in nursing homes and can lead to an increased need for hospital care and increased mortality [42,43]. Similarly, nosocomial outbreaks occur in hospitals and other health care settings [44]. In the United Kingdom, norovirus outbreaks have required the closure of wards to new admissions in attempts at outbreak control; these control measures are associated with significant costs (~$1 million per 1000 hospital beds). The morbidity of norovirus infection in military personnel adversely impacts the performance of duties during deployment or training, and the severity of infection can require the need for hospital care [45,46]. Finally, these viruses are being recognized increasingly as the cause of chronic diarrhea in patients who undergo transplantation (see later discussion).

Norovirus infection is a more common cause of traveler's diarrhea than has been recognized previously. In one study, it caused 17% of episodes of gastroenteritis and was the second most common cause of traveler's diarrhea after

Table 2
Frequency of norovirus infections in sporadic cases of acute gastroenteritis

Country [reference]	Years of study	Number of cases of gastroenteritis	Frequency of norovirus infection	Genogroup distribution of noroviruses	Population studied
Finland [26]	1993–1995	1477	21.2%	8% GI; 92% GII	Children <2 years of age in a rotavirus vaccine study
France [27]	1995–1998	414	14.0%	11% GI; 89% GII	Children <14 years of age presenting to an outpatient clinic
Australia [28]	1997–1999	638	11.4%	16% GI; 84% GII	Community study of persons 3 months to 48 years of age
Indonesia [29]	1997–1999	2788	8.9%	0% GI; 100% GII	14% sample from persons of all ages presenting for medical care
The Netherlands [30]	1998–1999	709	16.1%	Not reported	Community study of the general population
Australia [31]	1998–2002	1233	8.8%	5% GI; 95% GII	Hospitalized children <5 years of age
Vietnam [32]	1999–2000	1339 (448 rotavirus negative)	5.4%	6% GI; 94% GII	Hospitalized children <15 years of age
Spain [22]	2000–2001	310	12.9%	18% GI; 82% GII	Children <5 years of age
Germany [33]	2001–2002	217	20.7%	2% GI; 98% GII	Hospitalized children <16 years of age
Switzerland [34]	2001–2003	831	15.1%	Not reported	Community study of persons 6 months to 75 years of age

enterotoxigenic *Escherichia coli* [47]. Outbreaks of norovirus gastroenteritis are being recognized or are occurring with increasing frequency on cruise ships [39,48]. Attack rates as high as 30% have been observed among cruise ship passengers, and outbreaks have continued on as many as six successive cruise ship voyages [39]. Noroviruses were the only pathogen identified in cases of gastroenteritis in evacuees from Hurricane Katrina who were housed in crowded conditions in Houston, Texas [49].

TRANSMISSION

Noroviruses are transmitted primarily by the fecal–oral route. Fecal contamination of food, water, and fomites, as well as direct person-to-person spread, accounts for most outbreaks. Contamination of food may occur at any point during its production. For example, shellfish and raspberries that were contaminated at the site where these foods are harvested or produced have been implicated in outbreaks, whereas other foods, such as salads, cold foods, and sandwiches, have caused outbreaks after being contaminated by food handlers at the site of food preparation [50]. Virus transmission can occur during recreational activities, including canoeing, rafting, and football, either through consumption of contaminated water or by more direct exposure to ill participants [51]. There is a high rate (often >30%) of secondary attacks among contacts of infected persons, which often leads to amplification of an outbreak in closed settings, including hospital wards, cruise ships, and shelters. Continued transmission of norovirus infection can occur as the result of difficulties in eradicating these viruses from contaminated areas because of their relative resistance to many disinfectants. The multiple routes of transmission can make it difficult to institute interventions that interrupt transmission successfully [48]. This characteristic has led to the closure of hotels and cruise ships that were involved in serial norovirus outbreaks so that more extensive measures could be used to disinfect potentially contaminated areas [38,48,52].

Airborne transmission of noroviruses also occurs. Virus is present in vomitus, and the act of vomiting generates an infectious aerosol. Thus, norovirus transmission has been observed in persons who walked through an emergency room where a vomiting patient was being evaluated [53]. Another outbreak occurred in a restaurant where a norovirus-infected diner vomited; patrons who were sitting at other tables in the restaurant developed gastroenteritis in the next 1 or 2 days. The risk of infection was related inversely to the distance of a diner's table from the index case [54]. In both of these outbreaks, persons became ill without having direct contact with the index case or with the environment immediately around that case.

The norovirus infectious dose is low although few studies have examined this question systematically. Lindesmith and colleagues [55] infected volunteers with less than 10^4 viral genomes (measured as reverse-transcription polymerase chain reaction [RT-PCR] units) of Norwalk virus, and Le Guyader and colleagues [56] found 85 to 235 PCR units of norovirus in shellfish that were implicated in an outbreak of norovirus infection. One RT-PCR unit is estimated to be approximately 10 virions. Expert opinion has placed the infectious dose at less than 10 to 100 virions, and this assessment is supported by data from experimental human challenge studies that were presented at international meetings [57].

An unresolved question is the length of time that an infected individual remains infectious. Early studies identified virus shedding only in the first 100 hours after infection [58]. New, more sensitive molecular assays demonstrated that many infected persons have virus in their stools for several weeks after the resolution of symptoms [59,60].

Transmission can occur following recovery from symptomatic infection [61]. Thus, although public health guidelines recommend that food handlers not return to work for 48 to 72 hours following resolution of symptoms, it is reasonable to recommend stringent hand hygiene in the weeks following recovery from norovirus-associated illness [62]. This recommendation should apply not only to persons who work within the food industry but also to those who work in health care and other service industries that bring an individual into contact with large numbers of people.

CLINICAL MANIFESTATIONS

Norovirus infection is characterized by the sudden onset of vomiting or diarrhea or both symptoms. Human experimental infection studies with Norwalk virus show that the predominant symptom can vary from person to person; in one person it may be vomiting without diarrhea, whereas in another person it may be diarrhea without vomiting [4,59]. Emesis is a characteristic finding in outbreaks that are associated with norovirus infection (Table 3), but this symptom is less common in children who are younger than 1 year of age and in hospitalized patients [42,60]. Nausea, abdominal pain, abdominal cramps, anorexia, malaise, and low-grade fever also occur. Bloody diarrhea is not seen with norovirus infection. Asymptomatic infection occurred in up to one third of persons who were infected during experimental challenge studies [59].

The incubation period following exposure to norovirus is 1 to 2 days, and the illness duration that was observed in volunteer studies and many outbreaks has been short (1–3 days) [59]. These characteristics led Kaplan and colleagues [63] to develop clinical criteria for recognizing outbreaks of norovirus infection: a short incubation period (24–48 hours), a short symptomatic illness (12–60 hours), a high frequency (>50%) of vomiting, and absence of bacterial pathogens. More recent studies showed that norovirus illnesses can last for a longer period of time. In a community study that examined the natural history of norovirus infection in The Netherlands, the median duration of illness decreased with increasing age (6 days for <1 year of age versus 4–5 days for 1–11 years of age versus 3 days for ≥12 years of age) [60]. In a study of persons who were involved in 271 outbreaks in nursing homes and hospitals in the United Kingdom from 2002 to 2003, the median duration of illness was 2 days (range, 1–21 days); 75% of the illnesses resolved by 4 days [42]. Hospitalized patients had a longer median duration of illness of 3 days (75th percentile = 5 days). Forty percent of hospitalized patients

Table 3
Symptoms associated with norovirus illness

Study group [reference]	Age range	Percentage with symptom						
		Diarrhea	Vomiting	Nausea	Abdominal pain	Abdominal cramps	Fever
The Netherlands community study [60]	<1 year (n = 37)	95	59	30	11	41	24
	1–4 years (n = 32)	84	75	53	63	35	40
	5–11 years (n = 11)	74	95	76	90	52	48
	≥12 years (n = 11)	91	82	55	91	82	45
Norwalk virus challenge study [59]	18–50 years N = 28)	86	57	96	NR	86	32
Healthcare- associated outbreaks in Avon, England [42]	<5 years of age and hospitalized (n = 29)	79	48	NR	NR	NR	NR
	5–14 years of age and hospitalized (n = 10)	70	80	NR	NR	NR	NR
	15–64 years of age and hospitalized (n = 78)	83	58	NR	NR	NR	NR
	15–64 years of age and healthcare worker (n = 594)	66	71	NR	NR	NR	NR
	≥65 years of age and hospitalized (n = 537)	86	57	NR	NR	NR	NR
	≥75 years of age and in nursing home (n = 222)	82	69	NR	NR	NR	NR

Abbreviation: NR, not reported.

older than 80 years of age remained symptomatic after 4 days. Thus, norovirus-associated illness can last longer than was recognized previously.

Norovirus infections are self-limited, and healthy patients generally recover without sequelae; however, volume depletion with hypokalemia and renal insufficiency can occur, especially in elderly persons and patients who have underlying disease [64]. Severe disease, including disseminated intravascular coagulation, was observed in otherwise healthy soldiers who were exposed to significant environmental stresses [65]. Aspiration of vomitus may lead to death, as can worsening of underlying diseases [64]. Immunocompromised patients (eg, transplant recipients) may develop chronic diarrhea and shed virus for months to years [66,67]. Recipients of small bowel transplants are a special patient population in whom symptoms that are related to norovirus infection must be differentiated from allograft rejection [67].

Susceptibility to norovirus infection involves genetic resistance to infection and acquired immunity. Approximately 30 years ago, Parrino and colleagues [68] observed that some individuals were repeatedly susceptible to Norwalk virus infection, whereas a second group was repeatedly resistant. They postulated that a genetic factor might be responsible for susceptibility to infection. Recent studies showed that resistance of an individual to Norwalk virus infection correlates with his/her histo-blood group antigen expression. Secretor-negative individuals have nonfunctional *FUT2* genes and do not express a fucosyltransferase enzyme that is responsible for making H type-1 antigen that appears on the surface of their epithelial cells (Fig. 2). This antigen serves as a ligand for Norwalk virus VLPs and probably functions as the viral receptor [57,69]. Secretor-negative persons who do not express this antigen on their epithelial cells are uniformly resistant to Norwalk virus infection following experimental challenge [55,70]. Secretor-negative persons also were observed to be resistant to infection in an outbreak that involved a GII.4 norovirus strain [71]. Norovirus-binding specificities to histo-blood group antigens vary among the different viral strains [57]. As a result, secretor-negative individuals can be infected by at least some norovirus strains, as demonstrated by infection of a secretor-negative person following experimental challenge with the Snow Mountain virus [72].

Acquired immunity also plays a role in susceptibility to infection. Short-term resistance to reinfection occurs following rechallenge with the same strain 6 to 14 weeks later [67]. Immunity is strain specific, in that infection can be induced following challenge with a serologically distinct strain [73]. Repeated exposure also seems to lead to resistance to reinfection [74]. The mechanism of immunity is unclear. In some studies absence of serum antibody correlated with resistance to infection, whereas in other studies, decreased infection frequencies were associated with higher serum antibody levels [50]. If antibody is the mediator of immunity, this apparent paradox may be due to differences in the populations studied. In studies where antibody correlated with protection from infection, higher antibody levels may be due to recent or repeated infection of the population, whereas in studies where absence of antibody was associated with resistance to infection, the absence of antibody is likely due to

Model for NV susceptibility

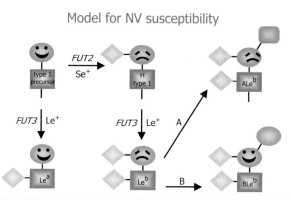

Fig. 2. Model for norovirus susceptibility. Synthetic pathway for blood group ABH and Lewis antigens. The H type-1 precursor is fucosylated on the terminal galactose sugar by the FUT2 enzyme in secretor-positive individuals. Another fucosyl-transferase, FUT3, adds a fucose to the N-acetyl glucosamine in Lewis positive individuals to make Lewis antigens (Le^a and Le^b). H-type 1 or Le^b sugars can be modified further to make A and B histoblood antigens. The antigens with smiling faces are absolutely (Le^a, H type-1 precursor) or relatively (B blood group) resistant to infection with Norwalk virus. Oval, galactose; diamond, fucose; rectangles, N acetyl glucos-amine (in α [rounded edges] or β [sharp edges] linkage to more proximal sugar). A (arrow) and B (arrow) represent the enzymes that modify Le^b to make A and B antigens, respectively.

genetic mechanisms that prevent infection, and thus, adaptive immune responses.

PATHOGENESIS

The pathogenesis of norovirus infections has been explored in experimental human infection studies. Biopsies obtained at the duodenojejunal junction from infected persons showed broadening and blunting of intestinal villi, epithelial cell disarray, crypt cell hyperplasia, cytoplasmic vacuolization, and infiltration of inflammatory cells into the lamina propria [75,76]. These histologic changes can be noted a few hours before the onset of symptomatic illness as well as in asymptomatically infected persons, and they also have been seen in symptomatically infected patients with small intestine transplants [76,77]. Increased apoptosis is seen in the superficial epithelial cells and in the lamina propria. The histopathologic changes are more prominent in proximal portions of the small intestine, although the distal small intestine also is involved. No histopathologic changes have been seen in the stomach [78]. Resolution of the pathologic changes occurs by 2 weeks in healthy subjects and at the time of virus clearance in patients who underwent an intestinal transplant [75,77].

The mechanisms that lead to symptomatic infection are unknown. No changes in intestinal adenylate cyclase activity occur, as is seen with toxin-mediated disease that is associated with *Vibrio cholerae* and some *E coli* infections [79]. Small intestinal brush border enzymatic activities (sucrase, trehalase, alkaline phosphatase) decrease in association with symptomatic infection and an associated transient carbohydrate malabsorption and steatorrhea occurs [75]. D-xylose absorption decreases by ~50% 2 days after inoculation and the decreased absorption persists for several days (even after resolution of illness) [76]. Gastric emptying is delayed, but the secretory function of the stomach (pepsin, hydrochloric acid, intrinsic factor) is not altered [80]. Attempts to measure interferon induction locally or systemically (serum) failed to demonstrate measurable responses to infection [81].

DIAGNOSIS

RT-PCR assays are the most common approach for establishing a diagnosis of norovirus infection [36]. Virus-specific primers are used to amplify conserved regions of the genome (usually in the polymerase or VP1 genes). Specificity of the amplification is established by hybridization with a virus-specific probe or by direct sequencing of the amplicons. No single primer pair can detect all norovirus strains because of the high sequence diversity, but more than 90% of strains can be detected using two separate primer pairs for genogroup I and II noroviruses [23]. GI- and GII-specific real-time RT-PCR assays reduce the time to identify virus in clinical samples [40].

Electron microscopy is used by many laboratories to screen stools for potential viral pathogens. This method is insensitive (<25%) compared with molecular detection assays [82]. Assay sensitivity can be increased by using specific antisera to aggregate viruses, which makes them easier to detect, but the antisera that are used in this assay are not widely available.

The identification of viral antigens in stools is another diagnostic approach. First-generation antigen-detection ELISA assays were too specific; these assays used hyperimmune sera produced to norovirus VLPs but only detected strains that were related closely to the immunizing VLPs [36]. More broadly reactive assays have been developed using monoclonal antibodies that recognize cross-reactive epitopes [83]. The sensitivity of one of these assays (Dako) is poor (39%–52%) when applied to individual specimens, but improves to 71% for identification of an outbreak when multiple stool samples are tested [82,84]. Another assay (Denka) has better sensitivity (80%) but poor specificity (69%) [84]. These antigen-detection assays are available in Europe, but are not approved for use in the United States.

Serologic assays also have been developed to detect immune responses to infecting norovirus strains. Because of the high seroprevalence against most norovirus strains in adults, diagnostic assays largely have relied on the use of paired sera that were collected at least 2 weeks apart; this makes the assay of more use for epidemiologic studies rather than for evaluation of the individual patient. Antibody responses are highest (largest fold increases, highest frequency of fourfold or greater increases) against virus strains that are related closely to the infecting strain, but heterologous responses also can be detected. The detection of virus-specific serum IgM or IgA is more strain specific and suggests recent infection, but these antibodies only become detectable more than 1 week following illness onset [36].

TREATMENT AND PREVENTION

Generally, norovirus-associated illness is mild and self-limited, so treatment is supportive (eg, rehydration, analgesics, antiemetics). Some patients become ill enough to require hospitalization for fluid and electrolyte replacement. Mortality is rare, but it has occurred as a result of aspiration or because of increased debility in chronically ill patients.

Prevention is based upon avoidance of contaminated foodstuffs and water, disinfection of virus-contaminated areas, and handwashing by health care providers and affected patients. Ill food handlers should not prepare food for 2 to 3 days after recovery from their illness, and should practice good hand hygiene after going back to work [62]. Raw shellfish consumption is a risk because illness has occurred after consumption of shellfish that met sanitary standards that are based upon microbial levels. Noroviruses are resistant to heat and to some standard disinfectants (eg, alcohols, quaternary ammonium) [85,86]. Sodium hypochlorite is effective at virus inactivation, and a combination of detergent and sodium hypochlorite solution is effective at cleaning contaminated surfaces [87,88].

CURRENT QUESTIONS AND FUTURE PROSPECTS

Recognition of the major importance of noroviruses as a cause of gastroenteritis in many different populations has increased significantly in the past decade. As rapid diagnostic assays become accessible in the near future, it will be important to determine if noroviruses cause chronic infections (as do animal caliciviruses) that are associated with arthritis, encephalitis, hepatitis, and myocarditis in addition to acute or chronic gastroenteritis. There is a great need for the development of effective inactivating agents; advances toward this need await methods to cultivate the human noroviruses. The development of an in vitro replication system for the Norwalk virus genome give hope that a culture system for virus may be developed soon [89]. Norovirus VLPs are being evaluated as a potential vaccine for prevention of norovirus infection or illness [90]. The three-dimensional structure of the Norwalk virus and key norovirus proteins that are required for replication have been solved, and these breakthroughs may lead to the development of antiviral agents that could be used for treatment or prophylaxis [91–93].

Acknowledgments

We thank Anne Hutson for help in preparation of Fig. 2. Norovirus research in our laboratories is supported by funding (N01-AI-25465, P01-AI-057788, and M01-RR-000188) from the National Institutes of Health.

References

[1] Zahorsky J. Hyperemesis hiemis or the winter vomiting disease. Arch Pediatr 1929;46: 391–5.
[2] Gordon I, Ingraham HS, Korns RF. Transmission of epidemic gastroenteritis to human volunteers by oral administration of fecal filtrates. J Exp Med 1947;86:409–22.
[3] Adler JL, Zickl R. Winter vomiting disease. J Infect Dis 1969;119(6):668–73.

[4] Dolin R, Blacklow NR, DuPont H, et al. Transmission of acute infectious nonbacterial gastroenteritis to volunteers by oral administration of stool filtrates. J Infect Dis 1971;123(3):307–12.

[5] Kapikian AZ, Wyatt RG, Dolin R, et al. Visualization by immune electron microscopy of a 27-nm particle associated with acute infectious nonbacterial gastroenteritis. J Virol 1972;10(5):1075–81.

[6] Jiang X, Graham DY, Wang K, et al. Norwalk virus genome cloning and characterization. Science 1990;250(4987):1580–3.

[7] Green KY, Ando T, Balayan MS, et al. Caliciviridae. In: van Regenmortel M, Fauquet CM, Bishop DHL, et al, editors. Virus taxonomy: 7th Report of the International Committee on Taxonomy of Viruses. Orlando (FL): Academic Press, Inc.; 2000. p. 725–35.

[8] Duizer E, Schwab KJ, Neill FH, et al. Laboratory efforts to cultivate noroviruses. J Gen Virol 2004;85(Pt 1):79–87.

[9] Wobus CE, Karst SM, Thackray LB, et al. Replication of norovirus in cell culture reveals a tropism for dendritic cells and macrophages. PLoS Biol 2004;2(12):e432.

[10] Hardy ME. Norovirus protein structure and function. FEMS Microbiol Lett 2005;253(1):1–8.

[11] Jiang X, Wang M, Graham DY, et al. Expression, self-assembly, and antigenicity of the Norwalk virus capsid protein. J Virol 1992;66(11):6527–32.

[12] Zheng DP, Ando T, Fankhauser RL, et al. Norovirus classification and proposed strain nomenclature. Virology 2006;346(2):312–23.

[13] Mounts AW, Ando T, Koopmans M, et al. Cold weather seasonality of gastroenteritis associated with Norwalk-like viruses. J Infect Dis 2000;181(Suppl 2):S284–7.

[14] Mead PS, Slutsker L, Dietz V, et al. Food-related illness and death in the United States. Emerg Infect Dis 1999;5(5):607–25.

[15] Vinje J, Altena SA, Koopmans MP. The incidence and genetic variability of small round-structured viruses in outbreaks of gastroenteritis in The Netherlands. J Infect Dis 1997;176(5):1374–8.

[16] Maguire AJ, Green J, Brown DW, et al. Molecular epidemiology of outbreaks of gastroenteritis associated with small round-structured viruses in East Anglia, United Kingdom, during the 1996–1997 season. J Clin Microbiol 1999;37(1):81–9.

[17] Fankhauser RL, Noel JS, Monroe SS, et al. Molecular epidemiology of "Norwalk-like viruses" in outbreaks of gastroenteritis in the United States. J Infect Dis 1998;178(6):1571–8.

[18] Iritani N, Seto Y, Haruki K, et al. Major change in the predominant type of "Norwalk-like viruses" in outbreaks of acute nonbacterial gastroenteritis in Osaka City, Japan, between April 1996 and March 1999. J Clin Microbiol 2000;38(7):2649–54.

[19] Fankhauser RL, Monroe SS, Noel JS, et al. Epidemiologic and molecular trends of "Norwalk-like viruses" associated with outbreaks of gastroenteritis in the United States. J Infect Dis 2002;186(1):1–7.

[20] Hamano M, Kuzuya M, Fujii R, et al. Epidemiology of acute gastroenteritis outbreaks caused by noroviruses in Okayama, Japan. J Med Virol 2005;77(2):282–9.

[21] Maunula L, Von Bonsdorff CH. Norovirus genotypes causing gastroenteritis outbreaks in Finland 1998–2002. J Clin Virol 2005;34(3):186–94.

[22] Buesa J, Collado B, Lopez-Andujar P, et al. Molecular epidemiology of caliciviruses causing outbreaks and sporadic cases of acute gastroenteritis in Spain. J Clin Microbiol 2002;40(8):2854–9.

[23] Blanton LH, Adams SM, Beard RS, et al. Molecular and epidemiologic trends of caliciviruses associated with outbreaks of acute gastroenteritis in the United States, 2000–2004. J Infect Dis 2006;193(3):413–21.

[24] Marshall JA, Dimitriadis A, Wright PJ. Molecular and epidemiological features of norovirus-associated gastroenteritis outbreaks in Victoria, Australia in 2001. J Med Virol 2005;75(2):321–31.

[25] van Duynhoven YT, de Jager CM, Kortbeek LM, et al. A one-year intensified study of outbreaks of gastroenteritis in The Netherlands. Epidemiol Infect 2005;133(1):9–21.

[26] Pang XL, Joensuu J, Vesikari T. Human calicivirus-associated sporadic gastroenteritis in Finnish children less than two years of age followed prospectively during a rotavirus vaccine trial. Pediatr Infect Dis J 1999;18(5):420–6.

[27] Bon F, Fascia P, Dauvergne M, et al. Prevalence of group A rotavirus, human calicivirus, astrovirus, and adenovirus type 40 and 41 infections among children with acute gastroenteritis in Dijon, France. J Clin Microbiol 1999;37(9):3055–8.

[28] Marshall JA, Hellard ME, Sinclair MI, et al. Incidence and characteristics of endemic Norwalk-like virus-associated gastroenteritis. J Med Virol 2003;69(4):568–78.

[29] Subekti DS, Tjaniadi P, Lesmana M, et al. Characterization of Norwalk-like virus associated with gastroenteritis in Indonesia. J Med Virol 2002;67(2):253–8.

[30] de Wit MA, Koopmans MP, Kortbeek LM, et al. Sensor, a population-based cohort study on gastroenteritis in the Netherlands: incidence and etiology. Am J Epidemiol 2001;154(7): 666–74.

[31] Kirkwood CD, Clark R, Bogdanovic-Sakran N, et al. A 5-year study of the prevalence and genetic diversity of human caliciviruses associated with sporadic cases of acute gastroenteritis in young children admitted to hospital in Melbourne, Australia (1998–2002). J Med Virol 2005;77(1):96–101.

[32] Hansman GS, Doan LT, Kguyen TA, et al. Detection of norovirus and sapovirus infection among children with gastroenteritis in Ho Chi Minh City, Vietnam. Arch Virol 2004;149(9):1673–88.

[33] Oh DY, Gaedicke G, Schreier E. Viral agents of acute gastroenteritis in German children: prevalence and molecular diversity. J Med Virol 2003;71(1):82–93.

[34] Fretz R, Herrmann L, Christen A, et al. Frequency of norovirus in stool samples from patients with gastrointestinal symptoms in Switzerland. Eur J Clin Microbiol Infect Dis 2005;24(3): 214–6.

[35] Wheeler JG, Sethi D, Cowden JM, et al. Study of infectious intestinal disease in England: rates in the community, presenting to general practice, and reported to national surveillance. The Infectious Intestinal Disease Study Executive. BMJ 1999;318(7190):1046–50.

[36] Atmar RL, Estes MK. Diagnosis of noncultivatable gastroenteritis viruses, the human caliciviruses. Clin Microbiol Rev 2001;14(1):15–37.

[37] Noel JS, Fankhauser RL, Ando T, et al. Identification of a distinct common strain of "Norwalk-like viruses" having a global distribution. J Infect Dis 1999;179(6):1334–44.

[38] Lopman B, Vennema H, Kohli E, et al. Increase in viral gastroenteritis outbreaks in Europe and epidemic spread of new norovirus variant. Lancet 2004;363(9410):682–8.

[39] Widdowson MA, Cramer EH, Hadley L, et al. Outbreaks of acute gastroenteritis on cruise ships and on land: identification of a predominant circulating strain of norovirus–United States, 2002. J Infect Dis 2004;190(1):27–36.

[40] Kageyama T, Shinohara M, Uchida K, et al. Coexistence of multiple genotypes, including newly identified genotypes, in outbreaks of gastroenteritis due to norovirus in Japan. J Clin Microbiol 2004;42(7):2988–95.

[41] Bull RA, Hansman GS, Clancy LE, et al. Norovirus recombination in ORF1/ORF2 overlap. Emerg Infect Dis 2005;11(7):1079–85.

[42] Lopman BA, Reacher MH, Vipond IB, et al. Clinical manifestation of norovirus gastroenteritis in health care settings. Clin Infect Dis 2004;39(3):318–24.

[43] Wu HM, Fornek M, Schwab KJ, et al. A norovirus outbreak at a long-term-care facility: the role of environmental surface contamination. Infect Control Hosp Epidemiol 2005;26(10): 802–10.

[44] Lopman BA, Reacher MH, Vipond IB, et al. Epidemiology and cost of nosocomial gastroenteritis, Avon, England, 2002–2003. Emerg Infect Dis 2004;10(10):1827–34.

[45] Arness MK, Feighner BH, Canham ML, et al. Norwalk-like viral gastroenteritis outbreak in US Army trainees. Emerg Infect Dis 2000;6(2):204–7.

[46] Bailey MS, Boos CJ, Vautier G, et al. Gastroenteritis outbreak in British troops, Iraq. Emerg Infect Dis 2005;11(10):1625–8.

[47] Ko G, Garcia C, Jiang ZD, et al. Noroviruses as a cause of traveler's diarrhea among students from the United States visiting Mexico. J Clin Microbiol 2005;43(12):6126–9.

[48] Isakbaeva ET, Widdowson MA, Beard RS, et al. Norovirus transmission on cruise ship. Emerg Infect Dis 2005;11(1):154–8.

[49] CDC. Norovirus outbreak among evacuees from hurricane Katrina–Houston, Texas, September 2005. MMWR Morb Mortal Wkly Rep 2005;54(40):1016–8.

[50] Schwab KJ, Estes MK, Atmar RL. Norwalk and other human caliciviruses: molecular characterization, epidemiology, and pathogenesis. In: Cary JW, Linz JE, Bhatnagar D, editors. Microbial foodborne diseases: mechanisms of pathogenicity and toxin synthesis. Lancaster (PA): Technomic Publishing Company, Inc.; 2000. p. 469–93.

[51] Becker KM, Moe CL, Southwick KL, et al. Transmission of Norwalk virus during a football game. N Engl J Med 2000;343(17):1223–7.

[52] Cheesbrough JS, Green J, Gallimore CI, et al. Widespread environmental contamination with Norwalk-like viruses (NLV) detected in a prolonged hotel outbreak of gastroenteritis. Epidemiol Infect 2000;125(1):93–8.

[53] Sawyer LA, Murphy JJ, Kaplan JE, et al. 25- to 30-nm virus particle associated with a hospital outbreak of acute gastroenteritis with evidence for airborne transmission. Am J Epidemiol 1988;127(6):1261–71.

[54] Marks PJ, Vipond IB, Carlisle D, et al. Evidence for airborne transmission of Norwalk-like virus (NLV) in a hotel restaurant. Epidemiol Infect 2000;124(3):481–7.

[55] Lindesmith L, Moe C, Marionneau S, et al. Human susceptibility and resistance to Norwalk virus infection. Nat Med 2003;9(5):548–53.

[56] Le Guyader FS, Neill FH, Dubois E, et al. A semiquantitative approach to estimate Norwalk-like virus contamination of oysters implicated in an outbreak. Int J Food Microbiol 2003;87(1–2):107–12.

[57] Hutson AM, Atmar RL, Estes MK. Norovirus disease: changing epidemiology and host susceptibility factors. Trends Microbiol 2004;12(6):279–87.

[58] Thornhill TS, Kalica AR, Wyatt RG, et al. Pattern of shedding of the Norwalk particle in stools during experimentally induced gastroenteritis in volunteers as determined by immune electron microscopy. J Infect Dis 1975;132(1):28–34.

[59] Graham DY, Jiang X, Tanaka T, et al. Norwalk virus infection of volunteers: new insights based on improved assays. J Infect Dis 1994;170(1):34–43.

[60] Rockx B, de Wit M, Vennema H, et al. Natural history of human *Calicivirus* infection: a prospective cohort study. Clin Infect Dis 2002;35(3):246–53.

[61] Patterson T, Hutchings P, Palmer S. Outbreak of SRSV gastroenteritis at an international conference traced to food handled by a post-symptomatic caterer. Epidemiol Infect 1993;111(1):157–62.

[62] CDC. Viral agents of gastroenteritis public health importance and outbreak management. MMWR Recomm Rep 1990;29(RR-5):1–24.

[63] Kaplan JE, Feldman R, Campbell DS, et al. The frequency of a Norwalk-like pattern of illness in outbreaks of acute gastroenteritis. Am J Public Health 1982;72(12):1329–32.

[64] Mattner F, Sohr D, Heim A, et al. Risk groups for clinical complications of norovirus infections: an outbreak investigation. Clin Microbiol Infect 2006;12(1):69–74.

[65] CDC. Outbreak of acute gastroenteritis associated with Norwalk-like viruses among British military personnel–Afghanistan, May 2002. MMWR Morb Mortal Wkly Rep 2002;51(22):477–9.

[66] Nilsson M, Hedlund KO, Thorhagen M, et al. Evolution of human calicivirus RNA in vivo: accumulation of mutations in the protruding P2 domain of the capsid leads to structural changes and possibly a new phenotype. J Virol 2003;77(24):13117–24.

[67] Kaufman SS, Chatterjee NK, Fuschino ME, et al. Characteristics of human calicivirus enteritis in intestinal transplant recipients. J Pediatr Gastroenterol Nutr 2005;40(3):328–33.

[68] Parrino TA, Schreiber DS, Trier JS, et al. Clinical immunity in acute gastroenteritis caused by Norwalk agent. N Engl J Med 1977;297(2):86–9.

[69] Hutson AM, Atmar RL, Marcus DM, et al. Norwalk virus-like particle hemagglutination by binding to h histo-blood group antigens. J Virol 2003;77(1):405–15.

[70] Hutson AM, Airaud F, LePendu J, et al. Norwalk virus infection associates with secretor status genotyped from sera. J Med Virol 2005;77(1):116–20.

[71] Thorven M, Grahn A, Hedlund KO, et al. A homozygous nonsense mutation (428G→A) in the human secretor (FUT2) gene provides resistance to symptomatic norovirus (GGII) infections. J Virol 2005;79(24):15351–5.

[72] Lindesmith L, Moe C, Lependu J, et al. Cellular and humoral immunity following Snow Mountain virus challenge. J Virol 2005;79(5):2900–9.

[73] Wyatt RG, Dolin R, Blacklow NR, et al. Comparison of three agents of acute infectious nonbacterial gastroenteritis by cross-challenge in volunteers. J Infect Dis 1974;129(6):709–14.

[74] Johnson PC, Mathewson JJ, DuPont HL, et al. Multiple-challenge study of host susceptibility to Norwalk gastroenteritis in US adults. J Infect Dis 1990;161(1):18–21.

[75] Agus SG, Dolin R, Wyatt RG, et al. Acute infectious nonbacterial gastroenteritis: intestinal histopathology. Histologic and enzymatic alterations during illness produced by the Norwalk agent in man. Ann Intern Med 1973;79(1):18–25.

[76] Schreiber DS, Blacklow NR, Trier JS. The mucosal lesion of the proximal small intestine in acute infectious nonbacterial gastroenteritis. N Engl J Med 1973;288(25):1318–23.

[77] Morotti RA, Kaufman SS, Fishbein TM, et al. Calicivirus infection in pediatric small intestine transplant recipients: pathological considerations. Hum Pathol 2004;35(10):1236–40.

[78] Widerlite L, Trier JS, Blacklow NR, et al. Structure of the gastric mucosa in acute infectious nonbacterial gastroenteritis. Gastroenterology 1975;38(3):425–30.

[79] Levy AG, Widerlite L, Schwartz CJ, et al. Jejunal adenylate cyclase activity in human subjects during viral gastroenteritis. Gastroenterology 1976;70(3):321–5.

[80] Meeroff JC, Schreiber DS, Trier JS, et al. Abnormal gastric motor function in viral gastroenteritis. Ann Intern Med 1980;92(3):370–3.

[81] Dolin R, Baron S. Absence of detectable interferon in jejunal biopsies, jejunal aspirates, and sera in experimentally induced viral gastroenteritis in man. Proc Soc Exp Biol Med 1975;150(2):337–9.

[82] Richards AF, Lopman B, Gunn A, et al. Evaluation of a commercial ELISA for detecting Norwalk-like virus antigen in faeces. J Clin Virol 2003;26(1):109–15.

[83] Parker TD, Kitamoto N, Tanaka T, et al. Identification of genogroup I and genogroup II broadly reactive epitopes on the norovirus capsid. J Virol 2005;79(12):7402–9.

[84] Burton-MacLeod JA, Kane EM, Beard RS, et al. Evaluation and comparison of two commercial enzyme-linked immunosorbent assay kits for detection of antigenically diverse human noroviruses in stool samples. J Clin Microbiol 2004;42(6):2587–95.

[85] Duizer E, Bijkerk P, Rockx B, et al. Inactivation of caliciviruses. Appl Environ Microbiol 2004;70(8):4538–43.

[86] Drinka PJ. Norovirus outbreaks in nursing homes. J Am Geriatr Soc 2005;53(10):1839–40.

[87] Keswick BH, Satterwhite TK, Johnson PC, et al. Inactivation of Norwalk virus in drinking water by chlorine. Appl Environ Microbiol 1985;50(2):261–4.

[88] Barker J, Vipond IB, Bloomfield SF. Effects of cleaning and disinfection in reducing the spread of norovirus contamination via environmental surfaces. J Hosp Infect 2004;58(1):42–9.

[89] Asanaka M, Atmar RL, Ruvolo V, et al. Replication and packaging of Norwalk virus RNA in cultured mammalian cells. Proc Natl Acad Sci U S A 2005;102(29):10327–32.

[90] Estes MK, Ball JM, Guerrero RA, et al. Norwalk virus vaccines: challenges and progress. J Infect Dis 2000;181(Suppl 2):S367–73.

[91] Prasad BV, Crawford S, Lawton JA, et al. Structural studies on gastroenteritis viruses. Novartis Found Symp 2001;238:26–46.

[92] Ng KK, Pendas-Franco N, Rojo J, et al. Crystal structure of Norwalk virus polymerase reveals the carboxyl terminus in the active site cleft. J Biol Chem 2004;279(16):16638–45.

[93] Zeitler CR, Estes MK, Prasad BVV. X-ray crystallographic structure of the Norwalk virus protease at 1.5 Å. J Virol 2006;80(10):5050–8.

Gastroenterol Clin N Am 35 (2006) 291–314

GASTROENTEROLOGY CLINICS
OF NORTH AMERICA

An Updated Review on *Cryptosporidium* and *Giardia*

David B. Huang, MD, PhD, MPH, A. Clinton White, MD*

Division of Infectious Diseases, Department of Medicine, Baylor College of Medicine,
One Baylor Plaza, 535EE, Houston, TX 77030, USA

CRYPTOSPORIDIOSIS (*CRYPTOSPORIDIUM HOMINIS*, *CRYPTOSPORIDIUM PARVUM*, AND OTHER SPECIES)

The genus *Cryptosporidium* was identified in mice during the early twentieth century [1]; however, the first human cases of cryptosporidiosis were described in 1976. In the early 1980s, cryptosporidiosis was identified as a cause of diarrhea in AIDS. Subsequent studies identified cases among animal handlers and children and as a cause of waterborne outbreaks of diarrhea. *Cryptosporidium* is recognized as an important cause of acute, self-limited diarrhea in normal hosts worldwide; of persistent diarrhea in developing countries; and of chronic diarrhea in immunocompromised hosts, such as patients who have AIDS.

The Parasite

Cryptosporidium is a genus of protozoan parasites within the subphylum Apicomplexa (which also includes the malaria parasites). Species names were based on the host species [2]. Most human isolates previously were believed to belong to a single species, *C parvum*. More recent molecular studies demonstrated that human *Cryptosporidium* isolates include several different genotypes. The bovine genotype commonly infects humans and cows, but also can infect other species, including mice. The human genotype naturally infects only people [3], and recently was renamed *C hominis* [3]. Similarly, the *Cryptosporidium* parasites that infect dogs and people have been reclassified as *C canis* [4]. Humans also can be infected with *C meleagridis*, *C felis*, and *C muris*. *C meleagridis*, formerly believed to infect birds mainly, has been identified in most large series and seems to cause about 1% of cases of human cryptosporidiosis.

    Cryptosporidium species can complete their entire lifecycle in a single host, with asexual and sexual reproductive cycles [1]. The lifecycle begins with ingestion of the infectious oocyst. For one bovine isolate, more than half of volunteers are infected with 10 oocysts [5]. The oocysts are activated in the stomach

Dr. White is a consultant and speaker for RoMark Laboratories, the company that developed nitazoxanide.

*Corresponding author. *E-mail address*: arthurw@bcm.tmc.edu (A.C. White).

0889-8553/06/$ – see front matter
doi:10.1016/j.gtc.2006.03.006   gastro.theclinics.com

and upper intestines to produce serine proteases and aminopeptidases, which allow the organisms to excyst and release infective sporozoites. Each sporozoite contains a specialized attachment organelle, the apical complex. The motile sporozoites bind to receptors on the surface of the intestinal epithelial cells and induce actin polymerization and protrusion of the epithelial cell membrane to engulf the parasite [6,7]. The cell membrane fuses to form the parasitophorous vacuole within the microvillus layer of the epithelial surface. The growing parasite is separated from the host cytoplasm by a dense band, which prevents free flow of materials between parasite and the host cell cytoplasm but contains several transporters [8]. The parasites enlarge into trophozoite forms, divide to form type I meronts, and rupture to release the motile merozoites, which bind to and are engulfed by other epithelial cells. In some cases, the merozoites differentiate into the sexual forms (micro- and macrogametocytes), which fuse to form the oocyst that contains four sporozoites.

Epidemiology

Cryptosporidium parasites have been found in every region of the world except Antarctica. Generally, infection is more common in warm, moist months. For example, cases in the United States peak in July through September. Most studies on the prevalence of infection have relied on detection of oocysts in fecal specimens that were submitted for parasitologic examination. Only 2426 to 3793 cases were reported each year in the United States from 1995 through 2002, but an estimated 300,000 persons in the United States are affected each year [9]. The difference assumes underreporting; however, the underuse of diagnostic tests and their poor sensitivity suggest that the higher estimate may be low. Overall, older surveys that did not involve patients who had HIV documented oocysts in 1% to 3% of specimens from industrialized countries of Europe and North America (mean, 2.3%) [10]. Most studies from developing countries document *Cryptosporidium* in at least 5% of diarrheal stools (mean, 12.7%) [10]. With improving diagnostic techniques more cases are being identified. For example, a survey of stool specimens that were submitted to a large commercial laboratory in the United States documented oocysts in specimens from 121 of 2896 (4.2%) individuals [11]. Similarly, a sensitive and specific polymerase chain reaction (PCR) method documented *Cryptosporidium* in 444 of 1779 (25%) cases of diarrhea in Uganda, including 22% of cases of acute diarrhea [12]. Similarly, oocysts were found in 83 of 445 (18.7%) children who had diarrhea by direct immunofluorescence in a study from Brazil [13]. Thus, the prevalence may be higher than suggested by earlier stool studies.

Serologic testing also has been used to determine the prevalence of cryptosporidiosis. Most of the assays have used unfractionated oocyst antigens using ELISA assays, but there also are purified and recombinant antigens. Most serosurveys have documented a seroprevalence of about 30% among United States adults, with higher rates associated with contact with contaminated water or animals [14]. Thirty-one percent of 803 children in Oklahoma were seropositive, with rates increasing with age [15]. Along the United States–Mexico border, seroprevalence rates were documented to be 82% to 89% [16]. That compares with rates of about 75% for children ages 11 to 13 in China and 64% for adults in urban Latin America. By contrast, more than 90% of children seroconverted during the first year of life in a Brazilian shantytown [17]. In recent intensive studies of a birth cohort in Lima, many diarrhea episodes associated with seroconversion never had organisms identifiable in stool. Overall, there is a significant disconnect between serologic studies and stool studies, which suggest that nearly half of cases of cryptosporidiosis will have negative stool studies [18]. Similar data has been noted in human challenge studies. In that case, infection was confirmed by PCR.

Cryptosporidium oocysts are hardy; if kept moist they remain infectious for more than 6 months. Oocysts can be killed by freezing, but *Cryptosporidium* oocysts are highly resistant to chlorination. Incubation of oocysts for up to 2 hours in household bleach failed to decrease infectivity [19]. Although oocysts are sensitive to hydrogen peroxide, ozone, and ultraviolet radiation, outbreaks have been associated with ozonated cider.

Surveys have demonstrated that most sources of drinking water are contaminated with oocysts before treatment [20], with 39% of apparently pristine sources contaminated [20]. More than 50 outbreaks of cryptosporidiosis have been linked to contaminated drinking water [21]. The largest documented outbreak occurred in Milwaukee in 1993 [22] with an estimated 403,000 people developing a diarrheal illness [23]. Many of the waterborne outbreaks, including the outbreak in Milwaukee, have been caused by *C hominis*. However, *C parvum* (bovine genotype) also has been associated with waterborne outbreaks, especially when linked to contamination with agricultural runoff.

Cryptosporidiosis also is associated with contaminated recreational water. Swimming in a public swimming pool was one of the main risk factors for cryptosporidiosis in Australia [24]. Outbreaks often were linked to fecal accidents [24]. The chlorine concentration in pool water is insufficient to disinfect the water.

Foodborne infection occurs less frequently, but it has been tied to contaminated apple cider, unpasteurized milk, chicken salad, and raw produce. Oocysts commonly are found on vegetables in developing countries. Oocysts have been identified frequently in shellfish from the Chesapeake Bay and in flies, but there is no good evidence of transmission to persons.

Because *Cryptosporidium* oocysts are infectious when shed, direct person-to-person spread is common, including outbreaks that are associated with contact with day care centers and nosocomial transmission. Contact with a person who had diarrhea was a major risk factor for cryptosporidiosis [24,25], and secondary transmission within households occurs commonly [26]. For example, Newman and colleagues [26] noted secondary cases in 18 of 31 households (58%) that involved 19% of household members. In day care–associated outbreaks, secondary transmission rates have ranged from 14% to 38% [27]. High rates of transmission also were noted in children during the Milwaukee outbreak, but only 5% of adult cases were associated with secondary transmission [22].

Cryptosporidiosis also is a cause of travel-associated diarrhea. *Cryptosporidium* has been linked to 2% of cases of traveler's diarrhea [28], but recent studies that used antigen-detection tests suggest that the numbers are closer to 10%. Most travel-associated cases of diarrhea are due to *C hominis* [29].

Cryptosporidiosis outbreaks have been linked to animal contact. Endemic cryptosporidiosis in England is caused mainly by *C parvum* [29]. There was a dramatic decrease in human cryptosporidiosis when animal contact was controlled during a foot-and-mouth disease epidemic [30].

Host immune status affects the epidemiology of cryptosporidiosis. In studies from resource-poor countries with heavy exposure, cryptosporidiosis is a disease of young children, which suggests the development of immunity [26,31–33]. Also, previous challenge or prechallenge immunity was associated with resistance to experimental infection [34,35]. *Cryptosporidium* is found in about 16% of patients who have AIDS and diarrhea [10]. For example, in a waterborne outbreak 104 of 339 (30.7%) persons who were infected with HIV developed cryptosporidiosis compared with 190 of 1392 (13.6%) HIV-negative participants [36]. Also, the infection rate among patients who had AIDS was proportional to the CD4 cell count; however, infection was not more frequent in patients who had HIV during the Milwaukee outbreak. Cryptosporidiosis also has been noted in other immunodeficient subjects, and primarily was associated with defects of the cell-mediated immune response.

Pathogenesis

Cryptosporidium tissue forms develop within parasitophorous vacuoles in the microvillus layer of the epithelial cells (Fig. 1). The organisms have a predilection for the distal small intestines (eg, terminal ileum) and proximal colon, but can be identified throughout the gut, the biliary tract, and even in the respiratory tract in immunodeficient hosts. Persistent cryptosporidiosis in children is associated with villous atrophy and a mild increase in lamina propria lymphocytes. Heavier infection in patients who have AIDS is associated with villous atrophy, crypt hyperplasia, and marked infiltration with lymphocytes, plasma cells, and even neutrophils [37–40].

Cryptosporidiosis characteristically presents with watery diarrhea and malabsorption. The diarrhea is believed to result from sodium malabsorption, electrogenic chloride secretion, and increased intestinal permeability. Epithelial cell infection is associated with activation of nuclear factor κB [41,42], which activates antiapoptotic mechanisms, but also leads to up-regulation of a proinflammatory cascade with increased expression of proinflammatory cytokines and markers of inflammation, including tumor necrosis factor α, interleukin (IL)-1, IL-8, and lactoferrin [43–45]. Chemokines, including IL-8 and IP-10, are produced by the infected epithelial cells [46]. Infection also up-regulates expression of cyclooxygenase 2, production of prostaglandins by the epithelial cells, and production of neuropeptides. Infection results in increased epithelial permeability, decreased sodium absorption, and chloride secretion.

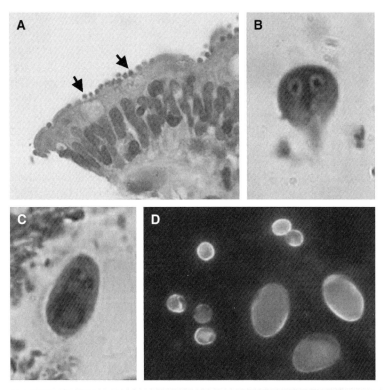

Fig. 1. (A) *Cryptosporidium*. The arrows indicate intracellular replication of *Cryptosporidium* within human small intestinal epithelial cells. (Courtesy of David Glembocki, MD and William A. Petri, MD, Charlottesville, VA.) [155]. (B) *Giardia* trophozoites stained with iron hematoxylin. The cell, which is 10 to 20 μm in length, has two nuclei with a large central karysome. (*From* http://www.dpd.cdc.gov/dpdx/HTML/Giardiasis.htm.) (C) *Giardia* cyst stained with iron hematoxylin. Note the size of the cyst, 8 to 12 lm in length, and that it has two nuclei. (*From* http://www.dpd.cdc.gov/dpdx/HTML/Giardiasis.htm.) (D) *Giardia* (*lower right*) and *Cryptosporidium* (*upper left*) labeled with immunofluorescent antibody. (*From* http:// www.dpd.cdc.gov/dpdx/HTML/Giardiasis.htm.)

Cryptosporidium infection causes increased intestinal permeability with decreased absorption of fluids and electrolytes as well as solute fluxes into the gut. The severity of cryptosporidiosis in patients who have AIDS and children correlates with altered intestinal permeability (as measured by ratios of excreted lactulose and mannitol in the urine) [38,47].

Cryptosporidium infection induces defects in the epithelial cell barrier function in vitro, which may be caused by proinflammatory cytokines, such as interferon (IFN)-γ [48]. Biopsies from infected intestines reveal increased epithelial cell apoptosis [37]. The organisms also may cause necrosis of the infected cells and loss of villous surface as demonstrated in human infection by tests of D-xylose malabsorption [38].

Host Response and Immunity

Cryptosporidiosis is self-limited in normal hosts and patients with HIV CD4 cell counts and preserved [49–51]. Furthermore, cryptosporidiosis can resolve in response to effective antiretroviral therapy and is associated with an influx of CD4 cells into the intestines [52]. Thus, CD4 cell function is important for clearance and prevention of infection.

IFN-γ is the key mediator of the immune response to *Cryptosporidium* as illustrated by studies of knockout mice [53,54]. Antigen-stimulated T cells from people who have recovered from cryptosporidiosis produce IFN-γ; however, only half of volunteers produced IFN-γ after experimental infection, and expression was limited to those with evidence of previous exposure (ie, seropositive before challenge or demonstrated resistance to infection) [55,56]. Similarly, IFN-γ was not detected in stools from Haitian children who had active cryptosporidiosis, despite the fact that they had self-limited disease [45]. Thus, other factors seem to be involved in limiting human infection after initial exposure. Control of infection was associated with expression of IL-15 in seronegative normal volunteers who were infected experimentally and in patients who had AIDS who were recovering from cryptosporidiosis in response to antiretrovirals [57]. This effect probably is mediated by activation of natural killer cells [58].

Clinical Manifestations

Symptoms of cryptosporidiosis develop after an incubation period of about 1 week. Diarrhea is the most common clinical presentation; however, there are significant differences in the clinical presentation that depend on the host population.

Immunocompetent Individuals in Developed Countries

Immunocompetent individuals usually present with watery diarrhea [23]. The median duration of illness is approximately 5 to 10 days. Other symptoms include abdominal cramps, nausea, vomiting, and fever [23]. Cryptosporidiosis also has been associated with respiratory symptoms. Often, there is a biphasic course with recurrent symptoms after initial resolution in up to 39% of cases [22,23,26]. Relapses may follow a diarrhea-free period of several days to weeks.

Milder or even asymptomatic infection also may be common as illustrated by the fact that seroconversion is more common than is clinically diagnosed disease in developed and developing countries [15,18,59]. For example, of the estimated 403,000 cases of disease in the Milwaukee outbreak only a minority of patients presented for clinical care [23]. Patients who were not diagnosed in the clinics were less severely ill, had a shorter duration of diarrhea, and often had negative stool tests compared with patients who had laboratory-confirmed disease.

Childhood Diarrhea in Resource-Poor Countries

The most common clinical manifestation of cryptosporidiosis in developing countries is childhood diarrhea [12,26,44,60,61]. In studies from Asia, Africa, and Latin America, cryptosporidiosis is common. Children usually present with an acute diarrhea similar to that seen with other enteric pathogens [62]. Fever, shortness of breath, and foul stools are noted in only a minority of cases. Up to 45% of the children develop diarrhea that persists beyond 14 days [26], which makes *Cryptosporidium* among the more common causes of persistent diarrhea in developing countries [12,26,62]. Persistent diarrhea is associated with an increased risk for recurrent episodes of diarrhea, weight loss, and premature death [63–66]. In children who have the onset of cryptosporidiosis before 1 year of age there is an association with poorer physical fitness and cognitive development years later [67]; however, it is not clear if this is more common with *Cryptosporidium* compared with other pathogens [68].

Cryptosporidiosis in HIV Infection

Before the advent of effective antiretroviral combinations cryptosporidiosis was diagnosed mainly in patients who had AIDS [50]; however, the prevalence of cryptosporidiosis in HIV has decreased dramatically with improvements in antiretroviral therapy. The clinical presentation of cryptosporidiosis in patients who have HIV is variable. Patients with CD4 cell counts above 180/μL present with a self-limited diarrhea that is similar to normal hosts [37,49–51]. Cryptosporidiosis can be mild and self-limited in patients who have advanced AIDS; however, most patients present with chronic diarrhea with frequent, foul smelling, bulky stools and weight loss. Some patients who have AIDS, primarily those with CD4 cell counts that are less than 50/μL, develop a voluminous watery diarrhea or cholera-like illness.

Biliary and respiratory tract involvement can occur in advanced AIDS [50,69]. Biliary tract involvement usually is noted in patients who have AIDS with CD4 cell counts that are less than 50/μL, and it is associated with a markedly shortened survival [50,69]. Biliary manifestations include acalculous cholecystitis, sclerosing cholangitis, or pancreatitis [50,69], which usually presents with right upper quadrant abdominal pain. Laboratory studies reveal elevated levels of alkaline phosphatase; often, bilirubin and transaminase levels also are elevated. Ultrasound examination may reveal dilation of the biliary duct or gallbladder thickening. Endoscopic retrograde cholecystopancreatogram evaluation usually is required to make the anatomic diagnosis. Biliary duct biopsies, examination of the bile, or stool studies may demonstrate the parasites.

Diagnosis

Traditionally, cryptosporidiosis has been diagnosed by microscopic examination of stool. Generally, stools should be preserved in 10% buffered formalin because fresh stool is infectious to laboratory personnel and polyvinyl alcohol interferes with staining [70]. Formalin-ethyl acetate concentration can improve the yield in cryptosporidiosis, but centrifugation speeds and time must be increased [70,71]. Oocysts are 4 to 6 μm in diameter, and are similar in size and shape to yeast (see Fig. 1). Traditional stool examinations usually miss the organism, but many laboratories only test for *Cryptosporidium* when requested to specifically. Thus, underdiagnosis is a significant problem.

Oocysts stain with modified acid-fast stains [70]; however, stool examination with acid-fast staining is insensitive and requires an oocyst concentration of more than 500,000/mL in formed stools [72,73]. Fluorescent stains (eg, auramine O, auramine-rhodamine) can be read more quickly than other acid-fast stains and may have improved sensitivity at the expense of false positive results [70].

Immunofluorescent assays (IFAs) that use monoclonal antibodies to the *Cryptosporidium* oocysts are used commonly (see Fig. 1). IFA is up to 10 times more sensitive than is acid-fast staining [73,74]. Some of the commercial IFAs (Merifluor *Cryptosporidium/Giardia*, Meridian Bioscience, Inc., Cincinnati, Ohio) also are sensitive and specific assays in giardiasis [73,74].

Antigen-detection assays are being used increasingly for stool diagnosis. Commercial kits for *Cryptosporidium* are available in ELISA and immunochromatographic formats. The ELISA kits for *Cryptosporidium* generally have performed well for the diagnosis of cryptosporidiosis with sensitivities ranging from 66% to 100% and excellent specificity [70,74,75]; however, pseudo-outbreaks have been reported because of false positive results. The immunochromatographic tests are rapid tests for *Cryptosporidium* and *Giardia* antigen [73,75]. The sensitivity is less than with other assays, but the specificity is excellent and the results are available in minutes [73,75]. Antigen assays have the advantage of not requiring the skills that are needed for microscopic identification. PCR tests for *C parvum* DNA also have been used to detect organisms. The sensitivity is much better than with the microscopic studies of stool [76]. Overall, the diagnosis of cryptosporidiosis remains problematic because of the limited availability of sensitive, specific, and easily performed assays. The result is that most laboratories miss most cases.

Management

Initial management of cryptosporidiosis should focus on the replacement of fluids and electrolytes. Oral rehydration is the preferred. Supportive care should include a lactose-free diet. Glutamine supplementation may improve fluid absorption [77]. Nutrition is important, and oral feeding is as effective as parenteral nutrition [78].

Antimotility agents are important adjuncts to therapy. Loperamide and diphenoxylate/atropine can decrease symptoms in mild to moderate disease. More potent opiates, including tincture of opium (paregoric), may work in patients who do not respond to milder agents. Octreotide can be effective in AIDS-associated diarrhea, but its cost is higher than other agents [79].

Among patients who have AIDS and chronic cryptosporidiosis, improvement in immune function with effective antiretroviral therapy can result in dramatic improvement in diarrhea [80–82]. Antiretroviral therapy should include one or more HIV protease inhibitors, because the protease inhibitors have anti-cryptosporidial activity in vitro and in animals [83]; however, cryptosporidiosis also can cause malabsorption of antiretroviral medications [84]. Several recent studies combined antiretroviral therapy with antiparasitic agents [82]. This approach should improve the response to both treatments.

Biliary involvement in cryptosporidiosis requires mechanical interventions. Patients who have calculous cholecystitis should be treated with cholecystectomy [85]. Sclerosing cholangitis usually can be treated by endoscopic retrograde cholangiopancreatography with sphincterotomy. Often, stenting is required [50].

Numerous studies have examined the role of antiparasitic therapy in cryptosporidiosis (Table 1). Nitazoxanide is a broad-spectrum antiparasitic drug that was approved in United States for treatment of cryptosporidiosis and giardiasis [86,87].

Two randomized trials were performed in patients who had cryptosporidiosis and were not infected with HIV. In a study of adults and children who had cryptosporidiosis that was performed in Egypt, diarrhea and oocyst shedding resolved significantly more rapidly with nitazoxanide. Studies were performed in Zambia on malnourished children who were hospitalized with chronic cryptosporidiosis [88]. Among HIV-negative children, diarrhea had resolved by day 7 in 14 of 25 (56%) who were treated with nitazoxanide compared with 5 of 22 (23%) who received placebo. Four HIV-negative children died; all received placebo. Among the HIV-infected children, there were no significant differences in clinical and parasitologic responses or in mortality with nitazoxanide treatment [88]. Nitazoxanide was studied in HIV-infected patients who had cryptosporidiosis in a randomized trial that was performed in Mexico [89]. Among patients who had CD4 cell counts of greater than 50/μL, 10 of 14 (71%) responded to nitazoxanide, 1 g/d, and 9 of 10 (90%) responded to nitazoxanide, 2 g/d, (compared with 3 of 15 [20%] who were treated with placebo); however, the response with nitazoxanide was no better than placebo for patients whose CD4 cell counts were less than or equal to 50/μL.

Paromomycin is a nonabsorbable aminoglycoside. Initial in vitro studies noted poor activity against *C parvum*. The first 12 published case series of patients who had AIDS and were treated with paromomycin included more than 300 patients with a response rate of 67% [50]. Three placebo-controlled trials examined the effects of paromomycin in patients who had AIDS and cryptosporidiosis. All three studies demonstrated limited complete response rates with few cures, but diarrhea improved more with the drug than with placebo [1].

Macrolide antibiotics have some activity against *Cryptosporidium*. Sáez-Lloren and colleagues [90] reported shorter duration of symptoms and oocyst shedding in children who were treated with spiramycin, 100 mg/kg/d; however, the results were not confirmed in a second trial [91]. Trials of spiramycin and azithromycin in patients who had AIDS did not show superior efficacy to placebo. Smith and colleagues [92] conducted a pilot study of paromomycin plus azithromycin in patients who had AIDS and chronic cryptosporidiosis. Overall, there was a 2-log decrease in oocyst shedding, but few patients were

Table 1
Treatment and side effect profile for available treatment of cryptosporidiosis and giardiasis

Drug	Adult dosage	Pediatric dosage	Side effects
Metronidazole	250 mg tid × 5–7 d	5 mg/kg tid × 7 d	Metallic taste; nausea; vomiting; dizziness; headache; disulfaram-like effect; neutropenia
Tinidazole	2 g, single dose	50 mg/kg, single dose	Metallic taste; nausea; vomiting; belching; dizziness; headache; disulfiram-like effect
Nitazoxanide	500 mg bid × 3 d	Age 1–2 yr: 100 mg bid × 3 d; Age 4–11 yr: 200 mg bid × 3 d	Abdominal pain; diarrhea; vomiting; headache; yellow-green discoloration of urine
Quinacrine	100 mg tid × 5–7 d	2 mg/kg tid × 7 d	Abdominal pain; diarrhea; dizziness; headache; loss of appetite; nausea; vomiting; yellow discoloration of the sclera; skin; and urine; toxic psychosis; darkening of the fingernails and toenails; exfoliative dermatitis
Furazolidone	100 mg qid × 7–10 d	2 mg/kg qid × 10 d	Hypersensitivity reaction; hypotension; urticaria; fever; arthralgia; morbilliform rash; nausea; vomiting; headache; malaise; brownish discoloration of urine; disulfiram-like effect; rarely reversible intravascular hemolysis
Albendazole	400 mg qd × 5 d	15 mg/kg/d × 5–7 d	Abnormal liver function tests; abdominal pain; nausea; vomiting; headache; dizziness; leukopenia
Paromomycin	500 mg tid × 5–10 d	30 mg/kg/d tid × 5–10 d	Abdominal pain; nausea; diarrhea; dizziness; rash; oto- and nephrotoxicity

Abbreviations: bid, twice a day; qd, every day; qid, four times a day; tid, three times a day.

cured. Rifaximin, a nonabsorbable rifamycin, also improved cryptosporidiosis in patients who had HIV [93].

Prevention

Water purification is an important public health measure. Generally, water purification should involve flocculation and filtration [20]. Ultraviolet radiation or ozonation, can disinfect contaminated water, but it is used rarely. Recreational waters, such as lakes, may pose a danger for compromised hosts, who should avoid untreated water. Swimming pools are an important source of infection. For individual use, water can be decontaminated by bringing it to a boil or by passing it through a filter with a 1-μm or smaller pore size. Generally, chlorine and iodine are ineffective. Although cryptosporidiosis can be transmitted within health care facilities, the risk is minimal with standard precautions.

GIARDIASIS

Giardia is a flagellated enteric protozoan that was recognized first in 1681 by Van Leeuwenhoek, who discovered this pathogen in his stool. In 1915, the parasite was named *Giardia* in honor of Professor A. Giard of Paris. The species name of *Giardia* is dependent on the morphology and the host of origin. Humans are believed to be infected by a single species, variably termed *G lamblia*, *G intestinalis*, or *G duodenalis*. Giardiasis is a major cause of waterborne and foodborne diarrhea throughout the world [94].

The Parasite

Giardia has a complex genome that consists of 1.2×10^7 base pairs of DNA and a GC content of 46% [94]. This protozoa is capable of undergoing antigenic variation of its cysteine-rich surface proteins through a palmitoylated process during human infection and during the encystation and the excystation cycle [95,96]. Antigenic variation protects this parasite from the activity of intestinal proteases, provides oxygen stability, and allows adaptation to different hosts. The clinical significance of *Giardia* antigenic variation is not known.

The *Giardia* lifecycle consists of two stages. The first stage involves the trophozoite (see Fig. 1), which has two anteriorly placed nuclei. The trophozoite is an aerotolerant anaerobe that requires glucose as a source of carbohydrate energy and divides by longitudinal binary fission every 9 to 12 hours. The trophozoite has a convex dorsal surface and a flat ventral surface that contains an adhesive disk that is made of microtubules and allows for attachment at the brush border of enterocytes. The trophozoite also has four pairs of posteriorly directed flagella that aid in locomotion and attachment to intestinal epithelium.

Cysts, which are 10 to 20 μm in length, are responsible for transmission of *Giardia* (see Fig. 1). Cysts are relatively resistant to chlorination and ozonolysis and can survive in cold surface water for several weeks to months. Specific environmental changes, including cholesterol starvation followed by alkaline pH and excess bile salts [97], result in down-regulation of trophozoite-specific genes and dipeptidyl peptidase IV–associated proteolysis [98]. These environmental stimuli result in the formation of specific encystment vesicles and transcription and secretion into the vesicles of cysteine-rich cyst wall proteins CWP-1 and CWP-2 [99]. A granule-specific protein regulates the Ca^{2+}-dependent degranulation of encystation-specific vesicles during the formation of the cyst wall.

Environmental stimuli, such as the presence of gastric acid and pancreatic enzymes, initiate the excystation process by way of cysteine protease activation and protein kinase A [100,101]. Excystation results in the release of a single trophozoite that contains four nuclei. This trophozoite divides twice and results in four daughter trophozoites. Trophozoites replicate and colonize the proximal small bowel by way of a ventral sucking disk.

Epidemiology

In the United States, *Giardia* is among the most commonly diagnosed parasitic enteric pathogens. *G lamblia* has been identified in 4% to 7% of stool specimens from patients in the United States who have diarrheal illness. In the mid-1990s, a United States epidemiologic survey identified 25,000 to 28,000 cases of giardiasis annually [102]; however, because of underreporting, estimates of annual giardiasis cases are likely to be 4 to 100 times that of reported cases.

Giardiasis affects persons of all ages and occurs during the late summer and fall months. The populations that are affected most frequently include children 0 to 5 years of age (children in day care and their close contacts), adults 31 to 40 years of age, backpackers, campers, hunters, and travelers to disease-endemic areas. A multicenter study of outpatient pediatric nondysenteric diarrhea in the United States found that *Giardia* was the cause of diarrhea in 15% of children [103]. In developing regions of the world, *Giardia* is one of the first enteric pathogens to infect infants, with a prevalence rate up to 30% in children who are younger than 10 years of age [104–108].

Giardia is acquired by ingestion of cysts from contaminated water and food and by person-to-person spread, especially persons with poor fecal-oral hygiene. *Giardia* and *Cryptosporidium* are the most common pathogens in outbreaks of diarrheal illness that are due to drinking water [109]. Recreational, surface, and well water can contain *Giardia* cysts. Backpackers may become infected if they do not treat water adequately (ie, faulty purification system or inadequate chlorination). A case control study in southwestern England showed that swallowing water while swimming, contact with recreational fresh water, drinking tap water, and eating lettuce were risk factors for developing giardiasis [110]. Person-to-person transmission occurs in groups who have poor fecal-oral hygiene. Among children in day care centers, *Giardia* cyst passage was documented to be as high as 50% [111]. Many of these infected children are asymptomatic and they can spread the cysts among household members. The *Giardia* cyst passage rate is as high as 20% among sexually active gay men [112]. *Giardia* cysts also were reported to be transmitted in commercial food establishments, corporate office settings, and small gatherings and were ingested among travelers to developing countries [113–115].

Pathogenesis

The pathogenesis of *Giardia* has been postulated to involve trophozoite direct damage to the intestinal brush border and mucosa, induction of a host immune response that results in the secretion of fluid and damage to the gut, alteration of bile content or duodenal flora, and apoptosis in the small intestinal epithelial cells. Disruption of the intestinal epithelial cell brush border may explain the lactose intolerance that develops commonly. In vitro studies showed that *Giardia* disrupts tight junctional zona occludens, increases permeability, and induces apoptosis in small intestinal epithelial cells [116]. Increased permeability of the small intestinal epithelial cells occurs by way of a myosin light chain kinase–dependent phosphorylation of F-actin [117,118]; however, mucosal invasion occurs rarely and no *Giardia* enterotoxin has been found.

Host Response and Immunity

Host immunity, which consists of humoral and cellular components, is important in the clearance and protection against reinfection of *Giardia*. Studies have demonstrated IgM and IgG antibody with complement to be lethal to *Giardia* trophozoites. In the intestinal lumen, however, where trophozoites are located, secretory IgA antibody is important in the temporal control of *Giardia*, probably by binding trophozoites, and thus, preventing this parasite from adhering to intestinal epithelial cells. The absence of secretory IgA is associated with the inability to clear *Giardia* infection and correlates with chronic giardiasis in humans [119]. In a murine model, IL-6 is important in the early control of giardiasis [120] and a secretory and systemic antibody response can be elicited to infection with *G lamblia* [121]. B-cell– and T-cell–deficient mice are unable to clear *Giardia* [122,123]. Similarly, patients who have antibody deficits (eg, common variable immunodeficiency and X-linked agammaglobulinemia) or reduced gastric acidity (eg, previous gastric surgery) have a predisposition to giardiasis. When infected, these patients may develop prolonged diarrhea, malabsorption, and abnormal small bowel histology which have characteristic spruelike lesions with marked flattening of the villi, crypt hypertrophy, and a dense mononuclear cell infiltration of the submucosa [124].

Clinical Manifestations

Giardiasis can result in asymptomatic illness, acute self-limiting diarrhea, or chronic diarrhea and malabsorption depending on host factor susceptibility and pathogen genotypic differences in virulence [125,126]. Infection may occur with oral ingestion with as few as 10 to 25 cysts. Among persons who ingest *Giardia* cysts, 5% to 15% pass cysts without symptoms, 25% to 50% develop acute self-limiting diarrhea, and 35% to 70% have no evidence of infection. The incubation period of giardiasis is 7 to 14 days. Symptoms of giardiasis include diarrhea (89%), malaise (84%), flatulence (74%), foul-smelling, greasy stools (72%), abdominal cramps (70%), bloating (69%), nausea (68%), anorexia (64%), and weight loss (64%) [112]. Other less commonly reported symptoms include urticaria (9%), constipation (9%), reactive arthritis, biliary tract disease, and gastric infection. The white blood cell count usually is normal and eosin-ophilia is absent. Patients may describe their stools as watery or greasy and foul smelling. Gross blood, pus, and mucus usually are absent.

Patients who have giardiasis often have symptoms for more than 7 to 10 days. Patients who develop persistent or chronic diarrhea, defined as diarrhea for more than 14 days, may have profound malaise, lassitude, occasional head-ache, diffuse abdominal and epigastric discomfort that is exacerbated by eating, and weight loss. Stools from patients who have chronic diarrhea often are greasy and foul smelling or frothy, yellowish, and frequently occur in small vol-umes. Periods of diarrhea may alternate with periods of constipation or normal bowel habits over a period of months until spontaneous resolution or an anti-microbial therapy is given.

Malabsorption may occur with chronic diarrhea that is due to giardiasis. Children who have symptomatic giardiasis may develop steatorrhea and mal-absorption of vitamin A, B_{12}, protein, D-xylose, and iron [127,128]. Lactase de-ficiency occurs in 20% to 40% of cases after *Giardia* infection and it may persist for several weeks after treatment [129]. The deleterious effects of chronic giar-diasis on growth and development are controversial. Studies suggest that pro-longed episodes of giardiasis in children with underlying poor nutrition result in deleterious effects, such as stunted growth, poor intestinal permeability, low weight and height for age, and decreased cognitive function compared with normal children who do not have giardiasis [68,130–134]. One study in Salva-dor, Brazil found that asymptomatic children who were infected with *Giardia* had impeded growth [135].

Diagnosis

Traditionally, the diagnosis of *Giardia* infection has depended on microscopic identification of the organism in stool. This requires an experienced microsco-pist and a specialized laboratory. Stool samples should be examined fresh or placed immediately in a preservative. Motile trophozoites may be seen in a saline wet mount of fresh liquid stool from a patient who has acute diarrheal illness. Cysts can be identified after iodine staining or after preservation in 10% buffered formalin or polyvinyl alcohol and subsequent trichrome or iron hematoxylin staining. Repeated samplings may be necessary. The yield of cysts may be increased with formalin-ether or zinc sulfate flotation concen-tration techniques [136,137]. Nevertheless, even under ideal conditions, organ-isms are identified in a single stool sample in only half of patients.

Giardia antigen detection by immunofluorescence ELISAs, nonenzymatic immunoassays (ImmunoCard STAT! *Cryptosporidium/Giardia* Rapid Assay, Meridian Bioscience, Inc.), and direct fluorescence antibody (DFA) tests are be-coming the standard diagnostic tests in the United States. Commercial antigenic detection tests are similar in cost to microscopy (O & P [stool examination] cost per specimen is approximately $72–$111, *Giardia* EIA $137–$188, and *Giardia* DFA $80–$126) with better reproducibility and more rapid return of results [74,138]. Antigen tests have a sensitivity of 85% to 98% and a specificity of

90% to 100% compared with microscopy [74,138–141]. A commonly used assay, ProSpecT (*Giardia* Microplate Assay, Remel, Lenexa, Kansas) detects cyst wall protein (CWP-1) by ELISA, and Merifluor DFA (Meridian Bioscience, Inc.) uses a fluorescein-tagged monoclonal antibody against *Giardia* (see Fig. 1). The Merifluor DFA has a reported sensitivity and specificity of 96% to 100% [74,139].

Other tests that may be used for the diagnosis of *Giardia* include the string test or EnteroTest (HDC Corporation, Milpitas, California), duodenal aspiration, duodenal biopsy, and anti-*Giardia* antibody. A string test that yields bile-stained mucus from the duodenum can be examined by wet mount for trophozoites. Although more invasive, duodenal aspiration and biopsy offer the advantage of examining for trophozoites and other enteric pathogens.

Management

The main treatments that are available for giardiasis include metronidazole, tinidazole, and nitazoxanide. Quinacrine, furazolidone, and albendazole are used less commonly. Table 1 shows the dosage and side effect profile for the available treatment for giardiasis.

Metronidazole has been first-line therapy for giardiasis although it never has been approved by the US Food and Drug Administration. The mechanism of action of metronidazole is reduction of its nitro group which accepts electrons from parasite ferredoxins; it subsequently binds to parasite DNA and causes trophozoite death [142]. An extensive systematic review of all randomized trials on the treatment of giardiasis showed that metronidazole has an improved parasitologic cure rate compared with most older treatments and placebo [143]. Several studies evaluated metronidazole on parasitologic cure, defined as a negative stool specimen. Although these studies used different dosages and different treatment times, metronidazole had a higher cure rate compared with the comparator treatment in most patients. Metronidazole in divided doses over 7 days has an efficacy of 80% to 95%; however, side effects are common and include metallic taste, nausea, headache, disulfiram-like effect, and neutropenia. Metronidazole is mutagenic in bacteria and is carcinogenic in mice and rats; it probably should be avoided during pregnancy.

Tinidazole is the second nitroimidazole drug to be approved in the United States for treatment of giardiasis, amebiasis, and trichomoniasis. Some authorities consider tinidazole as first-line therapy for giardiasis because it can be offered as a single-dose treatment. Tinidazole interferes with DNA synthesis. This drug offers an improved clinical cure rate when compared with other single-dose therapies, although the parasitologic cure rate is similar. A single dose of tinidazole is more effective than a single dose of metronidazole (97.5% versus 54%, respectively) and it is as effective as metronidazole given for 3 days [144]. When given as a single 2-g dose, tinidazole yields an efficacy of approximately 90% [145]. The side effect profile of tinidazole is similar to metronidazole but the side effects are less common, maybe because of the reduced dosing frequency. This drug is mutagenic in bacteria and is carcinogenic in mice, and it should be avoided in pregnancy.

Nitazoxanide (Alinia; Romark Pharmaceuticals, Tampa, Florida) was approved for the treatment of children who had giardiasis and cryptosporidiosis in 2003, and it subsequently was approved for the treatment of adults. Nitazoxanide has broad-spectrum coverage against many intestinal protozoa and helminths and some aerobic and anaerobic bacteria. The drug interferes with anaerobic energy metabolism by inhibiting the pyruvate-ferredoxin oxidoreductase enzyme–dependent electron transfer. Nitazoxanide, 500 mg twice a day for 3 days, was given to 87 patients who had giardiasis at a primary school in San Pedro Toliman, Queretaro, Mexico. Nitazoxanide had a parasitologic cure rate of 71% and was tolerated well [146]. Clinical trials in the pediatric population have yielded efficacy in the range of 70% to 85%; these cure rates are similar to metronidazole in direct comparison [147–149].

Quinacrine is an antimalarial agent that has an efficacy of more than 90%. Quinacrine, 8 mg/kg, divided in three dosages for 5 days, was equally effective as metronidazole in children who had giardiasis (100% in both groups) [150]. It has a significant side effect profile (see Table 1). This drug is no longer produced in the United States but it may be obtained from selective pharmacies (Panorama Pharmacy, Lake Balboa, California) and the Centers for Disease Control and Prevention. Furazolidone, a nitrofuran, has an efficacy of 80% to 85%. In a comparative study with metronidazole, furazolidone had a cure rate of 80% compared with 95% for metronidazole [150]. Like quinacrine it has a significant side effect profile. Albendazole, a broad-spectrum antihelminthic agent, was effective against *Giardia* in some, but not all, clinical trials. Albendazole binds to parasite tubulin, which inhibits its polymerization and microtubule-dependent glucose uptake. Albendazole has been given as a single dose at 600 mg and 800 mg with success rates of 62% and 75%, respectively. When albendazole, 400 mg for 3 days or 5 days, was given the treatment success increased to 81% and 95%, respectively. Albendazole, 400 mg for 5 days, was as effective as metronidazole, 125 mg three time daily for 5 days (97% cure rate) [151]. Albendazole is teratogenic in animals and should be avoided during pregnancy. Side effects include abdominal discomfort, nausea, vomiting, headache, dizziness, and reversible increases in hepatic transaminases.

For patients who are not cured by a single drug course or who relapse, switching to an agent from a different drug class usually is effective. Combination treatment with metronidazole and quinacrine was shown to be effective [152]. In pregnant women who have giardiasis, delayed therapy until after delivery or after the first trimester should be considered when disease is mild and hydration and nutrition can be maintained. In severe giardiasis, paromomycin, a nonabsorbed oral aminoglycoside, in an adult dosage of 500 mg three times a day for 5 to 10 days, has been given with an efficacy rate of 60% to 70% [153]. Metronidazole also probably can be given safely in the last two trimesters in pregnancy.

Prevention

Giardiasis may be prevented with the proper handling and treatment of food and water and with good personal hygiene (eg, thorough hand washing when using the toilet, playing with pets, or changing diapers) in communities. In endemic regions, uncooked foods that are prepared or washed with contaminated water should be avoided. Public water supplies should be subjected to chlorination, flocculation, sedimentation, and filtration [154]. Individual water supplies, such as for travelers or backpackers, should be boiled or filtered. Water filters with pores of 1 μm also may be used. *Giardia* and *Cryptosporidium* are relatively resistant to chlorine or iodine treatment. Avoidance of oral-anal and oral-genital sex may reduce the transmission of *Giardia* among sexually active homosexuals.

Treatment of healthy persons with asymptomatic carriage of *Giardia* is controversial and should be decided on a case-by-case basis. Treating all infected persons during an outbreak may be considered if strict hand washing and treatment of symptomatic children fail to control an outbreak of diarrhea. No immunoprophylactic strategy for giardiasis in humans exists.

References

[1] White AC Jr. Cryptosporidiosis (*Cryptosporidium hominis, Cryptosporidium parvum*, other species). In: Mandell GL, Bennett JE, Dolin R, editors. Principles and practice of infectious diseases. 6th edition. Philadelphia: Elsevier Churchill Livingstone; 2005. p. 3215–28.

[2] Xiao L, Fayer R, Ryan U, et al. Cryptosporidium taxonomy: recent advances and implications for public health. Clin Microbiol Rev 2004;17:72–97.

[3] Morgan-Ryan UM, Fall A, Ward LA, et al. *Cryptosporidium hominis* n. sp. (Apicomplexa: Cryptosporidiidae) from *Homo sapiens*. J Eukaryot Microbiol 2002;49:433–40.

[4] Fayer R, Trout JM, Xiao L, et al. *Cryptosporidium canis* n. sp. from domestic dogs. J Parasitol 2001;87:1415–22.

[5] Okhuysen PC, Chappell CL, Crabb JH, et al. Virulence of three distinct *Cryptosporidium parvum* isolates for healthy adults. J Infect Dis 1999;180:1275–81.

[6] Elliott DA, Coleman DJ, Lane MA, et al. *Cryptosporidium parvum* infection requires host cell actin polymerization. Infect Immun 2001;69:5940–2.

[7] Chen XM, Huang BQ, Splinter PL, et al. *Cryptosporidium parvum* invasion of biliary epithelia requires host cell tyrosine phosphorylation of cortactin via c-Src. Gastroenterology 2003;125:216–28.

[8] Griffiths JK, Balakrishnan R, Widmer G, et al. Paromomycin and geneticin inhibit intracellular *Cryptosporidium parvum* without trafficking through the host cell cytoplasm: implications for drug delivery. Infect Immun 1998;66:3874–83.

[9] Mead PS, Slutsker L, Dietz V, et al. Food-related illness and death in the United States. Emerg Infect Dis 1999;5:607–25.

[10] Bushen OY, Lima AA, Guerrant RL. Cryptosporidiosis. In: Guerrant RL, Walker DH, Weller PF, editors. Tropical infectious diseases. Principle, pathogens, and practice. 2nd edition. Philadelphia: Elsevier-Churchill Livingston; 2006. p. 1003–41.

[11] Amin OM. Seasonal prevalence of intestinal parasites in the United States during 2000. Am J Trop Med Hyg 2002;66:799–803.

[12] Tumwine JK, Kekitiinwa A, Nabukeera N, et al. *Cryptosporidium parvum* in children with diarrhea in Mulago Hospital, Kampala, Uganda. Am J Trop Med Hyg 2003;68:710–5.

[13] Pereira SJ, Ramirez NE, Xiao L, et al. Pathogenesis of human and bovine *Cryptosporidium parvum* in gnotobiotic pigs. J Infect Dis 2002;186:715–8.

[14] Frost FJ, Muller T, Craun GF, et al. Serological evidence of endemic waterborne cryptosporidium infections. Ann Epidemiol 2002;12:222–7.

[15] Kuhls TL, Mosier DA, Crawford DL, et al. Seroprevalence of cryptosporidial antibodies during infancy, childhood, and adolescence. Clin Infect Dis 1994;18:731–5.

[16] Leach CT, Koo FC, Kuhls TL, et al. Prevalence of *Cryptosporidium parvum* infection in children along the Texas-Mexico border and associated risk factors. Am J Trop Med Hyg 2000;62:656–61.

[17] Zu SX, Li JF, Barrett LJ, et al. Seroepidemiologic study of *Cryptosporidium* infection in children from rural communities of Anhui, China and Fortaleza, Brazil. Am J Trop Med Hyg 1994;51:1–10.

[18] Priest JW, Bern C, Roberts JM, et al. Changes in serum immunoglobulin G levels as a marker for *Cryptosporidium* sp. infection in Peruvian children. J Clin Microbiol 2005;43: 5298–300.

[19] Fayer R. Effect of sodium hypochlorite exposure on infectivity of *Cryptosporidium parvum* oocysts for neonatal BALB/c mice. Appl Environ Microbiol 1995;61:844–6.

[20] Rose JB, Huffman DE, Gennaccaro A. Risk and control of waterborne cryptosporidiosis. FEMS Microbiol Rev 2002;26:113–23.

[21] Dillingham RA, Lima AA, Guerrant RL. Cryptosporidiosis: epidemiology and impact. Microbes Infect 2002;4:1059–66.

[22] MacKenzie WR, Schell WL, Blair KA, et al. Massive outbreak of waterborne cryptosporidium infection in Milwaukee, Wisconsin: recurrence of illness and risk of secondary transmission. Clin Infect Dis 1995;21:57–62.

[23] MacKenzie WR, Hoxie NJ, Proctor ME, et al. A massive outbreak of cryptosporidium infection transmitted through the public water supply. N Engl J Med 1994;331:161–7.

[24] Puech MC, McAnulty JM, Lesjak M, et al. A statewide outbreak of cryptosporidiosis in New South Wales associated with swimming at public pools. Epidemiol Infect 2001;126: 389–96.

[25] Robertson B, Sinclair MI, Forbes AB, et al. Case-control studies of sporadic cryptosporidiosis in Melbourne and Adelaide, Australia. Epidemiol Infect 2002;128:419–31.

[26] Newman RD, Sears CL, Moore SR, et al. Longitudinal study of *Cryptosporidium* infection in children in northeastern Brazil. J Infect Dis 1999;180:167–75.

[27] Heijbel H, Slaine K, Seigel B, et al. Outbreak of diarrhea in a day care center with spread to household members: the role of *Cryptosporidium*. Pediatr Infect Dis J 1987;6:532–5.

[28] Jelinek T, Lotze M, Eichenlaub S, et al. Prevalence of infection with *Cryptosporidium parvum* and *Cyclospora cayetanensis* among international travellers. Gut 1997;41: 801–4.

[29] McLauchlin J, Amar C, Pedraza-Diaz S, et al. Molecular epidemiological analysis of *Cryptosporidium* spp. in the United Kingdom: results of genotyping *Cryptosporidium* spp. in 1,705 fecal samples from humans and 105 fecal samples from livestock animals. J Clin Microbiol 2000;38:3984–90.

[30] Hunter PR, Chalmers RM, Syed Q, et al. Foot and mouth disease and cryptosporidiosis: possible interaction between two emerging infectious diseases. Emerg Infect Dis 2003;9:109–12.

[31] Bern C, Hernandez B, Lopez MB, et al. The contrasting epidemiology of *Cyclospora* and *Cryptosporidium* among outpatients in Guatemala. Am J Trop Med Hyg 2000;63:231–5.

[32] Bern C, Ortega Y, Checkley W, et al. Epidemiologic differences between cyclosporiasis and cryptosporidiosis in Peruvian children. Emerg Infect Dis 2002;8:581–5.

[33] Perch M, Sodemann M, Jakobsen MS, et al. Seven years' experience with *Cryptosporidium parvum* in Guinea-Bissau, West Africa. Ann Trop Paediatr 2001;21:313–8.

[34] Okhuysen PC, Chappell CL, Sterling CR, et al. Susceptibility and serologic response of healthy adults to reinfection with *Cryptosporidium parvum*. Infect Immun 2000;68:1710–3.

[35] Chappell CL, Okhuysen PC, Sterling CR, et al. Infectivity of *Cryptosporidium parvum* in healthy adults with pre-existing anti-*C. parvum* serum IgG. Am J Trop Med Hyg 1999;60:157–64.

[36] Pozio E, Rezza G, Boshini A, et al. Clinical cryptosporidiosis and human immunodeficiency virus (HIV)-induced immunosuppression: findings from a longitudinal study of HIV-positive and HIV-negative former injection drug users. J Infect Dis 1997;176:969–75.

[37] Lumadue JA, Manabe YC, Moore RD, et al. A clinicopathologic analysis of AIDS-related cryptosporidiosis. AIDS 1998;12:2459–66.

[38] Goodgame RW, Kimball K, Ou C, et al. Intestinal function and injury in AIDS-related cryptosporidiosis. Gastroenterology 1995;108:1075–82.

[39] Greenberg PD, Koch J, Cello JP. Diagnosis of Cryptosporidium parvum in patients with severe diarrhea and AIDS. Dig Dis Sci 1996;41:2286–90.

[40] Genta RM, Chappell CL, White AC Jr, et al. Duodenal morphology and intensity of infection in AIDS-related cryptosporidiosis. Gastroenterology 1993;105:1769–75.

[41] McCole DF, Eckmann L, Laurent F, et al. Intestinal epithelial cell apoptosis following Cryptosporidium parvum infection. Infect Immun 2000;68:1710–3.

[42] Chen XM, Levine SA, Splinter PL, et al. Cryptosporidium parvum activates nuclear factor kappaB in biliary epithelia preventing epithelial cell apoptosis. Gastroenterology 2001;120:1774–83.

[43] Robinson P, Okhuysen PC, Chappell CL, et al. Expression of tumor necrosis factor alpha and interleukin 1 beta in jejuna of volunteers after experimental challenge with Crypotsporidium parvum correlates with exposure but not with symptoms. Infect Immun 2001;69:1172–4.

[44] Kirkpatrick BD, Daniels MM, Jean SS, et al. Cryptosporidiosis stimulates an inflammatory intestinal response in malnourished Haitian children. J Infect Dis 2002;186:94–101.

[45] Alcantara CS, Yang CH, Steiner TS, et al. Interleukin-8, tumor necrosis factor-alpha, and lactoferrin in immunocompetent hosts with experimental and Brazilian children with acquired cryptosporidiosis. Am J Trop Med Hyg 2003;68:325–8.

[46] Lacroix-Lamande S, Mancassola R, Naciri M, et al. Role of gamma interferon in chemokine expression in the ileum of mice and in a murine intestinal epithelial cell line after Cryptosporidium parvum infection. Infect Immun 2002;70:2090–9.

[47] Zhang Y, Lee B, Thompson M, et al. Lactulose-mannitol intestinal permeability test in children with diarrhea caused by rotavirus and cryptosporidium. Diarrhea Working Group, Peru. J Pediatr Gastroenterol Nutr 2000;31:16–21.

[48] Roche JK, Martins CA, Cosme R, et al. Transforming growth factor beta1 ameliorates intestinal epithelial barrier disruption by Cryptosporidium parvum in vitro in the absence of mucosal T lymphocytes. Infect Immun 2000;68:5635–44.

[49] Blanshard C, Jackson A, Shanson D, et al. Cryptosporidiosis in HIV-seropositive patients. Q J Med 1992;308:813–23.

[50] Hashmey R, Smith NH, Cron S, et al. Cryptosporidiosis in Houston, Texas. A report of 95 cases. Medicine (Baltimore) 1997;76:118–39.

[51] Manabe YC, Clark DP, Moore RD, et al. Cryptosporidiosis in patients with AIDS: correlates of disease and survival. Clin Infect Dis 1998;27:536–42.

[52] Schmidt W, Wahnschaffe U, Schafer M, et al. Rapid increase of mucosal CD4 T cells followed by clearance of intestinal cryptosporidiosis in an AIDS patient receiving highly active antiretroviral therapy. Gastroenterology 2001;120:984–7.

[53] Theodos CM, Sullivan KL, Griffiths JK, et al. Profiles of healing and nonhealing Cryptosporidium parvum infection in C57Bl/6 mice with functional B and T lymphocytes: the extent of gamma interferon modulation determines the outcome of infection. Infect Immun 1997;65:4761–9.

[54] Mead JR, You X. Susceptibility differences to Cryptosporidium parvum infection in two strains of gamma interferon knockout mice. J Parasitol 1998;84:1045–8.

[55] White AC Jr, Robinson P, Okhuysen PC, et al. Interferon-gamma expression in jejunal biopsies in experimental human cryptosporidiosis correlates with prior sensitization and control of oocyst excretion. J Infect Dis 2000;181:701–9.

[56] Gomez Morales MA, La Rosa G, Ludovisi A, et al. Cytokine profile induced by Cryptosporidium antigen in peripheral blood mononuclear cells from immunocompetent and immunosuppressed persons with cryptosporidiosis. J Infect Dis 1999;179:967–73.

[57] Robinson P, Okhuysen PC, Chappell CL, et al. Expression of IL-15 and IL-4 in IFN-gamma-independent control of experimental human *Cryptosporidium parvum* infection. Cytokine 2001;15:39–46.

[58] Dann SM, Wang HC, Gambarin KJ, et al. Interleukin-15 activates human natural killer cells to clear the intestinal protozoan cryptosporidium. J Infect Dis 2005;192: 1294–302.

[59] Frost FJ, Fea E, Gilli G, et al. Serological evidence of *Cryptosporidium* infections in southern Europe. Eur J Epidemiol 2000;16:385–90.

[60] Molbak K, Aaby P, Hojlyng N, et al. Risk factors for *Cryptosporidium* diarrhea in early childhood: a case-control study from Guinea-Bissau, West Africa. Am J Epidemiol 1994;139:734–40.

[61] Sallon S, el Showwa R, el Masri M, et al. Cryptosporidiosis in children in Gaza. Ann Trop Paediatr 1991;11:277–81.

[62] Sallon S, el-Shawwa R, Khalil M, et al. Diarrhoeal disease in children in Gaza. Ann Trop Med Parasitol 1994;88:175–82.

[63] Molbak K, Hojlyng N, Gottschau A, et al. Cryptosporidiosis in infancy and childhood mortality in Guinea Bissau, west Africa. BMJ 1993;307:417–20.

[64] Lima AA, Moore SR, Barboza MS Jr, et al. Persistent diarrhea signals a critical period of increased diarrhea burdens and nutritional shortfalls: a prospective cohort study among children in northeastern Brazil. J Infect Dis 2000;181:1643–51.

[65] Agnew DG, Lima AA, Newman RD, et al. Cryptosporidiosis in northeastern Brazilian children: association with increased diarrhea morbidity. J Infect Dis 1998;177: 754–60.

[66] Amadi B, Kelly P, Mwiya M, et al. Intestinal and systemic infection, HIV, and mortality in Zambian children with persistent diarrhea and malnutrition. J Pediatr Gastroenterol Nutr 2001;32:550–4.

[67] Guerrant DI, Moore SR, Lima AA, et al. Association of early childhood diarrhea and cryptosporidiosis with impaired physical fitness and cognitive function four-seven years later in a poor urban community in northeast Brazil. Am J Trop Med Hyg 1999;61: 707–13.

[68] Berkman DS, Lescano AG, Gilman RH, et al. Effects of stunting, diarrhoeal disease, and parasitic infection during infancy on cognition in late childhood: a follow-up study. Lancet 2002;359:564–71.

[69] Vakil NB, Schwartz SM, Buggy BP, et al. Biliary cryptosporidiosis in HIV-infected people after the waterborne outbreak of cryptosporidiosis in Milwaukee. N Engl J Med 1996;334:19–23.

[70] Arrowood MJ. Diagnosis. In: Fayer R, editor. *Cryptosporidium* and cryptosporidiosis. New York: CRC Press; 1997. p. 43–64.

[71] Clavel A, Arnal A, Sanchez E, et al. Comparison of 2 centrifugation procedures in the formalin-ethyl acetate stool concentration technique for the detection of *Cryptosporidium* oocysts. Int J Parasitol 1996;26:671–2.

[72] Weber R, Bryan R, Bishop H, et al. Threshold for detection of *Cryptosporidium* oocysts in human stool specimens: evidence for low sensitivity of current diagnostic methods. J Clin Microbiol 1991;29:963–5.

[73] Johnston SP, Ballard MM, Beach MJ, et al. Evaluation of three commercial assays for detection of *Giardia* and *Cryptosporidium* organisms in fecal specimens. J Clin Microbiol 2003;41:623–6.

[74] Garcia LS, Shimizu RY. Evaluation of nine immunoassay kits (enzyme immunoassay and direct fluorescence) for detection of *Giardia lamblia* and *Cryptosporidium parvum* in human fecal specimens. J Clin Microbiol 1997;35:1526–9.

[75] Garcia LS, Shimizu RY, Novak S, et al. Commercial assay for detection of *Giardia lamblia* and *Cryptosporidium parvum* antigens in human fecal specimens by rapid solid-phase qualitative immunochromatography. J Clin Microbiol 2003;41:209–12.

[76] McLauchlin J, Amar CF, Pedraza-Diaz S, et al. Polymerase chain reaction-based diagnosis of infection with *Cryptosporidium* in children with primary immunodeficiencies. Pediatr Infect Dis J 2003;22:329–35.

[77] Carneiro-Filho BA, Bushen OY, Brito GA, et al. glutamine analogues as adjunctive therapy for infectious diarrhea. Curr Infect Dis Rep 2003;5:114–9.

[78] Kotler DP, Francisco A, Clayton F, et al. Small intestinal injury and parasitic diseases in AIDS. Ann Intern Med 1990;113:444–9.

[79] Simon DM, Cello JP, Valenzuela J, et al. Multicenter trial of octreotide in patients with refractory acquired immunodeficiency syndrome-associated diarrhea. Gastroenterology 1995;108:1753–60.

[80] Carr A, Marriott D, Field A, et al. Treatment of HIV-1-associated microsporidiosis and cryptosporidiosis with combination antiretroviral therapy. Lancet 1998;351:256–61.

[81] Foudraine NA, Weverling GJ, van Grool T, et al. Improvement of chronic diarrhea in patients with advanced HIV-1 infection during potent antiretroviral therapy. AIDS 1998;12:35–41.

[82] Okhuysen PC, Robinson P, Nguyen MT, et al. Jejunal cytokine response in AIDS patients with chronic cryptosporidiosis and during immune reconstitution. AIDS 2001;15:802–4.

[83] Mele R, Gomez Morales MA, Tosini F, et al. Indinavir reduces *Cryptosporidium parvum* infection in both in vitro and in vivo models. Int J Parasitol 2003;33:757–64.

[84] Bushen OY, Davenport JA, Lima AB, et al. Diarrhea and reduced levels of antiretroviral drugs: improvement with glutamine or alanyl-glutamine in a randomized controlled trial in northeast Brazil. Clin Infect Dis 2004;38:1764–70.

[85] French AL, Beaudet LM, Benator DA, et al. Cholecystectomy in patients with AIDS—clinicopathologic correlations in 107 cases. Clin Infect Dis 1995;21:852–8.

[86] White CA Jr. Nitazoxanide: a new broad spectrum antiparasitic agent. Expert Rev Anti Infect Ther 2004;2:43–9.

[87] Huang DB, Chappell C, Okhuysen PC. Cryptosporidiosis in children. Semin Pediatr Infect Dis 2004;15:253–9.

[88] Amadi B, Mwiya M, Musuku J, et al. Effect of nitazoxanide on morbidity and mortality in Zambian children with cryptosporidiosis: a randomised controlled trial. Lancet 2002;360:1375–80.

[89] Rossignol JF, Hidalgo H, Feregrino M, et al. A double-'blind' placebo-controlled study of nitazoxanide in the treatment of cryptosporidial diarrhoea in AIDS patients in Mexico. Trans R Soc Trop Med Hyg 1998;92:663–6.

[90] Sáez-Llorens X, Odio CM, Umaña MA, et al. Spiramycin vs. placebo for treatment of acute diarrhea caused by *Cryptosporidium*. Pediatr Infect Dis J 1989;8:136–40.

[91] Wittenberg DF, Miller NM, van den Ende J. Spiramycin is not effective in treating cryptosporidium diarrhea in infants: results of a double-blind randomized trial. J Infect Dis 1989;159:131–2.

[92] Smith NH, Cron S, Valdez LM, et al. Combination drug therapy for cryptosporidiosis in AIDS. J Infect Dis 1998;178:900–3.

[93] Amenta M, Dalle Nogare ER, Colomba C, et al. Intestinal protozoa in HIV-infected patients: effect of rifaximin in *Cryptosporidium parvum* and *Blastocystis hominis* infections. J Chemother 1999;11:391–5.

[94] Adam RD. Biology of *Giardia lamblia*. Clin Microbiol Rev 2001;14:447–75.

[95] Nash TE. Surface antigenic variation in *Giardia lamblia*. Mol Microbiol 2002;45:585–90.

[96] Touz MC, Conrad JT, Nash TE. A novel palmitoyl acyl transferase controls surface protein palmitoylation and cytotoxicity in *Giardia lamblia*. Mol Microbiol 2005;58:999–1011.

[97] Lujan HD, Mowatt MR, Byrd LG, et al. Cholesterol starvation induces differentiation of the intestinal parasite *Giardia lamblia*. Proc Natl Acad Sci U S A 1996;93:7628–33.

[98] Svard SG, Hagblom P, Palm JE. *Giardia lamblia*—a model organism for eukaryotic cell differentiation. FEMS Microbiol Lett 2003;218:3–7.

[99] Touz MC, Nores MJ, Slavin I, et al. The activity of a developmentally regulated cysteine proteinase is required for cyst wall formation in the primitive eukaryote Giardia lamblia. J Biol Chem 2002;277:8474–81.

[100] Hetsko ML, McCaffery JM, Svard SG, et al. Cellular and transcriptional changes during excystation of Giardia lamblia in vitro. Exp Parasitol 1998;88:172–83.

[101] Ward W, Alvarado L, Rawlings ND, et al. A primitive enzyme for a primitive cell: the protease required for excystation of Giardia. Cell 1997;89:437–44.

[102] Furness BW, Beach MJ, Roberts JM. Giardiasis surveillance–United States, 1992–1997. MMWR CDC Surveill Summ 2000;49:1–13.

[103] Caeiro JP, Mathewson JJ, Smith MA, et al. Etiology of outpatient pediatric nondysenteric diarrhea: a multicenter study in the United States. Pediatr Infect Dis J 1999;18:94–7.

[104] Gilman RH, Brown KH, Visvesvara GS, et al. Epidemiology and serology of Giardia lamblia in a developing country: Bangladesh. Trans R Soc Trop Med Hyg 1985;79:469–73.

[105] Fraser D, Dagan R, Naggan L, et al. Natural history of Giardia lamblia and Cryptosporidium infections in a cohort of Israeli Bedouin infants: a study of a population in transition. Am J Trop Med Hyg 1997;57:544–9.

[106] Farthing MJ, Mata L, Urrutia JJ, et al. Natural history of Giardia infection of infants and children in rural Guatemala and its impact on physical growth. Am J Clin Nutr 1986;43:395–405.

[107] Gilman RH, Marquis GS, Miranda E, et al. Rapid reinfection by Giardia lamblia after treatment in a hyperendemic Third World community. Lancet 1988;1:343–5.

[108] Cifuentes E, Gomez M, Blumenthal U, et al. Risk factors for Giardia intestinalis infection in agricultural villages practicing wastewater irrigation in Mexico. Am J Trop Med Hyg 2000;62:388–92.

[109] Lee SH, Levy DA, Craun GF, et al. Surveillance for waterborne-disease outbreaks–United States, 1999–2000. MMWR Surveill Summ 2002;51:1–47.

[110] Stuart JM, Orr HJ, Warburton FG, et al. Risk factors for sporadic giardiasis: a case-control study in southwestern England. Emerg Infect Dis 2003;9:229–33.

[111] Thompson SC. Giardia lamblia in children and the child care setting: a review of the literature. J Paediatr Child Health 1994;30:202–9.

[112] Hill DR. Giardiasis. Issues in diagnosis and management. Infect Dis Clin North Am 1993;7:503–25.

[113] Mintz ED, Hudson-Wragg M, Mshar P, et al. Foodborne giardiasis in a corporate office setting. J Infect Dis 1993;167:250–3.

[114] Olsen SJ, MacKinnon LC, Goulding JS, et al. Surveillance for foodborne-disease outbreaks–United States, 1993–1997. MMWR CDC Surveill Summ 2000;49:1–62.

[115] Ekdahl K, Andersson Y. Imported giardiasis: impact of international travel, immigration, and adoption. Am J Trop Med Hyg 2005;72:825–30.

[116] Chin AC, Teoh DA, Scott KG, et al. Strain-dependent induction of enterocyte apoptosis by Giardia lamblia disrupts epithelial barrier function in a caspase-3-dependent manner. Infect Immun 2002;70:3673–80.

[117] Scott KG, Meddings JB, Kirk DR, et al. Intestinal infection with Giardia spp. reduces epithelial barrier function in a myosin light chain kinase-dependent fashion. Gastroenterology 2002;123:1179–90.

[118] Buret AG, Mitchell K, Muench DG, et al. Giardia lamblia disrupts tight junctional ZO-1 and increases permeability in non-transformed human small intestinal epithelial monolayers: effects of epidermal growth factor. Parasitology 2002;125:11–9.

[119] Char S, Cevallos AM, Yamson P, et al. Impaired IgA response to Giardia heat shock antigen in children with persistent diarrhoea and giardiasis. Gut 1993;34:38–40.

[120] Zhou P, Li E, Zhu N, et al. Role of interleukin-6 in the control of acute and chronic Giardia lamblia infections in mice. Infect Immun 2003;71:1566–8.

[121] Velazquez C, Beltran M, Ontiveros N, et al. *Giardia lamblia* infection induces different secretory and systemic antibody responses in mice. Parasite Immunol 2005;27:351–6.

[122] Stager S, Muller N. *Giardia lamblia* infections in B-cell-deficient transgenic mice. Infect Immun 1997;65:3944–6.

[123] Heyworth MF, Carlson JR, Ermak TH. Clearance of *Giardia muris* infection requires helper/inducer T lymphocytes. J Exp Med 1987;165:1743–8.

[124] Rosen FS, Cooper MD, Wedgwood RJ. The primary immunodeficiencies. N Engl J Med 1995;333:431–40.

[125] Haque R, Roy S, Kabir M, et al. *Giardia* assemblage a infection and diarrhea in Bangladesh. J Infect Dis 2005;192:2171–3.

[126] Eligio-Garcia L, Cortes-Campos A, Jimenez-Cardoso E. Genotype of *Giardia intestinalis* isolates from children and dogs and its relationship to host origin. Parasitol Res 2005;97:1–6.

[127] Solomons NW. Giardiasis: nutritional implications. Rev Infect Dis 1982;4:859–69.

[128] Gillon J. Clinical studies in adults presenting with giardiasis to a gastro-intestinal unit. Scott Med J 1985;30:89–95.

[129] Welsh JD, Poley JR, Hensley J, et al. Intestinal disaccharidase and alkaline phosphatase activity in giardiasis. J Pediatr Gastroenterol Nutr 1984;3:37–40.

[130] Sackey ME, Weigel MM, Armijos RX. Predictors and nutritional consequences of intestinal parasitic infections in rural Ecuadorian children. J Trop Pediatr 2003;49:17–23.

[131] Goto R, Panter-Brick C, Northrop-Clewes CA, et al. Poor intestinal permeability in mildly stunted Nepali children: associations with weaning practices and *Giardia lamblia* infection. Br J Nutr 2002;88:141–9.

[132] Newman RD, Moore SR, Lima AA, et al. A longitudinal study of *Giardia lamblia* infection in north-east Brazilian children. Trop Med Int Health 2001;6:624–34.

[133] Celiksoz A, Acioz M, Degerli S, et al. Effects of giardiasis on school success, weight and height indices of primary school children in Turkey. Pediatr Int 2005;47:567–71.

[134] Al-Mekhlafi MS, Azlin M, Nor Aini U, et al. Giardiasis as a predictor of childhood malnutrition in Orang Asli children in Malaysia. Trans R Soc Trop Med Hyg 2005;99:686–91.

[135] Prado MS, Cairncross S, Strina A, et al. Asymptomatic giardiasis and growth in young children, a longitudinal study in Salvador, Brazil. Parasitology 2005;131:51–6.

[136] Hiatt RA, Markell EK, Ng E. How many stool examinations are necessary to detect pathogenic intestinal protozoa? Am J Trop Med Hyg 1995;53:36–9.

[137] Mank TG, Zaat JO, Deelder AM, et al. Sensitivity of microscopy versus enzyme immunoassay in the laboratory diagnosis of giardiasis. Eur J Clin Microbiol Infect Dis 1997;16:615–9.

[138] Aldeen WE, Carroll K, Robison A, et al. Comparison of nine commercially available enzyme-linked immunosorbent assays for detection of *Giardia lamblia* in fecal specimens. J Clin Microbiol 1998;36:1338–40.

[139] Zimmerman SK, Needham CA. Comparison of conventional stool concentration and preserved-smear methods with Merifluor Cryptosporidium/Giardia Direct Immunofluorescence Assay and ProSpecT Giardia EZ Microplate Assay for detection of *Giardia lamblia*. J Clin Microbiol 1995;33:1942–3.

[140] Chan R, Chen J, York MK, et al. Evaluation of a combination rapid immunoassay for detection of *Giardia* and *Cryptosporidium* antigens. J Clin Microbiol 2000;38:393–4.

[141] Aziz H, Beck CE, Lux MF, et al. A comparison study of different methods used in the detection of *Giardia lamblia*. Clin Lab Sci 2001;14:150–4.

[142] Samuelson J. Why metronidazole is active against both bacteria and parasites. Antimicrob Agents Chemother 1999;43:1533–41.

[143] Zaat JO, Mank TG, Assendelft WJ. A systematic review on the treatment of giardiasis. Trop Med Int Health 1997;2:63–82.

[144] Nigam P, Kapoor KK, Kumar A, et al. Clinical profile of giardiasis and comparison of its therapeutic response to metronidazole and tinidazole. J Assoc Physicians India 1991;l39:613–5.

[145] Zaat JO, Mank T, Assendelft WJ. Drugs for treating giardiasis. Cochrane Database Syst Rev 2000;2:CD000217.

[146] Cabello RR, Guerrero LR, Munoz Garcia MR, et al. Nitazoxanide for the treatment of intestinal protozoan and helminthic infections in Mexico. Trans R Soc Trop Med Hyg 1997;91:701–3.

[147] Gilles HM, Hoffman PS. Treatment of intestinal parasitic infections: a review of nitazoxanide. Trends Parasitol 2002;18:95–7.

[148] Medical Letter. Nitazoxanide (Alinia): a new anti-protozoal agent. Med Lett Drugs Ther 2003;45:29–31.

[149] Ochoa TJ, White AC Jr. Nitazoxanide for treatment of intestinal parasites in children. Pediatr Infect Dis J 2005;24:641–2.

[150] Bassily S, Farid Z, Mikhail JW, et al. The treatment of *Giardia lamblia* infection with mepacrine, metronidazole and furazolidone. J Trop Med Hyg 1970;73:15–8.

[151] Hall A, Nahar Q. Albendazole as a treatment for infections with *Giardia duodenalis* in children in Bangladesh. Trans R Soc Trop Med Hyg 1993;87:84–6.

[152] Nash TE, Ohl CA, Thomas E, et al. Treatment of patients with refractory giardiasis. Clin Infect Dis 2001;33:22–8.

[153] Rotblatt MD. Giardiasis and amebiasis in pregnancy. Drug Intell Clin Parhm 1983;17:187–8.

[154] Jakubowski WS. Purple burps and the filtration of drinking water supplies. Am J Public Health 1988;78:123–5.

[155] Petri WA Jr. Therapy of intestinal protozoa. Trends Parasitol 2003;19:523–6.

GASTROENTEROLOGY CLINICS
OF NORTH AMERICA

An Update on Diagnosis, Treatment, and Prevention of *Clostridium difficile*–Associated Disease

Saima Aslam, MD[a,b,*], Daniel M. Musher, MD[a,b]

[a]Medical Service (Infectious Disease Section), Michael E. DeBakey Veterans Affairs Medical Center, Room 4B-370, 2002 Holcombe Boulevard, Houston, TX 77030, USA
[b]Departments of Medicine, Molecular Virology and Microbiology, Baylor College of Medicine, Room N1319, One Baylor Plaza, Houston, TX 77030, USA

*C*lostridium difficile* is the leading identified cause of nosocomial diarrhea associated with antibiotic therapy. About 3% to 29% of hospitalized patients who receive antibiotics develop diarrhea [1]. *Clostridium difficile* has been implicated as the causative organism in 10% to 25% of patients who have antibiotic-associated diarrhea, in 50% to 75% of those who have antibiotic-associated colitis, and in 90% to 100% of those who have antibiotic-associated pseudomembranous colitis [2,3]. Mortality of *Clostridium difficile*–associated disease ranges from 6% to 30% when pseudomembranous colitis is present [4–9]. The incidence of *Clostridium difficile* colitis has increased in the past decade, with a tenfold increase documented in Quebec [7], as has the proportion of patients who have severe, refractory, or recurrent disease [7–10]. Hospital costs attributable to this condition in the United States [11] and the United Kingdom [12] exceed $4000 per case.

HISTORY OF *CLOSTRIDIUM DIFFICILE* COLITIS

Pseudomembranous enterocolitis was first described in the 1950s and was initially attributed to *Staphylococcus aureus*, an organism that had become prevalent in hospitalized patients who had received antibiotics [13–17], or to *Candida albicans* [18]. In 1974, a prospective study of 200 patients treated with clindamycin detected diarrhea in 21% and pseudomembranous colitis in 10% [19].

Dr. Aslam has no conflict of interest. Dr. Musher's laboratory has received funds from Romark Laboratories for the study of nitazoxanide and is currently involved in studies of rifaximin, tolevamer, and tiacumicin B (OPT-80) under grant support from Salix Pharmaceuticals, Genzyme, and Optimer Pharma, respectively.

*Corresponding author. Infectious Disease Section, Michael E. DeBakey Veterans Affairs Medical Center, Room 4B-370, 2002 Holcombe Boulevard, Houston, TX 77030.
E-mail address: saslam@bcm.tmc.edu (S. Aslam).

0889-8553/06/$ – see front matter
doi:10.1016/j.gtc.2006.03.009

Published by Elsevier Inc.
gastro.theclinics.com

A toxin produced by a *Clostridium* species was proposed as the cause of clindamycin-induced ileocecitis in hamsters in 1977 [20]; later this toxin was isolated from stool samples of patients [21–23]. By 1978, however, *Clostridium difficile* clearly proved to be the etiologic agent of antibiotic-associated colitis [24].

MICROBIOLOGY AND EPIDEMIOLOGY

Clostridium difficile was first described in 1935 by Hall and O'Toole [25] as part of the normal flora of neonates. This organism is a gram-positive, spore-forming rod that is an obligate anaerobe. It is relatively large (2–17 μm in length) and grows well on a culture medium consisting of cycloserine, cefoxitin, and fructose agar in an egg-yolk agar base. Toxin A, toxin B, and the binary toxin of *Clostridium difficile* may each contribute to disease. Toxin A causes fluid secretion and intestinal inflammation when injected into the rodent intestine [26] and is a chemoattractant for neutrophils in vitro [27]. Toxins A and B activate the release of cytokines from monocytes [28]. It is unclear whether the binary toxin is pathogenic; however, recent studies have noted more severe disease in patients who have *Clostridium difficile* colitis whose infecting organism produced binary toxin [9,29]. The expression of the genes encoding toxins A and B is thought to be downregulated by the tcdC gene. A recent epidemic strain producing the binary toxin was also noted to have an 18–base pair partial deletion in the tcdC gene [9]. This partial deletion has been associated with increased levels of toxins A and B in the stool [30].

Clostridium difficile can be cultured from the stool of 3% of healthy adults [31]. Stool carriage rates reach 16% to 35% in hospitalized patients, with rates proportional to the duration of hospitalization and increasing with exposure to antibiotics [32–34]. Newly admitted patients who are colonized appear to be an important source of contagion in hospitals [34]. *Clostridium difficile* colitis may also occur in outpatients, although the incidence is low [35,36].

PATHOGENESIS AND IMMUNITY

The pathogenesis of *Clostridium difficile* colitis is complex and only partly understood. The congruence of debilitating diseases and antibiotic therapy (sometimes chemotherapy) in hospitalized patients is thought to alter the bacterial flora of the colon, thus creating conditions that favor new acquisition or proliferation of *Clostridium difficile* [3,37]. Individuals who acquire *Clostridium difficile* may be colonized or develop disease; the immune status of the host is an important determinant of the outcome. Patients who have more severe underlying illnesses are more likely to develop the disease [38]. Persons who carry *Clostridium difficile* without developing colitis have higher levels of serum antibody to toxin A than symptomatic patients [39,40] and are less likely to develop clinical disease [41]. For patients who develop colitis, higher levels of anti–toxin A antibody are associated with a shorter duration of illness and a decreased risk of recurrence [5,42].

CLINICAL FEATURES

The clinical presentation of *Clostridium difficile* colitis is variable. Some individuals who have toxigenic strains in stool remain asymptomatic. Patients who have symptoms can have disease that can range from diarrhea, colitis without pseudomembranes, pseudomembranous colitis, to fulminant colitis. Fig. 1 shows the typical endoscopic appearance and Fig. 2 shows the pathologic features of pseudomembranous colitis from *Clostridium difficile*. Mild to moderate disease is usually accompanied by lower abdominal cramping pain but can have an absence of systemic symptoms or physical findings. Moderate or severe colitis usually presents with profuse diarrhea, abdominal distention with pain, and in some cases, occult colonic bleeding. Also, systemic symptoms such as fever, nausea, anorexia, and malaise are usually present. Some patients have disease primarily in the cecum and right colon, presenting with marked leukocytosis and abdominal pain but little or no diarrhea. Fever and marked leukocytosis can occur in the absence of clinical symptoms [43]. Fulminant colitis has been reported in 1% to 3% of patients, leading to ileus, toxic megacolon, perforation, and death [44], although it appears that the number of patients who have life-threatening disease is now increasing [7,9,30]. The development of these life-threatening complications may be accompanied by a decrease in diarrhea due to loss of colonic muscular tone and ileus. Other complications of *Clostridium difficile* infection include chronic diarrhea and hypoalbuminemia with anasarca [45]. Polyarticular reactive arthritis following *Clostridium difficile* infection has also been described in the literature [46,47].

IMAGING STUDIES

Colonoscopic features for pseudomembranous colitis are pathognomonic for this disease, although when the disease is particularly severe, it can produce thickening of the colon wall that is recognizable by CT scan (see Fig. 1). On endoscopy, the colonic mucosa is studded with adherent raised yellowish plaques that can easily be dislodged. Pseudomembranes tend to be most pronounced in the rectosigmoid area [48]. In many cases, however, the findings are nonspecific and limited to erythema, edema, or friability of the colonic mucosa.

RISK FACTORS

The main prerequisite for *Clostridium difficile*–associated disease is antibiotic usage. Almost all cases are associated with prior antimicrobial usage or, at times, with chemotherapeutic agents that have antimicrobial activity. It seems that some antibiotics have a greater propensity to be causally associated with *Clostridium difficile* colitis than others, especially in recent data. These antibiotics include clindamycin, which has classically been associated with *Clostridium difficile* colitis [19,49,50]; third-generation cephalosporins [9,49–53]; and flouroquinolones [9,50,54–57]. Other risk factors that have been described include degree of severity of underlying illness [38], use of proton pump inhibitors

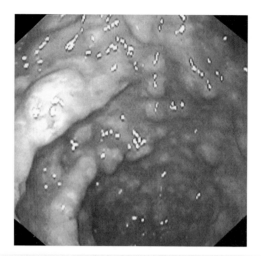

Fig. 1. Typical endoscopic appearance of pseudomembranous colitis due to *Clostridium difficile*. (Courtesy of Richard Goodgame, MD, Houston, TX.)

[58–61], gastrointestinal surgery [62], older patient age [63], prolonged hospital stay [49,64], stay in the ICU [63,64], and tube feeding [65].

DIAGNOSIS

Various methods are available to diagnose *Clostridium difficile*–associated disease. These methods include anaerobic culture on selective media, direct toxin testing for toxin A alone or for toxins A and B, detection of the cytopathic effect of

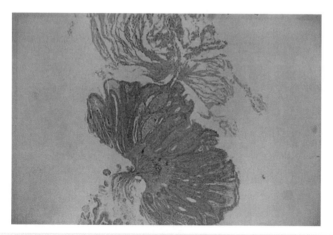

Fig. 2. Pathologic features of pseudomembranous colitis from *Clostridium difficile*. (Courtesy of Richard Goodgame, MD, Houston, TX.)

the toxins on cell culture assay, detection of *Clostridium difficile* antigen with subsequent toxin testing of positive samples, and nucleic acid amplification techniques.

The cell cytotoxicity assay has been regarded as the "gold standard" for the diagnosis of this infection. This method consists of inoculating stool filtrate onto a cell culture medium (cell lines used include Vero, human fibroblasts, and Hep 2) and observing the cytopathic effect of the toxins (mainly toxin B) that cause disruption of the cell cytoskeleton. The assay includes control wells that must document neutralization of the cytopathic effect by antitoxin if the result is to be reported as positive. The assay is very sensitive and can detect as little as 10 pg of toxin B. It is a labor-intensive process, and results take up to 48 to 72 hours. For these reasons, many laboratories have abandoned the cell culture assay in favor of commercially available enzyme immunoassay (EIA) kits.

Various EIAs are commercially available that use monoclonal antibodies to toxin A, toxins A and B, or the common antigen (glutamate dehydrogenase). These tests are easy to use, with a turn-around time of about 20 minutes, and may be batched. Early studies showed that EIAs have a lower sensitivity and specificity than cytotoxicity assays, although more recent studies show a much higher concordance between the cytotoxicity assay and the EIA for toxins A and B [66,67] when a single specimen is tested; this EIAs most likely can be used alone for the diagnosis of *Clostridium difficile* colitis.

Polymerase chain reaction amplification of toxin B gene for diagnosis of *Clostridium difficile* infection is also commercially available. Table 1 [68–78] describes the sensitivities and specificities of each test.

TREATMENT

The initial treatment for *Clostridium difficile* colitis was oral vancomycin. Later on, metronidazole was shown to be effective, perhaps equally so, but a strong preference to avoid the use of vancomycin in hospitalized patients, which was reinforced by several sets of therapeutic recommendations [79–81], led to increasing reliance on metronidazole. In 1997, the American Gastroenterology Association [82] published recommendations for treating *Clostridium difficile* colitis that included discontinuation of antibiotics, supportive nonspecific therapy,

Table 1
Reported sensitivities and specificities of various diagnostic tests for *Clostridium difficile*

Test	Sensitivity (%)	Specificity (%)	Reference
Cell cytotoxicity assay	92.7–100	99–100	[69–72]
Toxigenic culture	96.4	99.1	[69]
EIA for toxin A + B	66–96.2	93.5–100	[66,67,69,70,73–75]
EIA for toxin A	65.4–88.3	65.4–100	[69,75,76,80]
Real-time polymerase chain reaction	87–91.5	96–100	[77,78]

and addition of metronidazole for those who failed to respond within 2 to 3 days. Oral vancomycin was recommended for patients (1) who were critically ill, unable to tolerate metronidazole, pregnant, or younger than 10 years; (2) who failed initial therapy with metronidazole; or (3) whose organism proved to be metronidazole resistant. The past few years have witnessed an increase in the rate of failure of antimicrobial therapy [8,10,83]. Some patients simply fail to respond to conventional therapy and others promptly relapse after discontinuation of treatment. The Cochrane database found only nine well-designed randomized trials evaluating treatments for *Clostridium difficile* colitis [84].

Stopping the Offending Antibiotic
In earlier studies [4,85,86], 15% to 23% of patients who had *Clostridium difficile* colitis had spontaneous resolution of symptoms within 48 to 72 hours of stopping the offending antibiotic and without specific antimicrobial therapy. Continuation of systemic antibiotics has been associated with refractoriness to treatment [87]; however, because one cannot predict which patients will clear the infection spontaneously and because it is often not feasible to discontinue antibiotics, it is difficult to put this into practice.

Specific Therapy
Vancomycin
Oral vancomycin was used to treat "staphylococcal enterocolitis" and clindamycin-associated diarrhea before the discovery that *Clostridium difficile* was responsible for the disease [2,88,89]. Recognition of the role of this organism was followed by additional studies using vancomycin for treatment [86,90–93]. Doses of vancomycin ranging from 125 to 500 mg four times daily were found to be equally effective [93]. Subsequent studies showed cure rates with oral vancomycin ranging from 86% to 100% [2,4,85,94–96].

In vitro, *Clostridium difficile* is susceptible to vancomycin; the reported minimum inhibitory concentration (MIC) required to inhibit 90% of strains (MIC_{90}) is between 0.75 and 2 μg/mL [97–103]. A recent study [104] found that 3% of *Clostridium difficile* isolates had intermediate resistance to vancomycin (MIC, 4–16 μg/mL), but clinical correlation was not provided and other investigators have not confirmed these results. Orally administered vancomycin is minimally absorbed and has a stool concentration of up to 3100 μg/g [90], suggesting that the resistance reported to date is not clinically important.

Metronidazole
Treatment with metronidazole was initially shown to be effective for *Clostridium difficile* colitis in a nonrandomized fashion [105]. A randomized trial comparing metronidazole and vancomycin [85] in 92 patients for 10 days noted similar rates of response (88% for vancomycin and 90% for metronidazole) and recurrence (12% for vancomycin and 5% for metronidazole) within a 21-day follow-up period.

The apparent equivalence of these two drugs and ongoing concern over the selection of vancomycin-resistant bacteria, especially within hospitals, led the

Centers for Disease Control and Prevention to recommend that metronidazole be used as first-line therapy for *Clostridium difficile* colitis [82,106,107]. One study [4] reported a 98% response rate with 7% recurrences in 632 CDAD patients treated with metronidazole. A response rate of 90% to 98% with the use of metronidazole has been noted in other studies [85,108]; however, poorer response rates have been noted more recently [8,10,87]. In a prospective observational study, Musher and colleagues [8] found that 78% of all patients who were treated with metronidazole for documented *Clostridium difficile* colitis responded with a cessation of symptoms; 22% failed therapy. About one third of those who initially responded had a recurrence of disease within 60 days of completion of therapy. Thus, the overall cure rate was only 50%. In a study published at the same time, Pepin and colleagues [10] found remarkably similar results in Quebec Province, Canada. In vitro, the MIC$_{90}$ of metronidazole for *Clostridium difficile* ranges from 0.20 to 2.0 μg/mL (median, <1 μg/mL) [97,99–103]. Although in vitro resistance has recently been reported [109,110], no clinical correlation has been provided. The authors' results [8] and those of Sanchez and colleagues [111] show that the metronidazole susceptibility of *Clostridium difficile* in patients who have clinical treatment failure is similar to those who clinically respond to metronidazole therapy. Thus, it is unclear at present whether metronidazole resistance plays any role in treatment failure and recurrence.

After ingestion by healthy volunteers, metronidazole is completely absorbed from the gastrointestinal tract and has undetectable fecal concentrations [112,113]; however, levels of this drug in feces are significantly higher when stools are watery or semiformed than when they are solid and generally exceed the MIC for *Clostridium difficile* when diarrhea is present [114]. A correlation between fecal metronidazole concentrations and clinical outcome has not been reported, but if the high MICs of metronidazole for *Clostridium difficile* are correct, then resistance may become clinically relevant, especially because concentrations are so low after diarrhea has subsided.

Very limited data suggest that parenteral metronidazole might also be useful in treating *Clostridium difficile* colitis. In 3 patients who received intravenous metronidazole [114], fecal concentrations ranged from 6.3 to 24 μg/g of stool during acute illness but were significantly lower in formed stool. A retrospective review of 10 patients who had *Clostridium difficile* colitis initially treated with intravenous metronidazole [115] for a mean of 4 days revealed clinical improvement in 9. The authors used this approach successfully in patients who had toxic megacolon (Saima Aslam, MD and Daniel Musher, MD, unpublished data). To their knowledge, no trial has compared oral to intravenous metronidazole for the treatment of *Clostridium difficile* colitis.

Bacitracin, teicoplanin, fusidic acid

Bacitracin was successfully used to treat isolated cases of *Clostridium difficile* colitis in the 1980s [116] and was later compared with vancomycin in two randomized clinical trials [94,95]. There was no difference between the drugs in the rates of clinical response, which ranged between 76% and 100%.

Teicoplanin and fusidic acid, which are not available in the United States, have been shown to have similar efficacy to oral vancomycin [96,117] and metronidazole [118]. A European study [108] prospectively compared oral vancomycin, metronidazole, teicoplanin, and fusidic acid in 119 patients who had *Clostridium difficile* colitis and found 93% to 96% clinical cure rates for all regimens.

Nitazoxanide

Nitazoxanide has been approved for treating protozoan and helminthic infections [119–122] in the United States and has already been used to treat more than 5 million people around the world for these diseases. This drug blocks anaerobic metabolic pathways of microorganisms and is effective against *Clostridium difficile* in vitro (MIC_{90}, 0.06–0.5 µg/mL) [123,124]. In vivo, nitazoxanide prevents colitis after challenge of hamsters with *Clostridium difficile* [123], although it has not been shown to treat established disease. The authors recently completed two studies evaluating the use of nitazoxanide. One study identified 22 patients in whom *Clostridium difficile* colitis had plainly failed treatment with metronidazole or vancomycin. These patients had numerous comorbidities; persistent or recurrent colitis added to their debility, prolonging hospitalization or being associated with death. A prompt response to nitazoxanide was seen in 17 (77%) patients. Disease recurred in 6 of these 17 patients, 1 of whom was eventually treated successfully with this drug. Among the 5 (23%) patients whose symptoms persisted during a first course of nitazoxanide, subsequent courses of this drug eventually brought about a complete resolution of findings of colitis in 2. Thus, in aggregate, nitazoxanide produced a cure in 14 of 22 (64%) patients who had already failed other therapy, a response rate similar to that observed in the initial treatment of unselected hospitalized *Clostridium difficile* colitis patients with metronidazole [125]. In a prospective, double-blind, controlled study, the authors found that nitazoxanide is as effective as metronidazole in the treatment of *Clostridium difficile* colitis (in press). There were trends toward a greater rate of initial response among patients who received nitazoxanide and a better-sustained response, especially in those treated for 10 days with nitazoxanide, but the sample size was too small to demonstrate significant differences. A large, prospective, double-blind study comparing nitazoxanide with vancomycin is planned to begin soon.

Other drugs

Other drugs that are undergoing evaluation for the treatment of *Clostridium difficile* colitis include rifaximin (a nonabsorbable antimicrobial agent that has had excellent success in treating travelers' diarrhea and with in vitro activity against *Clostridium difficile*); tiacumicin B (OPT-80, a novel 18-membered macrocyclic antibiotic that is 8 to 10 fold as active as vancomycin against *Clostridium difficile* in vitro and has limited activity against the intestinal flora); ramoplanin; and rifalazil (a rifamycin). Most of these drugs are currently in phase II or III trials [126].

Non–antimicrobial treatments

Antiperistaltic agents such as loperamide and diphenoxylate should be avoided in *Clostridium difficile* colitis. Several case reports have linked the use of antiperistaltic agents in patients who have *Clostridium difficile* colitis with the development of toxic megacolon [127,128], probably because they delay excretion of toxin. Pooled human immunoglobulin (200–500 mg/kg) has been used with variable success to treat refractory disease in individual patients [129,130]. A monoclonal antibody to toxin A has shown promising results in experimental animals, and phase II studies in humans are currently in progress [131]. Colestipol and cholestyramine (anion exchange resins) bind the toxin produced by *Clostridium difficile* but lack clinical efficacy [132–134]; their potential is further compromised by the possibility that they also bind drugs that are used to treat the disease, such as vancomycin [135]. Tolevamer is a new polyanionic resin that binds *Clostridium difficile* toxins [136]; a randomized study comparing the efficacy of this polymer to that of antimicrobial treatment with metronidazole or vancomycin is under way. Anecdotal reports suggest that short courses of intravenous methylprednisolone may also effectively treat *Clostridium difficile* colitis [137]. The following list summarizes treatment recommendations for initial therapy.

1. Stop the offending antibiotic if possible (grade B).
2. Provide adequate fluid and electrolyte repletion.
3. Do not use antimotility agents.
4. If specific treatment is required, then use metronidazole, 500 mg orally every 6 to 8 hours for 7 to 10 days. Oral vancomycin at a dosage of 125 to 250 mg orally every 6 hours is a second-line alternative agent (grade A).
5. If the patient cannot tolerate oral medication, then metronidazole may be given intravenously, but switching to oral therapy is recommended after the patient is able to do so. In the case of ileus or toxic megacolon, the recommended treatment is intravenous metronidazole or vancomycin retention enemas (500 mg mixed in 100 mL of normal saline).
6. Vancomycin should be avoided unless metronidazole appears ineffective, the patient is pregnant or allergic to metronidazole, or true resistance is demonstrated.
7. In all cases, strict contact isolation of the patient is essential in controlling the spread of the disease to other patients (grade A).

RECURRENCES

Clostridium difficile colitis recurs after treatment in 8% to 50% of cases [4,85–87,91,94–96,105,108,138], and an increase in recurrent and refractory disease has recently been seen [7,8,10,83]. A single recurrence tends to be followed by repeated recurrences, perhaps in as many as 65% of cases [5,139,140]. New exposure to antibiotics, especially multiple antibiotics, is a significant risk factor for recurrence [87,140], as is age greater than 65 years [5,10], severity of underlying illness [5], a low serum albumin level (<2.5 g/dL) [87,141], stay in the ICU [141], and hospitalization for 16 to 30 days [10].

It was initially assumed that infection recurred because *Clostridium difficile* sporulated during treatment and germinated when treatment was completed. By using serotyping, polymerase chain reaction ribotyping, or chromosomal restriction endonuclease analysis, however, several reports [142–146] have implicated new strains of *Clostridium difficile* in a varying proportion of recurrences, suggesting that nosocomial reacquisition of hospital-associated strains is partly responsible for recurrent *Clostridium difficile* colitis. In the authors' experience, however, relapses occur so promptly after discontinuation of treatment that reinfection is exceedingly unlikely. Recurrence may also reflect a poor immune response during the initial infection. Antibody to *Clostridium difficile* toxin A appears in most patients by 3 days after colonization occurs [5,40]. A higher level of antitoxin antibody in the initial episode of *Clostridium difficile* colitis is associated with a decreased risk of recurrence [5,42].

TREATMENT OF RECURRENT DISEASE

Various strategies have been proposed to treat recurrent *Clostridium difficile* colitis. Longer courses of antimicrobial therapy are often given, although this approach is not needed to treat reinfection or expected to be effective against sporulating organisms. Vancomycin has been given in a "pulsed" dose or a "tapered" regimen, based on the concept that drug given every few days or in a decreasing dose would allow the *Clostridium difficile* spores to germinate and thus be susceptible to being killed by the antibiotic [147]; no reported data support this approach. A combination of vancomycin and rifampin has also been reported as an effective treatment in a few cases [148]. The authors' experience has been that repeated courses of metronidazole or vancomycin appear to have similar response rates of 70% to 78%, with further recurrences in an additional 25% [8].

With a better understanding of the pathogenesis of *Clostridium difficile* colitis, treatment has been directed to restoring a normal colonic ecosystem (which is presumably inimical to the growth of *Clostridium difficile*) or to bolstering the immune response. Stool infusions, in an effort to repopulate the colon with "normal" colonic flora, have been reported to be effective in refractory cases [149,150]. Such therapy lacks esthetic appeal, not to mention the risk of transferring communicable diseases.

There has also been growing interest in "probiotics"–the use of nonpathogenic organisms to repopulate the colonic microflora and, thus, presumably contain the growth of toxigenic *Clostridium difficile*. Agents that have been studied include a nontoxigenic strain of *Clostridium difficile* [151], *Saccharomyces boulardii*, and *Lactobacillus* spp [152,153]. The addition of *Saccharomyces boulardii* to vancomycin or metronidazole was studied in a prospective, double-blinded fashion [139]; in 60 patients who had recurrent *Clostridium difficile* colitis, there were fewer recurrences in patients who received *Saccharomyces boulardii* (35% versus 65%). Treatment with *Saccharomyces boulardii* did not, however, decrease recurrences in patients treated for their first episode of the disease. A placebo-controlled pilot study noted a trend toward a decreased rate of *Clostridium difficile* colitis in hospitalized patients who were given *Lactobacillus* and *Bifidobacterium* at the time that antibiotic therapy was initiated, although the results did not reach statistical significance [154]. A recent meta-analysis found that odds ratios from available randomized studies favored a role for probiotics over placebo [155], although their use has not yet become common practice.

Recurrent disease has also been treated with some success using pooled human immunoglobulin [130,156,157], which has been shown to contain IgG to toxins A and B in addition to having neutralizing capacity when measured in vitro using the cytotoxicity assay [129]. No prospective clinical trial has been reported. Based on the observation that recurrence is more likely in persons who lack anti–toxin A antibody, infusion of such an antibody or vaccination with a toxoid might be beneficial. The following list summarizes treatment recommendations for recurrent disease.

1. In case of a recurrence, a repeat course of metronidazole, 500 mg orally every 6 to 8 hours for 7 to 10 days, should be given. These patients may need prolonged treatment in case of a response (grade B).
2. After a second recurrence, oral vancomycin in a dose of 125 to 250 mg should be given every 6 hours (grade B).
3. In cases of recurrence or refractory disease, the use of probiotics should be considered.
4. There are no data to support certain practices such as coadministration of vancomycin and metronidazole, immune globulin, or steroids.
5. In all cases, strict contact isolation of the patient is essential in controlling the spread of the disease to other patients (grade A).

TREATMENT OF ASYMPTOMATIC PERSONS

Asymptomatic carriers of *Clostridium difficile* are at a relatively low risk of developing colitis [33,41], and treatment is not recommended. Asymptomatic colonized patients, however, may be a source for spread in hospitals [34], and attempts have been made to interrupt epidemics of *Clostridium difficile* colitis by treating such persons [158,159]. Treatment with oral vancomycin successfully suppresses the organism but may be followed by prolonged carriage [160]; metronidazole is ineffective. For these reasons and because asymptomatic persons, in general, are less likely to be sources of infection than those who have diarrhea, the authors do not regard treating them as an attractive option.

PREVENTIVE STRATEGIES

The implementation of a comprehensive infection control program that included strict application of universal precautions, periodic educational programs, phenolic disinfection for environmental cleaning, and strict handwashing was associated with a decrease in the rate of *Clostridium difficile* colitis from 155/y to 67/y in an acute care facility [161]. The use of hypochlorite solution as a disinfectant [162–164] and disposable rectal thermometers [165] may also decrease the risk of spread. Restrictive antibiotic policies [166,167]–for example, restricting clindamycin [168,169], cephalosporins [170–172], and gatifloxacin [56]–have been effective in reducing the rate of disease. The Society of Health Care Epidemiology recommends (1) antimicrobial use restriction after *Clostridium difficile* colitis occurs; (2) hand-washing with an antimicrobial agent or soap after contact with patients, their body substances, or contaminated environmental surfaces; (3) the use of gloves at all points of contact with patients and contaminated substances; (4) isolation of patients in privates rooms, especially if they are incontinent or have diarrhea; and (5) the use of disposable thermometers when the rate of *Clostridium difficile* infection is high [79].

The apparent role of immunity in controlling *Clostridium difficile* colitis has prompted research into the development of a vaccine. Various vaccines have been tested with some success in animal models, including a formalin inactivated *Clostridium difficile* toxoid vaccine [173]; live vaccines with *Vibrio cholerae* and *Salmonella typhimurium* acting as vector strains and expressing an attenuated toxin A [174,175]; and conjugate vaccines combining the nontoxic peptide of toxin A covalently with polysaccharides from pneumococcus, *Shigella flexneri*, and *Escherichia coli* [176]. A parenteral *Clostridium difficile* toxoid vaccine has been shown to be highly immunogenic in healthy human volunteers, and a trial is under way to test its efficacy in elderly patients and in those who have recurrent or relapsing *Clostridium difficile*–associated disease [177,178].

RECENT EPIDEMIC

An increase in the incidence of *Clostridium difficile* colitis has recently been noted in the United States and in Canada, with a greater propensity for more severe disease in addition to mortality [7,8,179,180]. This increase has been attributed to an epidemic strain of *Clostridium difficile* that has been denoted as strain B1 by means of restriction endonuclease analysis, NAP1 by way of pulsed-field gel electrophoresis, or toxinotype III [9,68]. This strain produces binary toxin, has an 18–base pair tcdC gene deletion and resistance to flouroquinolones. It has a 16 fold and 23 fold higher production of toxin A and toxin B, respectively, which may play a role in its hypervirulence [30]. The cumulative attributable mortality due to this strain in Quebec, Canada, was 16.7% with an additional 10.7 days spent in the hospital [180]. Patients who had the NAP1 strain in Canada were 2.3 times more likely to experience death, colectomy, or ICU admission [179].

SUMMARY

Clostridium difficile is an important cause of nosocomial morbidity and mortality and is implicated in recent epidemics. Data support the treatment of colitis with oral metronidazole in a dose of 1.0 to 1.5 g/d, with oral vancomycin as a second-line agent, not because its efficacy is questioned but because of environmental concerns. Nitazoxanide and other drugs are currently under intense study as alternatives. Treatment of asymptomatic patients is not recommended.

Current management strategies appear to be increasingly ineffective, especially for patients who experience multiple recurrences. Biotherapy and vaccination are currently being explored as treatment options for patients who have recurrent disease. Greater attention should be paid to hospital infection control policies and restriction of broad-spectrum antibiotics.

References

[1] McFarland LV. Diarrhea acquired in the hospital. Gastroenterol Clin North Am 1993;22(3):563–77.

[2] Bartlett JG. Clostridium difficile: clinical considerations. Rev Infect Dis 1990;12(Suppl 2): S243–51.

[3] Bartlett JG. Clinical practice. Antibiotic-associated diarrhea. N Engl J Med 2002;346(5): 334–9.

[4] Olson MM, Shanholtzer CJ, Lee JT Jr, et al. Ten years of prospective Clostridium difficile-associated disease surveillance and treatment at the Minneapolis VA Medical Center, 1982–1991. Infect Control Hosp Epidemiol 1994;15(6):371–81.

[5] Kyne L, Warny M, Qamar A, et al. Association between antibody response to toxin A and protection against recurrent *Clostridium difficile* diarrhoea. Lancet 2001;357(9251): 189–93.

[6] Moshkowitz M, Ben Baruch E, Kline Z, et al. Clinical manifestations and outcome of pseudomembranous colitis in an elderly population in Israel. Isr Med Assoc J 2004;6(4):201–4.

[7] Pepin J, Valiquette L, Alary ME, et al. Clostridium difficile-associated diarrhea in a region of Quebec from 1991 to 2003: a changing pattern of disease severity. CMAJ 2004;171(5): 466–72.

[8] Musher DM, Aslam S, Logan N, et al. Relatively poor outcome after treatment of *Clostridium difficile* colitis with metronidazole. Clin Infect Dis 2005;40(11):1586–90.

[9] Loo VG, Poirier L, Miller MA, et al. A predominantly clonal multi-institutional outbreak of Clostridium difficile-associated diarrhea with high morbidity and mortality. N Engl J Med 2005;353(23):2442–9.

[10] Pepin J, Alary ME, Valiquette L, et al. Increasing risk of relapse after treatment of *Clostridium difficile* colitis in Quebec, Canada. Clin Infect Dis 2005;40(11):1591–7.

[11] Kyne L, Hamel MB, Polavaram R, et al. Health care costs and mortality associated with nosocomial diarrhea due to Clostridium difficile. Clin Infect Dis 2002;34(3):346–53.

[12] Wilcox MH, Cunniffe JG, Trundle C, et al. Financial burden of hospital-acquired *Clostridium difficile* infection. J Hosp Infect 1996;34(1):23–30.

[13] Antibiotics, staphylococcal enteritis and pseudomembranous enterocolitis. N Engl J Med 1953;249(1):37–40.

[14] Lundsgaard-Hansen P, Senn A, Roos B, et al. Staphylococcic enterocolitis. Report of six cases with two fatalities after intravenous administration of N-(pyrrolidinomethvl) tetracycline. JAMA 1960;173:1008–13.

[15] Keidan SE, Sutherland IF. Staphylococcal pseudomembranous enterocolitis. Lancet 1954; 267(6848):1125–6.

[16] Williams E. Staphylococcal pseudomembranous enterocolitis complicating treatment with aureomycin. Lancet 1954;267(6846):999–1000.

[17] Friedell GH, Paige E. Pseudomembranous enterocolitis following antibiotic therapy for pneumonia: report of a case. Am J Clin Pathol 1954;24(10):1159–64.

[18] Baden WF. Staphylococcal and subsequent candida albicans enterocolitis complicating novobiocin therapy. Am J Obstet Gynecol 1957;74(1):47–52.

[19] Tedesco FJ, Barton RW, Alpers DH. Clindamycin-associated colitis. A prospective study. Ann Intern Med 1974;81(4):429–33.

[20] Bartlett JG, Onderdonk AB, Cisneros RL, et al. Clindamycin-associated colitis due to a toxin-producing species of Clostridium in hamsters. J Infect Dis 1977;136(5):701–5.

[21] Rifkin GD, Fekety FR, Silva J Jr. Antibiotic-induced colitis implication of a toxin neutralised by Clostridium sordellii antitoxin. Lancet 1977;2(8048):1103–6.

[22] Larson HE, Price AB. Pseudomembranous colitis: presence of clostridial toxin. Lancet 1977;2(8052–3):1312–4.

[23] Bartlett JG, Chang TW, Gurwith M, et al. Antibiotic-associated pseudomembranous colitis due to toxin-producing clostridia. N Engl J Med 1978;298(10):531–4.

[24] Bartlett JG, Moon N, Chang TW, et al. Role of Clostridium difficile in antibiotic-associated pseudomembranous colitis. Gastroenterology 1978;75(5):778–82.

[25] Hall IC, O'Toole E. Intestinal flora in new-born infants with a description of a new pathogenic anaerobe: Bacillus difficilis. Am J Dis Child 1935;48:390–402.

[26] Triadafilopoulos G, Pothoulakis C, O'Brien MJ, et al. Differential effects of Clostridium difficile toxins A and B on rabbit ileum. Gastroenterology 1987;93(2):273–9.

[27] Pothoulakis C, Sullivan R, Melnick DA, et al. Clostridium difficile toxin A stimulates intracellular calcium release and chemotactic response in human granulocytes. J Clin Invest 1988;81(6):1741–5.

[28] Miller PD, Pothoulakis C, Baeker TR, et al. Macrophage-dependent stimulation of T cell-depleted spleen cells by Clostridium difficile toxin A and calcium ionophore. Cell Immunol 1990;126(1):155–63.

[29] McEllistrem MC, Carman RJ, Gerding DN, et al. A hospital outbreak of Clostridium difficile disease associated with isolates carrying binary toxin genes. Clin Infect Dis 2005;40(2):265–72.

[30] Warny M, Pepin J, Fang A, et al. Toxin production by an emerging strain of Clostridium difficile associated with outbreaks of severe disease in North America and Europe. Lancet 2005;366(9491):1079–84.

[31] Viscidi R, Willey S, Bartlett JG. Isolation rates and toxigenic potential of Clostridium difficile isolates from various patient populations. Gastroenterology 1981;81(1):5–9.

[32] McFarland LV, Mulligan ME, Kwok RY, et al. Nosocomial acquisition of Clostridium difficile infection. N Engl J Med 1989;320(4):204–10.

[33] Johnson S, Clabots CR, Linn FV, et al. Nosocomial Clostridium difficile colonisation and disease. Lancet 1990;336(8707):97–100.

[34] Clabots CR, Johnson S, Olson MM, et al. Acquisition of Clostridium difficile by hospitalized patients: evidence for colonized new admissions as a source of infection. J Infect Dis 1992;166(3):561–7.

[35] Riley TV, Cooper M, Bell B, et al. Community-acquired Clostridium difficile-associated diarrhea. Clin Infect Dis 1995;20(Suppl 2):S263–5.

[36] Hirschhorn LR, Trnka Y, Onderdonk A, et al. Epidemiology of community-acquired Clostridium difficile-associated diarrhea. J Infect Dis 1994;169(1):127–33.

[37] Johnson S, Gerding DN. Clostridium difficile–associated diarrhea. Clin Infect Dis 1998;26(5):1027–34. [quiz: 1035–26].

[38] Kyne L, Sougioultzis S, McFarland LV, et al. Underlying disease severity as a major risk factor for nosocomial Clostridium difficile diarrhea. Infect Control Hosp Epidemiol 2002;23(11):653–9.

[39] Mulligan ME, Miller SD, McFarland LV, et al. Elevated levels of serum immunoglobulins in asymptomatic carriers of Clostridium difficile. Clin Infect Dis 1993;16(Suppl 4):S239–44.

[40] Kyne L, Warny M, Qamar A, et al. Asymptomatic carriage of Clostridium difficile and serum levels of IgG antibody against toxin A. N Engl J Med 2000;342(6):390–7.

[41] Shim JK, Johnson S, Samore MH, et al. Primary symptomless colonisation by Clostridium difficile and decreased risk of subsequent diarrhoea. Lancet 1998;351(9103):633–6.

[42] Warny M, Vaerman JP, Avesani V, et al. Human antibody response to Clostridium difficile toxin A in relation to clinical course of infection. Infect Immun 1994;62(2):384–9.

[43] Wanahita A, Goldsmith EA, Marino BJ, et al. Clostridium difficile infection in patients with unexplained leukocytosis. Am J Med 2003;115(7):543–6.

[44] Kelly CP, LaMont JT. Clostridium difficile infection. Annu Rev Med 1998;49:375–90.

[45] Bartlett JG. Antibiotic-associated diarrhea. Clin Infect Dis 1992;15(4):573–81.

[46] Jacobs A, Barnard K, Fishel R, et al. Extracolonic manifestations of *Clostridium difficile* infections. Presentation of 2 cases and review of the literature. Medicine (Baltimore) 2001;80(2):88–101.

[47] Veillard E, Guggenbuhl P, Bello S, et al. Reactive oligoarthritis in a patient with *Clostridium difficile* pseudomembranous colitis. Review of the literature. Rev Rhum Engl 1998;65(12): 795–8.

[48] Thielman NMWK. Mandell, Douglas and Bennett's principles and practices of infectious disease, vol 1. 6th edition. Philadelphia (PA): Elsevier; 2005.

[49] Palmore TN, Sohn S, Malak SF, et al. Risk factors for acquisition of Clostridium difficile-associated diarrhea among outpatients at a cancer hospital. Infect Control Hosp Epidemiol 2005;26(8):680–4.

[50] Muto CA, Pokrywka M, Shutt K, et al. A large outbreak of Clostridium difficile-associated disease with an unexpected proportion of deaths and colectomies at a teaching hospital following increased fluoroquinolone use. Infect Control Hosp Epidemiol 2005;26(3): 273–80.

[51] Schwaber MJ, Simhon A, Block C, et al. Factors associated with nosocomial diarrhea and Clostridium difficile-associated disease on the adult wards of an urban tertiary care hospital. Eur J Clin Microbiol Infect Dis 2000;19(1):9–15.

[52] McFarland LV, Surawicz CM, Stamm WE. Risk factors for *Clostridium difficile* carriage and C. difficile-associated diarrhea in a cohort of hospitalized patients. J Infect Dis 1990;162(3):678–84.

[53] Nelson DE, Auerbach SB, Baltch AL, et al. Epidemic Clostridium difficile-associated diarrhea: role of second- and third-generation cephalosporins. Infect Control Hosp Epidemiol 1994;15(2):88–94.

[54] Yip C, Loeb M, Salama S, et al. Quinolone use as a risk factor for nosocomial Clostridium difficile-associated diarrhea. Infect Control Hosp Epidemiol 2001;22(9):572–5.

[55] McCusker ME, Harris AD, Perencevich E, et al. Fluoroquinolone use and Clostridium difficile-associated diarrhea. Emerg Infect Dis 2003;9(6):730–3.

[56] Gaynes R, Rimland D, Killum E, et al. Outbreak of *Clostridium difficile* infection in a long-term care facility: association with gatifloxacin use. Clin Infect Dis 2004;38(5):640–5.

[57] Pepin J, Saheb N, Coulombe MA, et al. Emergence of fluoroquinolones as the predominant risk factor for Clostridium difficile-associated diarrhea: a cohort study during an epidemic in Quebec. Clin Infect Dis 2005;41(9):1254–60.

[58] Cunningham R, Dale B, Undy B, et al. Proton pump inhibitors as a risk factor for *Clostridium difficile* diarrhoea. J Hosp Infect 2003;54(3):243–5.

[59] Dial S, Alrasadi K, Manoukian C, et al. Risk of *Clostridium difficile* diarrhea among hospital inpatients prescribed proton pump inhibitors: cohort and case-control studies. CMAJ 2004;171(1):33–8.

[60] Dial S, Delaney JA, Barkun AN, et al. Use of gastric acid-suppressive agents and the risk of community-acquired Clostridium difficile-associated disease. JAMA 2005;294(23): 2989–95.

[61] Al-Tureihi FI, Hassoun A, Wolf-Klein G, et al. Albumin, length of stay, and proton pump inhibitors: key factors in Clostridium difficile-associated disease in nursing home patients. J Am Med Dir Assoc 2005;6(2):105–8.

[62] Thibault A, Miller MA, Gaese C. Risk factors for the development of Clostridium difficile-associated diarrhea during a hospital outbreak. Infect Control Hosp Epidemiol 1991;12(6):345–8.

[63] Brown E, Talbot GH, Axelrod P, et al. Risk factors for *Clostridium difficile* toxin-associated diarrhea. Infect Control Hosp Epidemiol 1990;11(6):283–90.

[64] Modena S, Bearelly D, Swartz K, et al. *Clostridium difficile* among hospitalized patients receiving antibiotics: a case-control study. Infect Control Hosp Epidemiol 2005;26(8): 685–90.

[65] Bliss DZ, Johnson S, Savik K, et al. Acquisition of *Clostridium difficile* and Clostridium difficile-associated diarrhea in hospitalized patients receiving tube feeding. Ann Intern Med 1998;129(12):1012–9.

[66] Lyerly DM, Neville LM, Evans DT, et al. Multicenter evaluation of the *Clostridium difficile* TOX A/B TEST. J Clin Microbiol 1998;36(1):184–90.

[67] Aldeen WE, Bingham M, Aiderzada A, et al. Comparison of the TOX A/B test to a cell culture cytotoxicity assay for the detection of *Clostridium difficile* in stools. Diagn Microbiol Infect Dis 2000;36(4):211–3.

[68] McDonald LC. Clostridium difficile: responding to a new threat from an old enemy. Infect Control Hosp Epidemiol 2005;26(8):672–5.

[69] Barbut F, Kajzer C, Planas N, et al. Comparison of three enzyme immunoassays, a cytotoxicity assay, and toxigenic culture for diagnosis of Clostridium difficile-associated diarrhea. J Clin Microbiol 1993;31(4):963–7.

[70] Snell H, Ramos M, Longo S, et al. Performance of the TechLab C. DIFF CHEK-60 enzyme immunoassay (EIA) in combination with the C. difficile Tox A/B II EIA kit, the Triage C. difficile panel immunoassay, and a cytotoxin assay for diagnosis of Clostridium difficile-associated diarrhea. J Clin Microbiol 2004;42(10):4863–5.

[71] O'Connor D, Hynes P, Cormican M, et al. Evaluation of methods for detection of toxins in specimens of feces submitted for diagnosis of Clostridium difficile-associated diarrhea. J Clin Microbiol 2001;39(8):2846–9.

[72] Doern GV, Coughlin RT, Wu L. Laboratory diagnosis of Clostridium difficile-associated gastrointestinal disease: comparison of a monoclonal antibody enzyme immunoassay for toxins A and B with a monoclonal antibody enzyme immunoassay for toxin A only and two cytotoxicity assays. J Clin Microbiol 1992;30(8):2042–6.

[73] Lozniewski A, Rabaud C, Dotto E, et al. Laboratory diagnosis of Clostridium difficile-associated diarrhea and colitis: usefulness of Premier Cytoclone A + B enzyme immunoassay for combined detection of stool toxins and toxigenic C. difficile strains. J Clin Microbiol 2001;39(5):1996–8.

[74] Alfa MJ, Swan B, VanDekerkhove B, et al. The diagnosis of Clostridium difficile-associated diarrhea: comparison of Triage C. difficile panel, EIA for Tox A/B and cytotoxin assays. Diagn Microbiol Infect Dis 2002;43(4):257–63.

[75] Arrow SA, Croese L, Bowman RA, et al. Evaluation of three commercial enzyme immunoassay kits for detecting faecal *Clostridium difficile* toxins. J Clin Pathol 1994;47(10):954–6.

[76] Bowman RA, Arrow S, Croese L, et al. Evaluation of an enzyme immunoassay kit for the detection of *Clostridium difficile* enterotoxin. Pathology 1994;26(4):480–1.

[77] van den Berg RJ, Bruijnesteijn van Coppenraet LS, Gerritsen HJ, et al. Prospective multicenter evaluation of a new immunoassay and real-time PCR for rapid diagnosis of Clostridium difficile-associated diarrhea in hospitalized patients. J Clin Microbiol 2005;43(10):5338–40.

[78] Guilbault C, Labbe AC, Poirier L, et al. Development and evaluation of a PCR method for detection of the *Clostridium difficile* toxin B gene in stool specimens. J Clin Microbiol 2002;40(6):2288–90.

[79] Gerding DN, Johnson S, Peterson LR, et al. Clostridium difficile-associated diarrhea and colitis. Infect Control Hosp Epidemiol 1995;16(8):459–77.

[80] Hospital Infection Control Practices Advisory Committee (HICPAC). Recommendations for preventing the spread of vancomycin resistance. Infect Control Hosp Epidemiol 1995;16(2):105–13.

[81] ASHP therapeutic position statement on the preferential use of metronidazole for the treatment of Clostridium difficile-associated disease. Am J Health Syst Pharm 1998;55(13):1407–11.

[82] Fekety R. Guidelines for the diagnosis and management of Clostridium difficile-associated diarrhea and colitis. American College of Gastroenterology, Practice Parameters Committee. Am J Gastroenterol 1997;92(5):739–50.

[83] Layton BAML, Gerding DN, Liedtke LA, et al. Changing patterns of *Clostridium difficile* disease: a report from infectious disease physicians. Paper presented at the 42nd Annual Meeting of the Infectious Disease Society of America. Boston, September 30–October 3, 2004.
[84] Bricker E, Garg R, Nelson R, et al. Antibiotic treatment for Clostridium difficile-associated diarrhea in adults. Cochrane Database Syst Rev 2005;1:CD004610.
[85] Teasley DG, Gerding DN, Olson MM, et al. Prospective randomised trial of metronidazole versus vancomycin for Clostridium-difficile-associated diarrhoea and colitis. Lancet 1983;2(8358):1043–6.
[86] Bartlett JG. Treatment of antibiotic-associated pseudomembranous colitis. Rev Infect Dis 1984;6(Suppl 1):S235–41.
[87] Nair S, Yadav D, Corpuz M, et al. *Clostridium difficile* colitis: factors influencing treatment failure and relapse—a prospective evaluation. Am J Gastroenterol 1998;93(10): 1873–6.
[88] Wallace JF, Smith RH, Petersdorf RG. Oral administration of vancomycin in the treatment of staphylococcal enterocolitis. N Engl J Med 1965;272:1014–5.
[89] Khan MY, Hall WH. Staphylococcal enterocolitis—treatment with oral vancomycin. Ann Intern Med 1966;65(1):1–8.
[90] Tedesco F, Markham R, Gurwith M, et al. Oral vancomycin for antibiotic-associated pseudomembranous colitis. Lancet 1978;2(8083):226–8.
[91] Silva J Jr, Batts DH, Fekety R, et al. Treatment of *Clostridium difficile* colitis and diarrhea with vancomycin. Am J Med 1981;71(5):815–22.
[92] Fekety R, Silva J, Buggy B, et al. Treatment of antibiotic-associated colitis with vancomycin. J Antimicrob Chemother 1984;14(Suppl D):97–102.
[93] Fekety R, Silva J, Kauffman C, et al. Treatment of antibiotic-associated *Clostridium difficile* colitis with oral vancomycin: comparison of two dosage regimens. Am J Med 1989;86(1): 15–9.
[94] Young GP, Ward PB, Bayley N, et al. Antibiotic-associated colitis due to Clostridium difficile: double-blind comparison of vancomycin with bacitracin. Gastroenterology 1985; 89(5):1038–45.
[95] Dudley MN, McLaughlin JC, Carrington G, et al. Oral bacitracin vs vancomycin therapy for Clostridium difficile-induced diarrhea. A randomized double-blind trial. Arch Intern Med 1986;146(6):1101–4.
[96] de Lalla F, Nicolin R, Rinaldi E, et al. Prospective study of oral teicoplanin versus oral vancomycin for therapy of pseudomembranous colitis and Clostridium difficile-associated diarrhea. Antimicrob Agents Chemother 1992;36(10):2192–6.
[97] Dzink J, Bartlett JG. In vitro susceptibility of *Clostridium difficile* isolates from patients with antibiotic-associated diarrhea or colitis. Antimicrob Agents Chemother 1980;17(4): 695–8.
[98] Biavasco F, Manso E, Varaldo PE. In vitro activities of ramoplanin and four glycopeptide antibiotics against clinical isolates of Clostridium difficile. Antimicrob Agents Chemother 1991;35(1):195–7.
[99] Wong SS, Woo PC, Luk WK, et al. Susceptibility testing of *Clostridium difficile* against metronidazole and vancomycin by disk diffusion and Etest. Diagn Microbiol Infect Dis 1999;34(1):1–6.
[100] Cheng SH, Chu FY, Lo SH, et al. Antimicrobial susceptibility of *Clostridium difficile* by E test. J Microbiol Immunol Infect 1999;32(2):116–20.
[101] Barbut F, Decre D, Burghoffer B, et al. Antimicrobial susceptibilities and serogroups of clinical strains of *Clostridium difficile* isolated in France in 1991 and 1997. Antimicrob Agents Chemother 1999;43(11):2607–11.
[102] Marchese A, Salerno A, Pesce A, et al. In vitro activity of rifaximin, metronidazole and vancomycin against *Clostridium difficile* and the rate of selection of spontaneously resistant mutants against representative anaerobic and aerobic bacteria, including ammonia-producing species. Chemotherapy 2000;46(4):253–66.

[103] Jamal WY, Mokaddas EM, Verghese TL, et al. In vitro activity of 15 antimicrobial agents against clinical isolates of Clostridium difficile in Kuwait. Int J Antimicrob Agents 2002;20(4):270–4.

[104] Pelaez T, Alcala L, Alonso R, et al. Reassessment of Clostridium difficile susceptibility to metronidazole and vancomycin. Antimicrob Agents Chemother 2002;46(6):1647–50.

[105] Cherry RD, Portnoy D, Jabbari M, et al. Metronidazole: an alternate therapy for antibiotic-associated colitis. Gastroenterology 1982;82(5 Pt 1):849–51.

[106] Preventing the Spread of Vancomycin Resistance—Report from the Hospital Infection Control Practices Advisory Committee. Federal Register 1994;59(94):25758–63.

[107] Gerding DN. Is there a relationship between vancomycin-resistant enterococcal infection and Clostridium difficile infection? Clin Infect Dis 1997;25(Suppl 2):S206–10.

[108] Wenisch C, Parschalk B, Hasenhundl M, et al. Comparison of vancomycin, teicoplanin, metronidazole, and fusidic acid for the treatment of Clostridium difficile-associated diarrhea. Clin Infect Dis 1996;22(5):813–8.

[109] Olsson-Liljequist B, Nord CE. In vitro susceptibility of anaerobic bacteria to nitroimidazoles. Scand J Infect Dis Suppl 1981;26:42–5.

[110] Brazier JS, Fawley W, Freeman J, et al. Reduced susceptibility of Clostridium difficile to metronidazole. J Antimicrob Chemother 2001;48(5):741–2.

[111] Sanchez JLGD, Olson MM, Johnson S. Metronidazole susceptibility in Clostridium difficile isolates recovered from cases of C. difficile-associated disease treatment failures and successes. Anaerobe 1999;5:205–8.

[112] Mattila J, Mannisto PT, Mantyla R, et al. Comparative pharmacokinetics of metronidazole and tinidazole as influenced by administration route. Antimicrob Agents Chemother 1983;23(5):721–5.

[113] Loft S, Dossing M, Poulsen HE, et al. Influence of dose and route of administration on disposition of metronidazole and its major metabolites. Eur J Clin Pharmacol 1986;30(4):467–73.

[114] Bolton RP, Culshaw MA. Faecal metronidazole concentrations during oral and intravenous therapy for antibiotic associated colitis due to Clostridium difficile. Gut 1986;27(10):1169–72.

[115] Friedenberg F, Fernandez A, Kaul V, et al. Intravenous metronidazole for the treatment of Clostridium difficile colitis. Dis Colon Rectum 2001;44(8):1176–80.

[116] Chang TW, Gorbach SL, Bartlett JG, et al. Bacitracin treatment of antibiotic-associated colitis and diarrhea caused by Clostridium difficile toxin. Gastroenterology 1980;78(6):1584–6.

[117] de Lalla F, Privitera G, Rinaldi E, et al. Treatment of Clostridium difficile-associated disease with teicoplanin. Antimicrob Agents Chemother 1989;33(7):1125–7.

[118] Wullt M, Odenholt I. A double-blind randomized controlled trial of fusidic acid and metronidazole for treatment of an initial episode of Clostridium difficile-associated diarrhoea. J Antimicrob Chemother 2004;54(1):211–6.

[119] Rossignol JF, Maisonneuve H. Nitazoxanide in the treatment of Taenia saginata and Hymenolepis nana infections. Am J Trop Med Hyg 1984;33(3):511–2.

[120] Rossignol JF, Hidalgo H, Feregrino M, et al. A double-'blind' placebo-controlled study of nitazoxanide in the treatment of cryptosporidial diarrhoea in AIDS patients in Mexico. Trans R Soc Trop Med Hyg 1998;92(6):663–6.

[121] Rossignol JF, Ayoub A, Ayers MS. Treatment of diarrhea caused by Giardia intestinalis and Entamoeba histolytica or E. dispar: a randomized, double-blind, placebo-controlled study of nitazoxanide. J Infect Dis 2001;184(3):381–4.

[122] Rossignol JF, Ayoub A, Ayers MS. Treatment of diarrhea caused by Cryptosporidium parvum: a prospective randomized, double-blind, placebo-controlled study of nitazoxanide. J Infect Dis 2001;184(1):103–6.

[123] McVay CS, Rolfe RD. In vitro and in vivo activities of nitazoxanide against Clostridium difficile. Antimicrob Agents Chemother 2000;44(9):2254–8.

[124] Dubreuil L, Houcke I, Mouton Y, et al. In vitro evaluation of activities of nitazoxanide and tizoxanide against anaerobes and aerobic organisms. Antimicrob Agents Chemother 1996;40(10):2266–70.

[125] Musher DM, Logan N, Hanill RJ, et al. Nitazoxanide in the treatment of *Clostridium difficile* colitis. Clinical Infectious Diseases, in press.

[126] Louie TJ. Treating *Clostridium difficile* in the future: what's coming? Paper presented at the Interscience Conference on Antimicrobial Agents and Chemotherapy. Washington DC: 2005.

[127] Trudel JL, Deschenes M, Mayrand S, et al. Toxic megacolon complicating pseudomembranous enterocolitis. Dis Colon Rectum 1995;38(10):1033–8.

[128] Elinav E, Planer D, Gatt ME. Prolonged ileus as a sole manifestation of pseudomembranous enterocolitis. Int J Colorectal Dis 2004;19(3):273–6.

[129] Salcedo J, Keates S, Pothoulakis C, et al. Intravenous immunoglobulin therapy for severe *Clostridium difficile* colitis. Gut 1997;41(3):366–70.

[130] Wilcox MH. Descriptive study of intravenous immunoglobulin for the treatment of recurrent *Clostridium difficile* diarrhoea. J Antimicrob Chemother 2004;53(5):882–4.

[131] Babcock GJMR, Coccia JA, Esshaki DJ, et al. Human monoclonal antibody against toxin A protects hamsters from *Clostridium difficile* disease. Paper presented at the 42nd Annual Meeting of the Infectious Disease Society of America. Boston, September 30–October 3, 2004.

[132] Bartlett JG, Chang TW, Onderdonk AB. Comparison of five regimens for treatment of experimental clindamycin-associated colitis. J Infect Dis 1978;138(1):81–6.

[133] Mogg GA, Arabi Y, Youngs D, et al. Therapeutic trials of antibiotic associated colitis. Scand J Infect Dis Suppl 1980;(Suppl 22):41–5.

[134] Mogg GA, George RH, Youngs D, et al. Randomized controlled trial of colestipol in antibiotic-associated colitis. Br J Surg 1982;69(3):137–9.

[135] Taylor NS, Bartlett JG. Binding of *Clostridium difficile* cytotoxin and vancomycin by anion-exchange resins. J Infect Dis 1980;141(1):92–7.

[136] Braunlin W, Xu Q, Hook P, et al. Toxin binding of tolevamer, a polyanionic drug that protects against antibiotic-associated diarrhea. Biophys J 2004;87(1):534–9.

[137] Cavagnaro C, Berezin S, Medow MS. Corticosteroid treatment of severe, non-responsive *Clostridium difficile* induced colitis. Arch Dis Child 2003;88(4):342–4.

[138] Bartlett JG, Tedesco FJ, Shull S, et al. Symptomatic relapse after oral vancomycin therapy of antibiotic-associated pseudomembranous colitis. Gastroenterology 1980;78(3):431–4.

[139] McFarland LV, Surawicz CM, Greenberg RN, et al. A randomized placebo-controlled trial of Saccharomyces boulardii in combination with standard antibiotics for *Clostridium difficile* disease. JAMA 1994;271(24):1913–8.

[140] Fekety R, McFarland LV, Surawicz CM, et al. Recurrent *Clostridium difficile* diarrhea: characteristics of and risk factors for patients enrolled in a prospective, randomized, double-blinded trial. Clin Infect Dis 1997;24(3):324–33.

[141] Fernandez A, Anand G, Friedenberg F. Factors associated with failure of metronidazole in Clostridium difficile-associated disease. J Clin Gastroenterol 2004;38(5):414–8.

[142] Johnson S, Adelmann A, Clabots CR, et al. Recurrences of *Clostridium difficile* diarrhea not caused by the original infecting organism. J Infect Dis 1989;159(2):340–3.

[143] O'Neill GL, Beaman MH, Riley TV. Relapse versus reinfection with Clostridium difficile. Epidemiol Infect 1991;107(3):627–35.

[144] Barbut F, Richard A, Hamadi K, et al. Epidemiology of recurrences or reinfections of Clostridium difficile-associated diarrhea. J Clin Microbiol 2000;38(6):2386–8.

[145] Tang-Feldman Y, Mayo S, Silva J Jr, et al. Molecular analysis of *Clostridium difficile* strains isolated from 18 cases of recurrent clostridium difficile-associated diarrhea. J Clin Microbiol 2003;41(7):3413–4.

[146] Noren T, Akerlund T, Back E, et al. Molecular epidemiology of hospital-associated and community-acquired *Clostridium difficile* infection in a Swedish county. J Clin Microbiol 2004;42(8):3635–43.

[147] McFarland LV, Elmer GW, Surawicz CM. Breaking the cycle: treatment strategies for 163 cases of recurrent Clostridium difficile disease. Am J Gastroenterol 2002;97(7):1769–75.

[148] Buggy BP, Fekety R, Silva J Jr. Therapy of relapsing Clostridium difficile-associated diarrhea and colitis with the combination of vancomycin and rifampin. J Clin Gastroenterol 1987;9(2):155–9.

[149] Persky SE, Brandt LJ. Treatment of recurrent Clostridium difficile-associated diarrhea by administration of donated stool directly through a colonoscope. Am J Gastroenterol 2000;95(11):3283–5.

[150] Aas J, Gessert CE, Bakken JS. Recurrent Clostridium difficile colitis: case series involving 18 patients treated with donor stool administered via a nasogastric tube. Clin Infect Dis 2003;36(5):580–5.

[151] Seal D, Borriello SP, Barclay F, et al. Treatment of relapsing Clostridium difficile diarrhoea by administration of a non-toxigenic strain. Eur J Clin Microbiol 1987;6(1):51–3.

[152] Pochapin M. The effect of probiotics on Clostridium difficile diarrhea. Am J Gastroenterol 2000;95(1 Suppl):S11–3.

[153] Wullt M, Hagslatt ML, Odenholt I. Lactobacillus plantarum 299v for the treatment of recurrent Clostridium difficile-associated diarrhoea: a double-blind, placebo-controlled trial. Scand J Infect Dis 2003;35(6–7):365–7.

[154] Plummer S, Weaver MA, Harris JC, et al. Clostridium difficile pilot study: effects of probiotic supplementation on the incidence of C. difficile diarrhoea. Int Microbiol 2004;7(1):59–62.

[155] D'Souza AL, Rajkumar C, Cooke J, et al. Probiotics in prevention of antibiotic associated diarrhoea: meta-analysis. BMJ 2002;324(7350):1361.

[156] Beales IL. Intravenous immunoglobulin for recurrent Clostridium difficile diarrhoea. Gut 2002;51(3):456.

[157] Leung DY, Kelly CP, Boguniewicz M, et al. Treatment with intravenously administered gamma globulin of chronic relapsing colitis induced by Clostridium difficile toxin. J Pediatr 1991;118. (4 Pt 1):633–7.

[158] Delmee M, Vandercam B, Avesani V, et al. Epidemiology and prevention of Clostridium difficile infections in a leukemia unit. Eur J Clin Microbiol 1987;6(6):623–7.

[159] Kerr RB, McLaughlin DI, Sonnenberg LW. Control of Clostridium difficile colitis outbreak by treating asymptomatic carriers with metronidazole. Am J Infect Control 1990;18(5):332–5.

[160] Johnson S, Homann SR, Bettin KM, et al. Treatment of asymptomatic Clostridium difficile carriers (fecal excretors) with vancomycin or metronidazole. A randomized, placebo-controlled trial. Ann Intern Med 1992;117(4):297–302.

[161] Zafar AB, Gaydos LA, Furlong WB, et al. Effectiveness of infection control program in controlling nosocomial Clostridium difficile. Am J Infect Control 1998;26(6):588–93.

[162] Kaatz GW, Gitlin SD, Schaberg DR, et al. Acquisition of Clostridium difficile from the hospital environment. Am J Epidemiol 1988;127(6):1289–94.

[163] Mayfield JL, Leet T, Miller J, et al. Environmental control to reduce transmission of Clostridium difficile. Clin Infect Dis 2000;31(4):995–1000.

[164] Wilcox MH, Fawley WN, Wigglesworth N, et al. Comparison of the effect of detergent versus hypochlorite cleaning on environmental contamination and incidence of Clostridium difficile infection. J Hosp Infect 2003;54(2):109–14.

[165] Brooks SE, Veal RO, Kramer M, et al. Reduction in the incidence of Clostridium difficile-associated diarrhea in an acute care hospital and a skilled nursing facility following replacement of electronic thermometers with single-use disposables. Infect Control Hosp Epidemiol 1992;13(2):98–103.

[166] McNulty C, Logan M, Donald IP, et al. Successful control of Clostridium difficile infection in an elderly care unit through use of a restrictive antibiotic policy. J Antimicrob Chemother 1997;40(5):707–11.

[167] Carling P, Fung T, Killion A, et al. Favorable impact of a multidisciplinary antibiotic management program conducted during 7 years. Infect Control Hosp Epidemiol 2003; 24(9):699–706.

[168] Pear SM, Williamson TH, Bettin KM, et al. Decrease in nosocomial Clostridium difficile-associated diarrhea by restricting clindamycin use. Ann Intern Med 1994;120(4):272–7.

[169] Climo MW, Israel DS, Wong ES, et al. Hospital-wide restriction of clindamycin: effect on the incidence of Clostridium difficile-associated diarrhea and cost. Ann Intern Med 1998;128(12 Pt 1):989–95.

[170] O'Connor KA, Kingston M, O'Donovan M, et al. Antibiotic prescribing policy and *Clostridium difficile* diarrhoea. QJM 2004;97(7):423–9.

[171] Wilcox MH, Freeman J, Fawley W, et al. Long-term surveillance of cefotaxime and piperacillin-tazobactam prescribing and incidence of *Clostridium difficile* diarrhoea. J Antimicrob Chemother 2004;54(1):168–72.

[172] Khan R, Cheesbrough J. Impact of changes in antibiotic policy on Clostridium difficile-associated diarrhoea (CDAD) over a five-year period in a district general hospital. J Hosp Infect 2003;54(2):104–8.

[173] Torres JF, Lyerly DM, Hill JE, et al. Evaluation of formalin-inactivated *Clostridium difficile* vaccines administered by parenteral and mucosal routes of immunization in hamsters. Infect Immun 1995;63(12):4619–27.

[174] Ryan ET, Butterton JR, Smith RN, et al. Protective immunity against *Clostridium difficile* toxin A induced by oral immunization with a live, attenuated Vibrio cholerae vector strain. Infect Immun 1997;65(7):2941–9.

[175] Ward SJ, Douce G, Figueiredo D, et al. Immunogenicity of a Salmonella typhimurium aroA aroD vaccine expressing a nontoxic domain of *Clostridium difficile* toxin A. Infect Immun 1999;67(5):2145–52.

[176] Pavliakova D, Moncrief JS, Lyerly DM, et al. *Clostridium difficile* recombinant toxin A repeating units as a carrier protein for conjugate vaccines: studies of pneumococcal type 14, Escherichia coli K1, and Shigella flexneri type 2a polysaccharides in mice. Infect Immun 2000;68(4):2161–6.

[177] Aboudola S, Kotloff KL, Kyne L, et al. *Clostridium difficile* vaccine and serum immunoglobulin G antibody response to toxin A. Infect Immun 2003;71(3):1608–10.

[178] Sougioultzis S, Kyne L, Drudy D, et al. *Clostridium difficile* toxoid vaccine in recurrent C. difficile-associated diarrhea. Gastroenterology 2005;128(3):764–70.

[179] Eggertson L. Quebec strain of C. difficile in 7 provinces. CMAJ 2006;174(5):607–8.

[180] Pepin J, Valiquette L, Cossette B. Mortality attributable to nosocomial Clostridium difficile-associated disease during an epidemic caused by a hypervirulent strain in Quebec. CMAJ 2005;173(9):1037–42.

Gastroenterol Clin N Am 35 (2006) 337–353

GASTROENTEROLOGY CLINICS
OF NORTH AMERICA

New Insights and Directions in Travelers' Diarrhea

Herbert L. DuPont, MD[a,b,c,*]

[a]St. Luke's Episcopal Hospital, 6270 Bertner Avenue, Houston, TX 77030, USA
[b]Department of Medicine, Baylor College of Medicine, One Baylor Plaza,
Houston, TX 77030, USA
[c]Center for Infectious Diseases, University of Texas–Houston School of Public Health,
1200 Herman Pressler, Houston, TX 77225, USA

The first systematic study of diarrhea of international travelers was performed by Kean and his associates [1–4]. The research team defined frequency of disease occurrence and provided the first clinical description of the illness. The rate of illness among persons who move from industrialized regions to developing countries with reduced hygiene has remained constant over the more than 50 years since the descriptions by Kean and colleagues.

This article focuses on the risk for diarrhea among persons who travel to various regions of the world, the etiologic agents that are involved and the sources of infection, the host factors that influence disease risk, the clinical features and complications of the illness, and available prevention strategies. The article concludes with a discussion of potential areas of future research as we try to prevent or treat enteric disease better in international travelers.

Much of the information that is related to each topic is presented in tables, which include a summary of available information and associated references.

EPIDEMIOLOGY

The world can be divided into three general regions, depending upon the level of local hygiene and rates of diarrhea in travelers and infant populations that live in the region [5]. Within countries in each risk category, there are pockets that show highly variable rates of illness that are related to special hygienic conditions. The often high-risk regions of the world include Latin America, Africa,

This work was supported in part by grants from Public Health Service (grant DK 56338) which funds the Texas Gulf Coast Digestive Diseases Center; NIH NCRR to the University of Texas GCRC: General Clinical Research Center, Grant M01-RR 02558 and NIH NIAID R01 AI54948.

The author has consulted with, received honoraria for speaking, and received research grants that were administered through his academic institution from Salix Pharmaceutical Company, Raleigh, North Carolina, which licenses rifaximin. He also has received an honorarium for advising IOMAI who is developing a transcutaneously applied vaccine for enterotoxigenic *Escherichia coli*.

*6720 Bertner Avenue, MC 1-164, Houston, TX 77030. E-mail address: hdupont@sleh.com

0889-8553/06/$ – see front matter
doi:10.1016/j.gtc.2006.03.008

and southern Asia. The expected low-risk areas include the United States, Canada, Western Europe, Japan, Australia, and New Zealand. The regions that typically show an intermediate risk for enteric disease among international travelers include certain Caribbean islands (eg, Jamaica), the Middle East, some northern Mediterranean areas, China, and Russia. The expected rates of diarrhea among international travelers according to visited region are outlined in Table 1.

Considering that 50 million persons cross international boundaries from industrialized to developing countries each year and that diarrhea develops in an average of 40%, approximately 20 million new cases of travelers' diarrhea occur annually. The rate of diarrhea is approximately 15% for the intermediate-risk areas; for travelers from one low-risk area to a second low-risk area, diarrhea rates are approximately 4%. Illness rates approach zero if these persons do not leave their home area. Persons who travel from one low-risk region to a second low-risk region generally eat all of their meals at public eating establishments and often show other characteristics (see Table 1) that put them at risk for enteric symptoms and low rates of diarrhea [6]. This baseline rate of approximately 4% also is noted in persons from high-risk regions who visit low-risk areas, as is seen when Mexicans visit the United States [7,8].

Table 1
Diarrhea risk in persons traveling from hygienic areas of the industrialized world to other regions of the world

Region	Expected rate of illness	Comment
Latin America, southern Asia, and Africa	40%	Food is contaminated heavily with fecal coliforms and contains enteropathogens [12–14] in these areas; water may be more important in viral gastroenteritis [9].
Less hygienic Caribbean islands, some northern Mediterranean regions, the Middle East, China and Russia	15%	Rates of illness are more spotty and many groups of travelers experience no enteric disease during travel to these areas.
United States, Canada, Western Europe, Japan, Australia, and New Zealand	4%	All meals are consumed at public restaurants, a subset drink more alcohol than customary and common stress of travel may influence rates of enteric symptoms; this rate of illness also is seen in persons from high-risk regions who spend time in the low-risk industrialized regions [6].

Data from DuPont HL, Ericsson CD. Prevention and treatment of traveler's diarrhea. N Engl of Med 1993;328(25):1821–7; and Steffen R. Epidemiologic studies of traveler's diarrhea, severe gastrointestinal infections, and cholera. Rev Infect Dis 1986;8(Suppl 2):S122–30.

MICROBIAL, ENVIRONMENTAL, AND HOST FACTORS

Three general factors contribute to the occurrence of enteric disease among international travelers. The first is the presence of a fully virulent microbe that is capable of producing illness in the environment with disease transmission facilitated by reduced environmental hygiene; this allows the microbe to grow to doses that are sufficient to produce disease. Travelers commonly worry about safety of water during their trips, which may be justified during the rainy seasons in some developing regions in Latin America where diarrheagenic viruses may be found [9] or in other areas where drinking water has been implicated in parasitic diarrhea [10,11]. Although water presents an occasional risk for illness, food is the principal source of bacterial enteropathogens and travelers' diarrhea in most areas of the world [12–14]. The food items of greatest concern are those that contain moisture and remain at room temperature for periods of time. For example, the hot sauces that remain in dishes on the tabletops in many countries commonly are contaminated with fecal coliforms and enteric pathogens, despite a low pH [12].

Travelers' diarrhea seems to be a series of small and poorly defined outbreaks among persons who consume contaminated food [15]. Although food is contaminated widely in developing regions, it is obvious to those of us in travel medicine that not all subjects in developing areas are at equal risk for developing diarrhea. The known host factors that influence susceptibility to illness are identified in Table 2. The best studied host risk factors are country of origin and region visited; highest rates of illness are noted when persons from highly industrialized areas spend time in areas with reduced hygiene. Not surprisingly, the number of errors that travelers make in food and beverage selection can be related to diarrhea rates [16]. Although it is not known if being careful with food and beverage selection is an effective way to prevent disease, it is known that most travelers are not informed or are not motivated to exercise care in what they consume.

The author and colleagues found increased rates of acute diarrhea in a subset of United States male students who drank excessive amounts of alcohol while in Mexico, whereas female students who reported consuming the same number of drinks did not show increased rates of illness [17]. Our interpretation of this is that only the interviewed women accurately reported their levels of consumption, whereas the men had heavier consumption of alcohol than reported.

Based on studies with volunteers and experimental challenge with bacterial enteropathogens the author and colleagues [18] had anticipated that the widespread use of proton pump inhibitor (PPI) drugs for gastroesophageal disease would be associated with high rates of diarrhea among international travelers. In reality, this class of drugs seems to predispose travelers minimally to enteric infection and diarrheal illness, presumably because of the intermittent alteration of gastric pH. One study linked susceptibility to *Campylobacter* diarrhea with the chronic use of PPIs [19].

Genetic factors seem to contribute importantly to susceptibility to enteric infectious diseases. This may explain the observation that subgroups report

Table 2
Microbial, environmental, and host factors that relate to susceptibility and occurrence of diarrhea in travelers

The microbe	The environment	The host	References
Virulent enteropathogen	High-risk region: reduced hygiene	Traveling from a low-risk industrialized region	[6]
	Exposure to enteropathogen in food or beverage	Toddler or adolescent with less controlled diet	[6,80]
	Dose of pathogen ingested	Eating from street vendors, selection of more dangerous foods and beverages[a], and consuming excessive quantities of alcohol	[12–14, 16]
		Regular use of proton pump inhibitor drug	[19]
		Genetic susceptibility	[21,81]

[a]Drinking nonbottled beverages, that are not hot or eating moist foods that are maintained at room temperature.

developing recurrent illness, whereas relatives and spouses show low rates of disease. In a group of travelers to India and Mexico, the author and colleagues found that fecal levels of inflammatory cytokines, including interleukin (IL)-8, were elevated in subjects who had bacterial diarrhea [20]. Jiang and colleagues [21] subsequently found that host polymorphism in the promoter (−251 position) region of the IL-8 gene was associated with increased rates of travelers' diarrhea that was due to noninvasive, but inflammatory, enteroaggregative *Escherichia coli* (EAEC). The polymorphism seems to be a nonspecific host risk factor that identifies persons with increased susceptibility to inflammatory forms of enteric bacterial infection, including EAEC and antibiotic-associated *Clostridium difficile* diarrhea [22]. Other uncharacterized host genetic factors are likely to be involved in predisposing subjects to enteric infections.

ETIOLOGY

The most important causes of travelers' diarrhea are bacterial agents (Table 3), which usually are responsible for about 80% of cases as determined by direct study of pathogen identification [23–25] and by showing clinical improvement to antibacterial therapy in subjects without a definable pathogen [26–29]. Diarrheagenic *E coli*, including enterotoxigenic *E coli* (ETEC) and EAEC, explain approximately half of the cases of disease that are studied in Latin America, Africa, and many parts of Asia [23,25,30]. Ciprofloxacin-resistant *Campylobacter* are important causes of illness in travelers to Thailand [31,32]. Norwalk virus or a norovirus can be found commonly in international travelers who have diarrhea, especially when illness is complicated by vomiting; it may explain up to 17% of total diarrheal illness [33]. Parasitic agents are not found commonly in cases of travelers' diarrhea although they may be more important for travelers to Nepal [34,35] or Russia [10] and in subjects

Table 3
Etiologic agents in travelers' diarrhea by region of the world

Etiologic agent	Region of the world	References
Diarrheagenic *Escherichia coli*[a]	All regions, particularly important in travelers to Latin America and Africa	[23,25]
Wide variety of bacterial enteropathogens	All regions	[23,25]
Invasive bacterial enteropathogen[b]	All regions, more common in Asia	[25,31,32,82]
Ciprofloxacin-resistant *Campylobacter*	All regions, highest rates reported in Thailand and Spain	[31,32,83]
Noroviruses	All regions, special problem of passengers on cruise ships	[33,84]
Giardia	Russia, all regions of the world	[10]
Cryptosporidium	Russia, all regions of the world	[10]
Cylospora cayetanensis	Nepal, Haiti, Peru, all regions of the world	[34]

Entamoeba histolytica and *Microsporidium* spp are unusual causes of diarrhea in international travelers.
  [a]ETEC and EAEC.
  [b]*Shigella, Campylobacter,* and *Salmonella.*

from diverse world regions who have persistent diarrhea, defined as illness lasting 2 weeks or longer [36].

CLINICAL ILLNESS

Illness typically occurs during the first week after entering the host country. The average illness consists of the passing of 7 to 13 watery stools over the first 2 days [37]. Fever and passage of blood and mucus were seen in 1% to 3% of patients who had travelers' diarrhea in Mexico, Egypt, and Morocco [38–40]. Febrile dysenteric illness is more common in persons who travel to Asia and occurs in approximately 10% of cases of diarrhea. Vomiting is the important clinical manifestation of enteric illness of travelers in about 10% of cases; it typically is due to viruses or to ingestion of preformed toxin of *Staphylococcus aureus* or *Bacillus cereus.*

COMPLICATIONS

The most common complication of travelers' diarrhea is a temporary disability that lasts about 24 hours per illness episode [41]. Considering the frequency of the illness in international travelers to high-risk regions and the duration of the average trip, this disruption of activities represents a major public health problem. Perhaps an even greater concern is the less common chronic intestinal complaints that can be found in a subset of travelers who experienced enteric disease during previous visits to developing regions.

Persistent enteric symptoms occur in 2% to 18% of travelers who had an initial bout of diarrhea [36]. This may relate to occult parasitic infection [35], idiopathic Brainerd diarrhea [42], unmasked inflammatory bowel disease [43], celiac disease [44], or to postinfectious irritable bowel syndrome (PI-IBS) [45]. The connection between travelers' and bacterial diarrhea and PI-IBS is becoming strong. Between 5% and 30% of patients who have "IBS" had the onset of their symptoms following an acute bout of apparently infectious diarrheal disease.

Travelers' diarrhea, largely caused by bacterial enteropathogens, predisposes patients to new-onset PI-IBS with rates between 4% [46] and 10% [45]. The rate may be highest for those who are infected with fully virulent and invasive bacterial enteropathogens that produce an inflammatory enterocolitis [47]. Like other forms of IBS, PI-IBS occurs more commonly in women, but there may be features that make it an identifiable syndrome. Although anxiety or depression is found in approximately one quarter of patients who have PI-IBS, psychiatric illness is seen in more than half of IBS patients who do not have PI-IBS [48]. PI-IBS is nearly always a diarrhea-predominant form of illness [49,50]. When a group of patients was followed for 6 years after making the diagnosis, only 40% had recovered to normal bowel habits [50].

Potential factors in the pathogenesis of PI-IBS diarrhea are outlined in Table 4. A pathologic host response follows infection by a fully virulent enteropathogen—usually, but not always, a bacterial agent. The host response includes the development of intestinal enteroendocrine or enterochromaffin cell that produces 5-hydroxytryptamine (5-HT). Mucosal stimulation of T lymphocytes can be found in these patients, which is associated with the release of various proinflammatory cytokines and the inhibition of anti-inflammatory cytokines. Persistent inflammation may lead to IgE response with secondary changes. The results of the various changes seem to be visceral hypersensitivity with heightened pain sensations, small bowel stasis that often leads to bacterial overgrowth, and small bowel permeability defects. Genetic factors may predispose to diarrhea-predominant IBS, which relate to the disease pathogenesis. A functional polymorphism in the serotonin transporter gene has been related to the development of IBS [51], and some patients who have IBS show a reduced frequency of the high producer genotypes for anti-inflammatory cytokine IL-10 [52]. If future studies confirm the importance of chronic intestinal complications and PI-IBS in patients who have travelers' diarrhea, prevention strategies will be given greater emphasis.

PREVENTION OF DISEASE

Prevention of travelers' diarrhea should be attempted in persons who are to be put at high risk. Although of unproven value, it may be possible to educate travelers about the avoidance of usually high-risk foods and the selection of often low-risk foods while in unhygienic settings. Cooked foods that are served steaming hot invariably are safe; bacterial enteropathogens can be expected to be inactivated when exposed to temperatures of at least 59°C [53]. Other usually safe foods include those with minimal moisture content (eg, bread), fruits and vegetables that have been peeled, and items that contain high concentrations of sugar (eg, syrup, jelly, jam, and honey).

Table 4
Pathogenesis of postinfectious irritable bowel syndrome

Initial event	Initial host response	Secondary events	Downstream events	Resultant disease
Enteric infection with virulent enteropathogen (Campylobacter, diarrheagenic E coli[a], Shigella, rotavirus, or parasites)	Inflammation of the gut	Cytokine release: ↑ IL-1β, IL-2, TNF; ↓ IL-10	Persistent inflammation	Smooth muscle alterations with: small bowel hypomotility with ↓ housekeeper waves; gut hypersensitivity resulting in ↑ visceral perception; and ↑ small bowel permeability
	↑ intestinal enteroendocrine cells ↑ intestinal T-lymphocytes	Mast cell degranulation Serotonin release	IgE and related mediators released Release of 5-hydroxytryptamine	

Abbreviation: TNF, tumor necrosis factor.
[a] ETEC and EAEC.
Data from Refs. [47–49,85–98].

Showing that antibacterial drugs prevented travelers' diarrhea during travel to high-risk regions was the first evidence that it was caused by preventable bacterial pathogens [1,2,4]. The prophylactic use of antibiotics in the 1950s and 1960s was widespread in the United States and Europe. In a survey that was conducted in 1957, approximately 35% of travelers who left Mexico City to return to the United States reported having taken prophylactic antibacterial drugs [4]. The British Olympic team credited chemoprophylaxis as a major reason for their good health during competition at the Mexico City Olympics in 1968 [54].

During a Consensus Development Conference that was held at the National Institutes of Health in 1985 it was recommended that chemoprophylaxis not be used with absorbed drugs because of systemic side effects, and because widespread use of the drugs would encourage the development of resistance and limit the future use of these drugs for the treatment of extraintestinal infection [55]. Nonantibiotic chemoprophylactic agents, including bismuth subsalicylate (BSS) and the probiotic *Lactobacillus* GG, provided a measure of disease prevention (Table 5). BSS that was taken in a dosage of two tablets (263 mg BSS per tablet) with each meal and at bedtime (eight tablets per day or 2.1 g of BSS) prevented 65% of cases of disease that otherwise would have occurred [56]. *Lactobacillus* GG was less effective in preventing diarrhea [57,58].

Rifaximin is the most useful chemoprophylactic drug for travelers' diarrhea prevention. One to three 200-mg dosages with daily meals while in a high-risk

Table 5
Decreasing the occurrence of diarrhea while traveling to high-risk areas

Approach	Comment	References
Careful food and beverage selection	Uncertain effectiveness, requires education on restricted pattern of beverage or food consumption	[16]
Bismuth subsalicylate	65% effective in preventing diarrhea, will turn tongues and stools black (harmless bismuth salt), occasionally tinnitus; dosage is two tablets with three daily meals and at bedtime (eight 263-mg BSS tablets each day) while in the region at risk	[56]
Probiotics	*Lactobacillus* GG most effective probiotic tested; provides 12% to 45% protection in preventing diarrhea[a]	[57,58]
Rifaximin	72% to 77% effective in preventing diarrhea, no side effects identified, effective in a single 200-mg dosage with first daily meal; recommended dose 200 mg twice a day with meals while in region at risk	[59]

[a]Protection rate indicates the level of disease prevention in those expected to become ill and is calculated by the formula: % attack rate in placebo group minus % attack rate in the active drug group divided by % attack rate in the placebo group times 100.

region prevented more than 70% of cases that would occurred without the preventive drug [59]. An accompanying editorial attempted to identify a subset of persons who could be encouraged to take the drug as a preventive measure during international travel: those on a tight schedule (eg, musicians, diplomats, lecturers, and athletes), those with a history of disease during travel (indicating increased susceptibility), and those who request prophylaxis [60]. A group that was not mentioned but that probably is appropriate for prophylaxis with rifaximin are persons who have immunosuppressive diseases or treatment or those who have unstable medical conditions, such as insulin-dependent diabetes and heart failure [5].

Two questions about the routine use of rifaximin to prevent diarrhea during international travel remain before recommending this approach to all international travelers. Will the drug provide protection against mucosally invasive bacterial enteropathogens (eg, *Shigella* and *Campylobacter*) and will rifaximin chemoprophylaxis prevent the development of PI-IBS in persons who travel internationally? Concerning the first question, there is reason to believe that rifaximin will prevent invasive forms of bacterial enteric infection. Preventing an infection before mucosal penetration has occurred should be easier than treating an established intramucosal infection. In support of the argument, Taylor and colleagues [61] demonstrated that rifaximin was effective in preventing experimental shigellosis by a fully virulent strain of *S flexneri* in a volunteer model of shigellosis. The author and colleagues are conducting a study to evaluate the effectiveness of rifaximin in preventing travelers' diarrhea in Thailand, where the prevalent pathogen is ciprofloxacin-resistant *Campylobacter* [31,32]. Regarding the prevention of PI-IBS by chemoprophylaxis, rifaximin effectively prevents diarrheal disease, and the author and colleagues showed that subjects who develop PI-IBS invariably experienced diarrheal illness during international travel [45]. Thus, it is likely that rifaximin will be effective in preventing PI-IBS by preventing diarrheal occurrence.

TREATMENT

Because of the predictable occurrence of bacterial diarrheal in international travelers and with data showing the effectiveness of antibacterial therapy in shortening the disease, all travelers to high-risk regions should be armed with medication for the self-treatment of potential illness. The various forms of effective treatment for travelers' diarrhea are detailed in Tables 6 and 7. Rifaximin, the previously tested safe and poorly absorbed (<0.4%) rifamycin, effectively shortens nondysenteric travelers' diarrhea when given orally in a dosage of 200 mg three times a day for 3 days. The absorbable fluoroquinolones and azalide, azithromycin, are equally effective in nondysenteric watery diarrhea providing that they are active in vitro to the infecting bacterium. With concern that travelers might develop uncommon febrile dysenteric diarrhea unresponsive to rifaximin, some travel medicine clinics have preferentially prescribed an absorbed fluoroquinolone such as ciprofloxacin for international travelers. Ciprofloxacin is not invariably effective for the therapy of febrile

Table 6
Antibacterial self-treatment of travelers' diarrhea

Therapy	Dose and comment	References
Rifaximin 200 mg TID for 3 days (nine 200-mg tablets)	As effective as absorbed agents for afebrile, nondysenteric travelers' diarrhea (>90% of the illness); general use makes public health sense to prevent widespread occurrence of resistance to drugs that are important in treating extraintestinal infections.	[28]
Fluoroquinolone-ciprofloxacin 500 mg BID or 750 mg QD or levofloxacin 500 mg QD for 1–3 days[a]	Effective in most regions of the world. Treatment failures occur commonly because of resistant strains of Campylobacter.	[68–70,99,100]
Azithromycin 1000 mg as a single dose or 500 mg initially and then 250 mg for 1–3 days[a]	Not as rapidly effective as the fluoroquinolones but show high rates of in vitro activity against all bacterial enteric pathogens, including ciprofloxacin-resistant Campylobacter	[31,97]

Abbreviations: BID, twice a day; QD, every day; TID, three times a day.
[a]Traveler takes a second dose the next morning or next two mornings depending upon degree of clinical improvement.

Table 7
Clinical trials that examined effectiveness of combined therapy: loperamide for rapid relief of symptoms plus curative antibacterial drugs

Therapy	Destination and major pathogens Encountered	Comment	References
Ofloxaxin plus loperamide	Mexico, diarrheagenic E coli[a]	Added effect by both drugs; ofloxacin has been replaced in the United States by related levofloxacin.	[68,69]
Ciprofloxacin plus loperamide	Egypt, ETEC	Loperamide offered only minimal value	[101]
Ciprofloxacin plus loperamide	Thailand, invasive bacterial pathogens[b] and ETEC	Loperamide offered only minimal value	[102]
Azithromycin plus loperamide	Mexico, diarrheagenic E coli[a]	Additive effect was seen by both drugs	Unpublished data[c]
Rifaximin plus loperamide	Mexico, diarrheagenic E coli[a]	Additive effect was seen by both drugs	Unpublished data[d]

Dose of loperamide to use is 4 mg (two capsules) initially followed by 2 mg (one capsule) after each unformed stool passed, not to exceed 8 mg (four capsules) per day for no more than 48 hours.
[a]EAEC and ETEC.
[b]Shigella, Campylobacter, and Salmonella.
[c]C.D. Ericsson, The University of Texas Medical School at Houston, Houston, TX.
[d]H.L. DuPont.

dysenteric diarrhea, which may be due to resistant strains of *Campylobacter* [62–66]. Although diarrhea that is secondary to ciprofloxacin-resistant *Campylobacter* strains produces self-limiting illness, the duration of symptoms can be shortened by azithromycin therapy [32]. Also, one of the newer fluoroquinolones may be active against these resistant strains in view of their differing activity against *Campylobacter* [67]. Public health concerns favor the widespread and preferential use of rifaximin for the self-treatment of travelers' diarrhea to minimize the development of resistance by endogenous bacteria (eg, *Streptococcus pneumoniae*) to absorbed drugs that are important in the therapy of extraintestinal infection (eg, pneumonia). Seasoned travelers can be given two prescriptions: one for nine 200-mg tablets of rifaximin and one for four 250-mg tablets of azithromycin. When the traveler experiences the common form of watery diarrhea without fever or dysentery, he or she takes the rifaximin and saves the azalide for future trips. In the rare event that fever with diarrhea develops and bloody stools are passed, the azithromycin can be taken.

Some travel medicine authorities who rely on fluoroquinolones prescribe a single dose for self-treatment of travelers' diarrhea [68–70]. In the author's unit in Mexico, patients have been seen who had travelers' diarrhea that failed to respond to one dose of a fluoroquinolone. The situation seems to be similar to that of another mucosal surface process, urinary tract infection (UTI). In UTIs and in bacterial diarrhea, including travelers' diarrhea, a single-dose treatment of an absorbed drug often is effective but treatment failures rarely will be seen. The author's current approach for self-treatment of travelers' diarrhea with absorbed fluoroquinolone or azithromycin is an initial single dose; the subject can take a second or third dosage on day two or three as needed with incomplete response. In this author's experience 20% of subjects require more than one dose when the absorbable drugs are used.

FUTURE DIRECTIONS

The most important line of future research is to work with local governments, tour operators, or hotels and restaurants to make the environment into which travelers move safer (Table 8). Working with the Jamaican Ministry of Health, Robert Steffen and the author helped to develop countrywide education and surveillance programs at the principal airport and in the resort hotels; diarrhea rates decreased by more than 70% over 6 years [71,72]. If countries do not wish to work on this problem it will be possible for organizations, such as the International Society of Travel Medicine, to work directly with hotels and restaurants in high-risk areas to assure the use of hygienic standards in food preparation and storage without guaranteeing the safety of the food [73].

Future studies should focus on improved treatment options for travelers' diarrhea. Although loperamide provides immediate antidiarrheal effects while antibacterial drugs lead to disease cure in most cases, loperamide can lead to posttreatment constipation. The newer antisecretory drugs [74–76] should be combined with antibacterial treatment to see if they provide additive and more physiologic antidiarrheal affects.

Table 8
Future directions of research to control travelers' diarrhea

Area for development	Comments	References
Food safety and detection	It is not known if it is possible to decrease illness by modifying food and beverage selection; if effective, innovative methods of modifying selection patterns among travelers should be developed. Methods of detection of pathogens or coliforms in food may be possible.	[12–14,16]
Rapidly effective treatment	Combining curative antibacterial drugs with rapidly acting agents that are used to improve symptoms may provide optimal disease management and return travelers to routine activities more rapidly	[68,69,101,102]
Chemoprophylaxis	Rifaximin is a near ideal drug for preventing travelers' diarrhea with efficacy, low frequency of side effects, or development of resistance; studies underway to determine if drug effectively prevents invasive forms of diarrhea and PI-IBS.	[59]
Immunoprophylaxis	Inexpensive, effective, and safe vaccines that are directed to the most common agents in travelers' diarrhea (eg, enteroxigenic E coli) to reduce occurrence of diarrhea, and possibly, PI-IBS	[79]

Newer uses of chemoprophylaxis may provide optimal approaches to preventing travelers' diarrhea during high-risk travel. Other dosage regimens of rifaximin should be tried using larger or intermittent dosages during high-risk travel. Perhaps rifaximin would be optimally effective in preventing diarrhea and PI-IBS when given in a single large daily dose (~600 mg).

As persons remain in an area of risk they develop protective immunity against prevalent pathogens [37]. This seems to relate primarily to immunity against ETEC infections [77]. The observations that natural immunity develops with exposure has encouraged the development of ETEC vaccines. One safe and effective ETEC vaccine preparation uses whole ETEC cells plus the binding subunit of cholera toxin—related to the binding subunit of the heat labile enterotoxin (LT) of ETEC—which is given in two oral dosages [78]. A novel approach in the immunoprophylaxis of travelers' diarrhea uses ETEC LT as an immunizing agent and as an adjuvant that is administered by skin patch after minor abrasion of the skin's stratum corneum [79]. The transcutaneously applied vaccine presents its antigens to epidermal Langerhans cells, which leads to immunogenic and protective responses to LT-producing

ETEC. Working with Johns Hopkins University, the author's group is planning field trials of the patch ETEC vaccine in US students in Mexico, Guatemala, and Peru.

References

[1] Kean BH. The diarrhea of travelers to Mexico. Summary of five-year study. Ann Intern Med 1963;59:605–14.

[2] Kean BH, Schaffner W, Brennan RW. The diarrhea of travelers. V. Prophylaxis with phthalylsulfathiazole and neomycin sulphate. JAMA 1962;180:367–71.

[3] Kean BH, Waters S. The diarrhea of travelers. I. Incidence in travelers returning to the United States from Mexico. AMA Arch Ind Health 1958;18(2):148–50.

[4] Kean BH, Waters SR. The diarrhea of travelers. III. Drug prophylaxis in Mexico. N Engl J Med 1959;261(2):71–4.

[5] DuPont HL, Ericsson CD. Prevention and treatment of traveler's diarrhea. N Engl J Med 1993;328(25):1821–7.

[6] Steffen R. Epidemiologic studies of travelers' diarrhea, severe gastrointestinal infections, and cholera. Rev Infect Dis 1986;8(Suppl 2):S122–30.

[7] Dandoy S. The diarrhea of travelers: incidence in foreign students in the United States. Calif Med 1966;104(6):458–62.

[8] Ryder RW, Wells J, Gangarosa EJ. A study of travelers' diarrhea in foreign visitors to the United States. J Infect Dis 1977;136:605–7.

[9] Deetz T, Smith EM, Goyal SM, et al. Occurrence of rota-and enteroviruses in drinking and environmental water in a developing nation. Water Res 1984;18:567–71.

[10] Jokipii L, Pohjola S, Jokipii AM. Cryptosporidiosis associated with traveling and giardiasis. Gastroenterology 1985;89(4):838–42.

[11] Sterling CR, Ortega YR. Cyclospora: an enigma worth unraveling. Emerg Infect Dis 1999;5(1):48–53.

[12] Adachi JA, Mathewson JJ, Jiang ZD, et al. Enteric pathogens in Mexican sauces of popular restaurants in Guadalajara, Mexico, and Houston, Texas. Ann Intern Med 2002;136(12):884–7.

[13] Tjoa WS, DuPont HL, Sullivan P, et al. Location of food consumption and travelers' diarrhea. Am J Epidemiol 1977;106(1):61–6.

[14] Wood LV, Ferguson LE, Hogan P, et al. Incidence of bacterial enteropathogens in foods from Mexico. Appl Environ Microbiol 1983;46(2):328–32.

[15] Paredes P, Campbell-Forrester S, Mathewson JJ, et al. Etiology of travelers' diarrhea on a Caribbean island. J Travel Med 2000;7(1):15–8.

[16] Kozicki M, Steffen R, Schar M. "Boil it, cook it, peel it or forget it": does this rule prevent travellers' diarrhoea? Int J Epidemiol 1985;14(1):169–72.

[17] Huang DB, Sanchez AP, Triana E, et al. United States male students who heavily consume alcohol in Mexico are at greater risk of travelers' diarrhea than their female counterparts. J Travel Med 2004;11(3):143–5.

[18] DuPont HL, Formal SB, Hornick RB, et al. Pathogenesis of *Escherichia coli* diarrhea. N Engl J Med 1971;285(1):1–9.

[19] Neal KR, Scott HM, Slack RC, et al. Omeprazole as a risk factor for campylobacter gastroenteritis: case-control study. BMJ 1996;312(7028):414–5.

[20] Greenberg DE, Jiang ZD, Steffen R, et al. Markers of inflammation in bacterial diarrhea among travelers, with a focus on enteroaggregative *Escherichia coli* pathogenicity. J Infect Dis 2002;185(7):944–9.

[21] Jiang ZD, Okhuysen PC, Guo DC, et al. Genetic susceptibility to enteroaggregative *Escherichia coli* diarrhea: polymorphism in the interleukin-8 promoter region. J Infect Dis 2003;188(4):506–11.

[22] Jiang Z-D, DuPont H, Garey K, et al. A common polymorphism in the interleukin 8 gene promoter is associated with *Clostridium difficile* diarrhea. Am J Gastroenterol 2006;101:1–5.

[23] Adachi JA, Jiang ZD, Mathewson JJ, et al. Enteroaggregative *Escherichia coli* as a major etiologic agent in traveler's diarrhea in 3 regions of the world. Clin Infect Dis 2001;32(12): 1706–9.

[24] Caeiro JP, Estrada-Garcia MT, Jiang ZD, et al. Improved detection of enterotoxigenic *Escherichia coli* among patients with travelers' diarrhea, by use of the polymerase chain reaction technique. J Infect Dis 1999;180(6):2053–5.

[25] Jiang ZD, Lowe B, Verenkar MP, et al. Prevalence of enteric pathogens among international travelers with diarrhea acquired in Kenya (Mombasa), India (Goa), or Jamaica (Montego Bay). J Infect Dis 2002;185(4):497–502.

[26] DuPont H, Ericsson CD, DuPont MW. Emporiatric enteritis: lessons learned from US students in Mexico. Amer Clin Climatol Assoc Trans 1986;97:32–42.

[27] DuPont HL, Ericsson CD, Mathewson JJ, et al. Five versus three days of ofloxacin therapy for traveler's diarrhea: a placebo-controlled study. Antimicrob Agents Chemother 1992;36(1):87–91.

[28] DuPont HL, Jiang ZD, Ericsson CD, et al. Rifaximin versus ciprofloxacin for the treatment of traveler's diarrhea: a randomized, double-blind clinical trial. Clin Infect Dis 2001;33(11): 1807–15.

[29] DuPont HL, Reves RR, Galindo E, et al. Treatment of travelers' diarrhea with trimethoprim/ sulfamethoxazole and with trimethoprim alone. N Engl J Med 1982;307(14):841–4.

[30] Steffen R, Mathewson JJ, Ericsson CD, et al. Travelers' diarrhea in West Africa and Mexico: fecal transport systems and liquid bismuth subsalicylate for self-therapy. J Infect Dis 1988;157(5):1008–13.

[31] Hoge CW, Gambel JM, Srijan A, et al. Trends in antibiotic resistance among diarrheal pathogens isolated in Thailand over 15 years. Clin Infect Dis 1998;26(2):341–5.

[32] Kuschner RA, Trofa AF, Thomas RJ, et al. Use of azithromycin for the treatment of *Campylobacter* enteritis in travelers to Thailand, an area where ciprofloxacin resistance is prevalent. Clin Infect Dis 1995;21(3):536–41.

[33] Ko G, Garcia C, Jiang ZD, et al. Noroviruses as a cause of traveler's diarrhea among students from the United States visiting Mexico. J Clin Microbiol 2005;43(12): 6126–9.

[34] Shlim DR, Hoge CW, Rajah R, et al. Persistent high risk of diarrhea among foreigners in Nepal during the first 2 years of residence. Clin Infect Dis 1999;29(3):613–6.

[35] Taylor DN, Connor BA, Shlim DR. Chronic diarrhea in the returned traveler. Med Clin North Am 1999;83(4):1033–52.

[36] DuPont HL, Capsuto EG. Persistent diarrhea in travelers. Clin Infect Dis 1996;22(1):124–8.

[37] DuPont HL, Haynes GA, Pickering LK, et al. Diarrhea of travelers to Mexico. Relative susceptibility of United States and Latin American students attending a Mexican University. Am J Epidemiol 1977;105(1):37–41.

[38] Ericsson CD, Patterson TF, DuPont HL. Clinical presentation as a guide to therapy for travelers' diarrhea. Am J Med Sci 1987;294(2):91–6.

[39] Haberberger RL Jr, Mikhail IA, Burans JP, et al. Travelers' diarrhea among United States military personnel during joint American-Egyptian armed forces exercises in Cairo, Egypt. Mil Med 1991;156(1):27–30.

[40] Mattila L. Clinical features and duration of traveler's diarrhea in relation to its etiology. Clin Infect Dis 1994;19(4):728–34.

[41] von Sonnenburg F, Tornieporth N, Waiyaki P, et al. Risk and aetiology of diarrhoea at various tourist destinations. Lancet 2000;356(9224):133–4.

[42] Mintz ED, Weber JT, Guris D, et al. An outbreak of Brainerd diarrhea among travelers to the Galapagos Islands. J Infect Dis 1998;177(4):1041–5.

[43] Yanai-Kopelman D, Paz A, Rippel D, et al. Inflammatory bowel disease in returning travelers. J Travel Med 2000;7(6):333–5.

[44] Landzberg BR, Connor BA. Persistent diarrhea in the returning traveler: think beyond persistent infection. Scand J Gastroenterol 2005;40(1):112–4.

[45] Okhuysen PC, Jiang ZD, Carlin L, et al. Post-diarrhea chronic intestinal symptoms and irritable bowel syndrome in North American travelers to Mexico. Am J Gastroenterol 2004;99(9):1774–8.

[46] Ilnyckyj A, Balachandra B, Elliott L, et al. Post-traveler's diarrhea irritable bowel syndrome: a prospective study. Am J Gastroenterol 2003;98(3):596–9.

[47] Thornley JP, Jenkins D, Neal K, et al. Relationship of *Campylobacter* toxigenicity in vitro to the development of postinfectious irritable bowel syndrome. J Infect Dis 2001;184(5): 606–9.

[48] Dunlop SP, Jenkins D, Spiller RC. Distinctive clinical, psychological, and histological features of postinfective irritable bowel syndrome. Am J Gastroenterol 2003;98(7): 1578–83.

[49] Gwee KA, Leong YL, Graham C, et al. The role of psychological and biological factors in postinfective gut dysfunction. Gut 1999;44(3):400–6.

[50] Neal KR, Barker L, Spiller RC. Prognosis in post-infective irritable bowel syndrome: a six-year follow up study. Gut 2002;51(3):410–3.

[51] Yeo A, Boyd P, Lumsden S, et al. Association between a functional polymorphism in the serotonin transporter gene and diarrhoea predominant irritable bowel syndrome in women. Gut 2004;53(10):1452–8.

[52] Gonsalkorale WM, Perrey C, Pravica V, et al. Interleukin 10 genotypes in irritable bowel syndrome: evidence for an inflammatory component? Gut 2003;52(1):91–3.

[53] Bandres JC, Mathewson JJ, DuPont HL. Heat susceptibility of bacterial enteropathogens. Implications for the prevention of travelers' diarrhea. Arch Intern Med 1988;148(10): 2261–3.

[54] Owen JR. Diarrhoea at the Olympics. BMJ 1968;4(631):645.

[55] Gorbach S, Edelman R. Travelers' diarrhea: National Institutes of Health Consensus Development Conference. Rev Inf Dis 1986;8(Suppl 2):S109–233.

[56] DuPont HL, Ericsson CD, Johnson PC, et al. Prevention of travelers' diarrhea by the tablet formulation of bismuth subsalicylate. JAMA 1987;257(10):1347–50.

[57] Hilton E, Kolakowski P, Singer C, et al. Efficacy of *Lactobacillus* GG as a diarrheal preventive in travelers. J Travel Med 1997;4(1):41–3.

[58] Oksanen PJ, Salminen S, Saxelin M, et al. Prevention of travellers' diarrhoea by *Lactobacillus* GG. Ann Med 1990;22(1):53–6.

[59] DuPont HL, Jiang ZD, Okhuysen PC, et al. A randomized, double-blind, placebo-controlled trial of rifaximin to prevent travelers' diarrhea. Ann Intern Med 2005;142(10):805–12.

[60] Gorbach SL. How to hit the runs for fifty million travelers at risk. Ann Intern Med 2005;142(10):861–2.

[61] Taylor D, McKenzie R, Durbin A, et al. Double-blind, placebo-controlled trial to evaluate the use of rifaximin (200 mg TID) to prevent diarrhea in volunteers challenged with *Shigella flexneri* 2a (2457T). Presented at the American Society of Tropical Medicine and Hygiene 53rd Annual Meeting. Miami, November 7–11, 2004.

[62] Ciprofloxacin resistance in *Campylobacter jejuni*: case-case analysis as a tool for elucidating risks at home and abroad. J Antimicrob Chemother 2002;50(4):561–8.

[63] Kassenborg HD, Smith KE, Vugia DJ, et al. Fluoroquinolone-resistant *Campylobacter* infections: eating poultry outside of the home and foreign travel are risk factors. Clin Infect Dis 2004;38(Suppl 3):S279–84.

[64] Murphy GS Jr, Echeverria P, Jackson LR, et al. Ciprofloxacin- and azithromycin-resistant *Campylobacter* causing traveler's diarrhea in US troops deployed to Thailand in 1994. Clin Infect Dis 1996;22(5):868–9.

[65] Nelson JM, Smith KE, Vugia DJ, et al. Prolonged diarrhea due to ciprofloxacin-resistant campylobacter infection. J Infect Dis 2004;190(6):1150–7.

[66] Sanders JW, Isenbarger DW, Walz SE, et al. An observational clinic-based study of diarrheal illness in deployed United States military personnel in Thailand: presentation and outcome of *Campylobacter* infection. Am J Trop Med Hyg 2002;67(5):533–8.

[67] Krausse R, Ullmann U. In vitro activities of new fluoroquinolones against *Campylobacter jejuni* and *Campylobacter coli* isolates obtained from humans in 1980 to 1982 and 1997 to 2001. Antimicrob Agents Chemother 2003;47(9):2946–50.

[68] Ericsson CD, DuPont HL, Mathewson JJ. Optimal dosing of ofloxacin with loperamide in the treatment of non-dysenteric travelers' diarrhea. J Travel Med 2001;8(4):207–9.

[69] Ericsson CD, DuPont HL, Mathewson JJ. Single dose ofloxacin plus loperamide compared with single dose or three days of ofloxacin in the treatment of traveler's diarrhea. J Travel Med 1997;4(1):3–7.

[70] Salam I, Katelaris P, Leigh-Smith S, et al. Randomised trial of single-dose ciprofloxacin for travellers' diarrhoea. Lancet 1994;344(8936):1537–9.

[71] Ashley DV, Walters C, Dockery-Brown C, et al. Interventions to prevent and control food-borne diseases associated with a reduction in traveler's diarrhea in tourists to Jamaica. J Travel Med 2004;11(6):364–7.

[72] Steffen R, Collard F, Tornieporth N, et al. Epidemiology, etiology, and impact of traveler's diarrhea in Jamaica. JAMA 1999;281(9):811–7.

[73] Steffen R, DuPont HL, Ericsson CD. The future of travelers' diarrhea: directions for research. In: Ericsson C, DuPont HL, Steffen R, editors. Travelers' diarrhea. Hamilton (Ontario): B.C. Decker, Inc.; 2003. p. 310–5.

[74] DiCesare D, DuPont HL, Mathewson JJ, et al. A double blind, randomized, placebo-controlled study of SP-303 (Provir) in the symptomatic treatment of acute diarrhea among travelers to Jamaica and Mexico. Am J Gastroenterol 2002;97(10):2585–8.

[75] DuPont HL, Ericsson CD, Mathewson JJ, et al. Zaldaride maleate, an intestinal calmodulin inhibitor, in the therapy of travelers' diarrhea. Gastroenterology 1993;104(3):709–15.

[76] Salazar-Lindo E, Santisteban-Ponce J, Chea-Woo E, et al. Racecadotril in the treatment of acute watery diarrhea in children. N Engl J Med 2000;343(7):463–7.

[77] DuPont HL, Olarte J, Evans DG, et al. Comparative susceptibility of Latin American and United States students to enteric pathogens. N Engl J Med 1976;295(27):1520–1.

[78] Peltola H, Siitonen A, Kyronseppa H, et al. Prevention of travellers' diarrhoea by oral B-subunit/whole-cell cholera vaccine. Lancet 1991;338(8778):1285–9.

[79] Guerena-Burgueno F, Hall ER, Taylor DN, et al. Safety and immunogenicity of a prototype enterotoxigenic *Escherichia coli* vaccine administered transcutaneously. Infect Immun 2002;70(4):1874–80.

[80] Steffen R, van der Linde F, Gyr K, et al. Epidemiology of diarrhea in travelers. JAMA 1983;249(9):1176–80.

[81] Hutson AM, Airaud F, LePendu J, et al. Norwalk virus infection associates with secretor status genotyped from sera. J Med Virol 2005;77(1):116–20.

[82] Black RE. Epidemiology of travelers' diarrhea and relative importance of various pathogens. Rev Infect Dis 1990;12(Suppl 1):S73–9.

[83] Saenz Y, Zarazaga M, Lantero M, et al. Antibiotic resistance in *Campylobacter* strains isolated from animals, foods, and humans in Spain in 1997–1998. Antimicrob Agents Chemother 2000;44(2):267–71.

[84] Gunn RA, Terranova WA, Greenberg HB, et al. Norwalk virus gastroenteritis aboard a cruise ship: an outbreak on five consecutive cruises. Am J Epidemiol 1980;112(6):820–7.

[85] Barbara G, Stanghellini V, De Giorgio R, et al. Activated mast cells in proximity to colonic nerves correlate with abdominal pain in irritable bowel syndrome. Gastroenterology 2004;126(3):693–702.

[86] Bearcroft CP, Perrett D, Farthing MJ. Postprandial plasma 5-hydroxytryptamine in diarrhoea predominant irritable bowel syndrome: a pilot study. Gut 1998;42(1):42–6.

[87] Coates MD, Mahoney CR, Linden DR, et al. Molecular defects in mucosal serotonin content and decreased serotonin reuptake transporter in ulcerative colitis and irritable bowel syndrome. Gastroenterology 2004;126(7):1657–64.

[88] D'Anchino M, Orlando D, De Feudis L. *Giardia lamblia* infections become clinically evident by eliciting symptoms of irritable bowel syndrome. J Infect 2002;45(3):169–72.

[89] Dunlop SP, Jenkins D, Neal KR, et al. Randomized, double-blind, placebo-controlled trial of prednisolone in post-infectious irritable bowel syndrome. Aliment Pharmacol Ther 2003;18(1):77–84.

[90] Gwee KA, Collins SM, Read NW, et al. Increased rectal mucosal expression of interleukin 1beta in recently acquired post-infectious irritable bowel syndrome. Gut 2003;52(4): 523–6.

[91] Gwee KA, Graham JC, McKendrick MW, et al. Psychometric scores and persistence of irritable bowel after infectious diarrhoea. Lancet 1996;347(8995):150–3.

[92] Ji S, Park H, Lee D, et al. Post-infectious irritable bowel syndrome in patients with *Shigella* infection. J Gastroenterol Hepatol 2005;20(3):381–6.

[93] Marshall JK, Thabane M, Garg AX, et al. Intestinal permeability in patients with irritable bowel syndrome after a waterborne outbreak of acute gastroenteritis in Walkerton, Ontario. Aliment Pharmacol Ther 2004;20(11–12):1317–22.

[94] Neal KR, Hebden J, Spiller R. Prevalence of gastrointestinal symptoms six months after bacterial gastroenteritis and risk factors for development of the irritable bowel syndrome: postal survey of patients. BMJ 1997;314(7083):779–82.

[95] Parry SD, Stansfield R, Jelley D, et al. Is irritable bowel syndrome more common in patients presenting with bacterial gastroenteritis? A community-based, case-control study. Am J Gastroenterol 2003;98(2):327–31.

[96] Rodriguez LA, Ruigomez A. Increased risk of irritable bowel syndrome after bacterial gastroenteritis: cohort study. BMJ 1999;318(7183):565–6.

[97] Spiller RC, Jenkins D, Thornley JP, et al. Increased rectal mucosal enteroendocrine cells, T lymphocytes, and increased gut permeability following acute *Campylobacter* enteritis and in post-dysenteric irritable bowel syndrome. Gut 2000;47(6):804–11.

[98] Wang LH, Fang XC, Pan GZ. Bacillary dysentery as a causative factor of irritable bowel syndrome and its pathogenesis. Gut 2004;53(8):1096–101.

[99] Adachi JA, Ericsson CD, Jiang ZD, et al. Azithromycin found to be comparable to levofloxacin for the treatment of US travelers with acute diarrhea acquired in Mexico. Clin Infect Dis 2003;37(9):1165–71.

[100] Wistrom J, Jertborn M, Hedstrom SA, et al. Short-term self-treatment of travellers' diarrhoea with norfloxacin: a placebo-controlled study. J Antimicrob Chemother 1989;23(6): 905–13.

[101] Taylor DN, Sanchez JL, Candler W, et al. Treatment of travelers' diarrhea: ciprofloxacin plus loperamide compared with ciprofloxacin alone. A placebo-controlled, randomized trial. Ann Intern Med 1991;114(9):731–4.

[102] Petruccelli BP, Murphy GS, Sanchez JL, et al. Treatment of traveler's diarrhea with ciprofloxacin and loperamide. J Infect Dis 1992;165(3):557–60.

Gastroenterol Clin N Am 35 (2006) 355–365

GASTROENTEROLOGY CLINICS
OF NORTH AMERICA

ELSEVIER
SAUNDERS

Probiotics in the Prevention and Treatment of Gastrointestinal Infections

Elizabeth S. Huebner, MD[a], Christina M. Surawicz, MD[b],*

[a]Division of Gastroenterology, University of Washington School of Medicine, Box 356424, 1959 NE Pacific Street, Seattle, WA 98195-6424, USA
[b]Department of Medicine, Section of Gastroenterology, Harborview Medical Center, 325 9th Avenue, Seattle, WA 98104, USA

Although the use of probiotics has gained popularity in recent years, the concept dates back almost a century. Metchnikoff [1] described the potential health benefits of lactic acid bacteria in 1908 and advocated their use to promote health and prolong life. Reports later surfaced in the veterinary literature, with the use of microorganisms as supplements in animal feed. Over the past few decades there has been increasing interest in the use of probiotics in humans. In 2001, an expert panel defined these substances as "live microorganisms which, when administered in adequate amounts, confer a health benefit on the host" [2].

This concept is particularly appealing in the setting of gastrointestinal (GI) infections, when the balance of endogenous microflora may become disrupted. Probiotics have been given in an attempt to maintain or restore the normal microflora, and thus, to promote colonization resistance and prevent the overgrowth of pathogenic microorganisms. Proposed mechanisms by which this might occur include competition for nutrients, stimulation of immunity, inhibition of mucosal adherence, and production of antimicrobial substances [3]. Studies in the pediatric population evaluated the use of probiotics in acute diarrhea and several other disease states. Recently, some evidence has supported a role for probiotics in adult GI infections, including *Helicobacter pylori*, traveler's diarrhea, antibiotic-associated diarrhea, recurrent *Clostridium difficile*–associated disease, and pancreatitis.

HELICOBACTER PYLORI

Infection with *H pylori* is associated with several GI conditions, including chronic gastritis, peptic ulcer disease, gastric adenocarcinoma, and gastric mucosa-associated lymphoid tissue lymphoma. Because of concern for increasing

*Corresponding author. E-mail address: surawicz@u.washington.edu (C.M. Surawicz).

0889-8553/06/$ – see front matter
doi:10.1016/j.gtc.2006.03.005
gastro.theclinics.com

antibiotic resistance, alternate options for eradication of this organism have been explored, including the use of probiotics.

Perhaps the best studied are *Lactobacillus* species, which can tolerate a low pH, and thus, may reside transiently in the stomach. Several in vitro and animal studies showed inhibition of *H pylori* by these organisms, with proposed mechanisms of action including lactic acid production [4], induction of cell autolysis [5], antibiotic production [6], and decreased binding to gastric mucosa [7,8]. Several human studies also suggested a suppressive effect. Michetti and colleagues [9] enrolled 20 volunteers who were infected with *H pylori* into a study that compared *L johnsonii* La1 plus omeprazole or *L johnsonii* La1 with placebo; they found a marked decrease in urea breath test values in both groups. Values remained low 6 weeks after treatment, although biopsies showed persistent infection. Other groups have found similar results with this strain in asymptomatic adults [10] and children [11], which suggested a decrease in bacterial load with probiotic therapy. When given in combination with clarithromycin, La1 decreased *H pylori* density in the gastric antrum and corpus when compared with placebo, although it did not improve the eradication rate [12]. In a separate study, *L johnsonii* LC1 led to slight improvement in the severity and activity of antral gastritis, as well as an increase in mucus thickness [13].

Several additional species also seem to decrease the bacterial load of *H pylori*. Linsalata and colleagues [14] compared therapy with *L brevis* (CD2) with placebo in *H pylori*–positive patients who had dyspepsia. They found a decrease in urea breath test values, as well as a significant decrease in gastric ornithine decarboxylase activity and polyamine biosynthesis. Another group gave yogurt containing *L acidophilus* La5 or *Bifidobacterium lactis* Bb12 to 59 adult volunteers who were infected with *H pylori*; they found a decrease in urease activity, compared with placebo, after 6 weeks of therapy [15]. Cats and colleagues [16] found that administration of *L casei* strain Shirota led to a trend toward decreased urease activity that was not statistically significant. Sakamoto and colleagues [17] found improvement in urea breath test results after treatment with *L gasseri* OLL2716 (LG21). This study also showed improvement in serum pepsinogen assays, which suggested a reduction of gastric mucosal inflammation. A study of *L gasseri* OLL2716 in children, however, did not demonstrate a benefit [18].

Other studies have shown a favorable role for probiotics in improving the eradication rate of *H pylori*. Canducci and colleagues [19] enrolled 120 *H pylori*–positive individuals into a study of standard therapy with rabeprazole, clarithromycin, and amoxicillin combined with *L acidophilus* or placebo. They found a significant improvement in eradication with *L acidophilus* (88% versus 72%). Another group found similar results using yogurt that contained *Lactobacillus* and *Bifidobacterium* plus traditional triple therapy, with eradication rates of 91% (compared with 78% with triple therapy alone) in the intention-to-treat analysis [20]; however, the per-protocol eradication rates were similar in both groups. In children, the addition of *L casei* DN-114 001 to standard treatment with omeprazole, amoxicillin, and clarithromycin led to improvement in

H pylori eradication (84.6% versus 57.5% without probiotics) [21]. *L casei* was studied as a second-line therapy in patients who were resistant to an initial course of treatment for *H pylori*; it led to slight improvement in eradication over that seen with a 10-day course of quadruple therapy alone [22]. Wendakoon and colleagues [23] studied yogurt that contained several *Lactobacillus* species, but they did not find an effect on *H pylori* eradication. Urea breath test values were not reported in this study; therefore, it is unclear whether the bacterial load may have been decreased.

Several studies suggested a reduction in side effects related to traditional eradication therapy with probiotic supplementation. *Lactobacillus* GG led to improvement in several symptoms, including nausea, bloating, taste disturbance, and diarrhea [24,25]. Another group found a lower frequency of diarrhea and taste disturbance with the use of *Lactobacillus* GG, *Saccharomyces boulardii*, or a combination of *Lactobacillus* species when compared with placebo, with no significant difference between groups [26]. Improved tolerability also was found with *Bacillus clausii* [27]. In a separate study that used a combination of several probiotics, however, there was no significant difference in the frequency of new or aggravated symptoms in the treatment group compared with placebo [28].

In summary, several lactobacillus species have shown efficacy at decreasing the bacterial load of *H pylori* in controlled trials, although their effect on eradication remains unclear. Probiotics may have an adjunctive role in reducing the side effects that are associated with traditional eradication therapy.

TRAVELER'S DIARRHEA

Acute diarrhea develops in approximately 20% to 60% of travelers to developing countries, and is the most common illness that is experienced by these individuals. Although many organisms can be responsible, enterotoxigenic *Escherichia coli* seem to be the most common. Although most cases are self-limited, symptoms can result in substantial morbidity and disruption of travel plans. Because travelers may find it difficult to avoid exposure to causative organisms, prophylaxis is a desirable alternative. Several investigators have evaluated the use of probiotics in this setting.

One study of Austrian travelers showed a modest, dose-dependent reduction in the incidence of diarrhea with prophylactic ingestion of the yeast *S boulardii*. In this study, 28.7% of individuals who received high-dose therapy had diarrhea compared with 39.1% who received placebo. The protective effect varied geographically, with the highest benefit occurring in travelers to North Africa and Turkey [29]. In travelers to Egypt, a mixture of *L acidophilus, Bifidobacterium bifidum, L bulgaricus,* and *S thermophilus* also reduced the frequency of diarrhea (43% versus 71%) [30]. Oksanen and colleagues [31] compared *Lactobacillus* GG with placebo in travelers to Turkey, and found a reduction in diarrhea (23.9% versus 39.5% in the placebo group). Another placebo-controlled trial of *Lactobacillus* GG in United States travelers also showed a modest effect, with diarrhea developing in 3.9% per day at risk compared with 7.4% in the placebo group [32].

Other studies have failed to show a beneficial effect. In 50 United States travelers to Mexico, prophylactic ingestion of a mixture of *L acidophilus* and *L bulgaricus* was not effective in reducing the frequency or duration of new-onset diarrhea [33]. In a study of British soldiers who were deployed to Belize, there was no significant difference in the prevalence of diarrhea between groups that received *L fermentum* strain KLD, *L acidophilus*, or placebo (25.0%, 29.7%, and 27.7%, respectively.) Studies have shown conflicting results, and it is premature to recommend the routine use of probiotics for prevention of traveler's diarrhea.

ANTIBIOTIC-ASSOCIATED DIARRHEA

Diarrhea is a common complication of antimicrobial therapy and occurs in 5% to 39% of patients [34]. The result is longer hospital stays, an increased incidence of other nosocomial infections, and a higher cost of care. Although the underlying pathogenesis is not understood completely, it is postulated that disruption of the normal fecal flora leads to overgrowth of opportunistic pathogens, alteration in the metabolic function of the flora, and diarrhea. *C difficile* is responsible for approximately 26% to 50% of cases [34]. Several probiotics have been studied in the prevention of antibiotic-associated diarrhea (AAD), with the strongest evidence supporting a role for *Lactobacillus* GG and *S boulardii* [35,36].

The use of *Lactobacillus* GG has been evaluated in adults and children. In adults who were treated with erythromycin, fewer cases of diarrhea occurred in those who took yogurt that contained *Lactobacillus* GG than in controls [37]. This organism also led to a decreased incidence of AAD in children who received antibiotics for respiratory infections (5% compared with 16% in the placebo group) [38]. Another study in the pediatric population found similar results [39]; however, a 14-day course of *Lactobacillus* GG did not reduce the rate of AAD in a study of 267 hospitalized adults who were receiving antibiotics [40].

Other lactobacilli preparations, including a combination of *L acidophilus* and *L bulgaricus* (Lactinex), have failed to show convincing results. When coadministered to 98 patients who were receiving ampicillin this preparation failed to demonstrate significant improvement [41]. Likewise in a small study of pediatric patients who were receiving amoxicillin, Lactinex did not prevent diarrhea consistently [42]. Another study found variable results in patients who had neomycin-associated diarrhea, with lot-to-lot variations in lactobacillus preparations [43].

S boulardii demonstrated efficacy in the prevention of AAD in several controlled trials. In a French study, AAD occurred in 4% of outpatients who were receiving *S boulardii* compared with 17% who were receiving placebo [44]. A United States study of 180 hospitalized patients showed AAD rates of 9% with *S boulardii* compared with 22% with placebo [45]. In hospitalized patients who were receiving β-lactam antibiotics, AAD rates of 7% were reported with prophylactic *S boulardii* (versus 15% with placebo) [46]. Diarrhea also was reduced with this organism in a study of critically ill tube-fed patients [47], as well as in patients who were receiving antibiotics for eradication of *H pylori* [48]; however, a British study of 69 hospitalized patients failed to demonstrate efficacy [49]. Recently, a randomized controlled trial showed a decreased risk for AAD with *S boulardii* in the pediatric population [50].

Other organisms have shown modest efficacy in small trials. In one study, the use of *Enterococcus faecium* SF68 led to AAD in 9% of patients (compared with 27% with placebo) [51]. Another group found similar results with this strain, with AAD rates of 3% compared with 18% in the placebo group [52]. Bifidobacteria also demonstrated some benefit, with reduction in gastrointestinal discomfort in patients who were receiving clindamycin [53] and lower stool weight and frequency in those who were receiving erythromycin [54]. Larger studies of these organisms are necessary before adopting their use.

In conclusion, controlled trials support the use of probiotics for the prevention of antibiotic-associated diarrhea, with the strongest evidence in favor of *Lactobacillus* GG and *S boulardii*. Their role in the treatment of this condition remains to be determined.

RECURRENT *CLOSTRIDIUM DIFFICILE*–ASSOCIATED DIARRHEA

C difficile is a gram-positive bacteria that produces two toxins (A and B) that lead to diarrhea and colitis. Although an initial episode usually responds to antibiotic therapy, recurrent disease can develop in up to one third of patients. In this setting, multiple recurrences are common and can be difficult to treat. Although several probiotics have been studied in the treatment of recurrent *C difficile*–associated disease (RCDAD), only *S boulardii* demonstrated efficacy in randomized controlled trials.

Initial work in an animal model of RCDAD found *S boulardii* to be effective [55]. This led to an open trial in humans, in which 11 of 13 patients who received *S boulardii* plus vancomycin had no further recurrences [56]. In another uncontrolled trial, 5 of 7 patients who had renal failure and RCDAD showed improvement following treatment with this organism [57]. In an initial randomized trial, recurrences occurred in 9 of 26 (34%) patients who had RCDAD following therapy with *S boulardii*, compared with 22 of 34 (65%) who received placebo [58]. A subsequent trial showed similar efficacy in patients who were treated with *S boulardii* plus high-dose vancomycin (2 g/d). Three of 18 patients (17%) had a recurrence, compared with 7 of 14 patients (50%) in the placebo group; however, no significant difference was found in subgroups of patients who took lower doses of vancomycin or metronidazole [59].

Lactobacillus GG also showed efficacy in RCDAD, although only in uncontrolled trials. In one report of five patients who were treated with this organism, four had an immediate response and no further relapses, and the fifth responded to two courses of therapy [60]. Additional trials reported efficacy in two of four children [61] and five of nine adults [62]. Although a preliminary report of a controlled trial suggested efficacy, no final report has been published [63]. A small randomized, controlled trial evaluated *L plantarum* 299v therapy in RCDAD, but it was not powered adequately to show a significant benefit [64].

Several alternate approaches to the treatment of RCDAD have been attempted. Several reports described benefit with stool donation, which can be administered by rectal infusion [65], fecal enema [66], colonoscopy [67], or nasogastric tube [68]. One group studied the rectal instillation of a mixture of aerobic and anaerobic bacteria, and found loss of *C difficile* and its toxin from the stool of six patients who had RCDAD [69]. This treatment led to bowel colonization by *Bacteroides* species. Oral administration of nontoxigenic strains of *C difficile* also was effective in a report of two patients [70]. Because these therapies only have been evaluated in small numbers of patients and in uncontrolled studies, their use should be considered investigational at this time.

In summary, although several probiotics have been evaluated in the management of RCDAD, the strongest evidence supports the use of *S boulardii*. Additional controlled trials are indicated.

PANCREATITIS

In patients who have severe acute pancreatitis, necrosis and infection contribute to poor outcomes and increased mortality. Probiotics have been used in this setting in the hopes of reducing bacterial translocation, and thus, preventing secondary pancreatic infections. Animal models of acute pancreatitis showed a reduction in bacterial translocation with the use of *L plantarum* 299v [71] and *S boulardii* [72]. In a human study, the use of live *L plantarum* 299v resulted in reduced rates of pancreatic infection, with abscess formation occurring in 1 of 22 patients compared with 7 of 23 patients who received an inactivated preparation [73]. More recently, these investigators evaluated a preparation of four different lactobacilli species, and found a trend toward lower incidence of multiorgan failure, septic complications, and mortality that was not statistically significant [74]. Although initial trials seem to be promising, controlled trials are not available. A larger multicenter trial is investigating the infectious complications of acute pancreatitis using a multispecies probiotic preparation [75].

ACUTE DIARRHEA IN INFANTS AND CHILDREN

The use of probiotics for the prevention and treatment of acute diarrhea in the pediatric population was reviewed recently by Vanderhoof and Young [76]. Several placebo-controlled studies showed efficacy for *Lactobacillus* GG in reducing the severity and duration of acute diarrhea. A meta-analysis of 18 studies concluded that probiotic therapy shortens the duration of acute diarrheal illness in children by approximately 1 day [77]. Placebo-controlled studies also suggest a benefit for *Lactobacillus* GG in the prevention of community-acquired acute diarrhea, and for combination probiotic therapy in the prevention of nosocomial diarrhea [76].

SUMMARY

Probiotics have been studied in a variety of GI infections, and are an appealing concept given their favorable safety profiles. Several placebo-controlled trials indicated that lactobacilli have a suppressive effect on *H pylori* infection. Although some studies reported improvement in *H pylori* eradication, others failed to confirm this. Controlled trials support the use of *Lactobacillus* GG and *S boulardii* for the prevention of AAD, and have demonstrated the effectiveness of *S boulardii* as adjunctive therapy for RCDAD. Several placebo-controlled trials showed a reduction in the severity and duration of acute diarrhea in children with use of *Lactobacillus* GG. Studies of probiotics for the prevention of traveler's diarrhea yielded conflicting results, and their routine use cannot be recommended in this setting. Preliminary evidence suggests a potential role for reducing secondary pancreatic infections, although conclusive evidence is not available at this time. Additional clinical trials are indicated to define the role of probiotics further before widespread use can be recommended.

References

[1] Metchnikoff E. The prolongation of life. London: Putnam's Sons; 1908.
[2] FAO/WHO. Evaluation of health and nutritional properties of probiotics in food including powder milk with live lactic acid bacteria. Expert Consultation Report: Cordoba, Argentina: Food and Agriculture Organization of the United Nations and World Health Organization, October 2001.
[3] Rolfe RD. The role of probiotic cultures in the control of gastrointestinal health. J Nutr 2000;183:396S–402S.
[4] Aiba Y, Suzuki N, Kabir AMA, et al. Lactic acid-mediated suppression of *Helicobacter pylori* by the oral administration of *Lactobacillus salivarius* as a probiotic in a gnotobiotic murine model. Am J Gastroenterol 1998;93(11):2097–101.
[5] Lorca GL, Wadström T, Font de Valdez G, et al. *Lactobacillus acidophilus* autolysins inhibit *Helicobacter pylori* in vitro. Curr Microbiol 2001;42(1):39–44.
[6] Pinchuk IV, Bressollier P, Verneuil B, et al. In vitro anti-*Helicobacter pylori* activity of the probiotic strain *Bacillus subtilis* 3 is due to secretion of antibiotics. Antimicrob Agents Chemother 2001;45(11):3156–61.
[7] Nam H, Ha M, Bae O, Lee Y. Effect of *Weissella confusa* strain PL9001 on the adherence and growth of *Helicobacter pylori*. Appl Environ Microbiol 2002;68(9):4642–5.
[8] Mukai T, Asasaka T, Sato E, et al. Inhibition of binding of *Helicobacter pylori* to the glycolipid receptors by probiotic *Lactobacillus reuteri*. FEMS Immunol Med Microbiol 2002;32(2):105–10.
[9] Michetti P, Dorta G, Wiesel PH, et al. Effect of whey-based culture supernatant of *Lactobacillus acidophilus (johnsonii)* La on *Helicobacter pylori* infection in humans. Digestion 1999;60(3):203–9.
[10] Gotteland M, Cruchet S. Suppressive effect of frequent ingestion of *Lactobacillus johnsonii* La1 on *Helicobacter pylori* colonization in asymptomatic volunteers. J Antimicrob Chemother 2003;51(5):1317–9.
[11] Cruchet S, Obregon MC, Salazar G, et al. Effect of the ingestion of a dietary product containing *Lactobacillus johnsonii* La1 on *Helicobacter pylori* colonization in children. Nutrition 2003;19(9):716–21.
[12] Felley CP, Corthesy-Theulaz I, Rivero JL, et al. Favourable effect of an acidified milk (LC-1) on *Helicobacter pylori* gastritis in man. Eur J Gastroenterol Hepatol 2001;13(1):25–9.
[13] Pantoflickova D, Corthesy-Theulaz I, Dorta G, et al. Favourable effect of regular intake of fermented milk containing *Lactobacillus johnsonii* on *Helicobacter pylori*-associated gastritis. Aliment Pharmacol Ther 2003;18(8):805–13.
[14] Linsalata M, Russo F, Berloco P, et al. The influence of *Lactobacillus brevis* on ornithine decarboxylase activity and polyamine profiles in *Helicobacter pylori*-infected gastric mucosa. Helicobacter 2004;9(2):165–72.
[15] Wang KY, Li SN, Liu CS, et al. Effects of ingesting *Lactobacillus*- and *Bifidobacterium*-containing yogurt in subjects with colonized *Helicobacter pylori*. Am J Clin Nutr 2004;80(3):737–41.

[16] Cats A, Kuipers EJ, Bosschaert MA, et al. Effect of frequent consumption of a *Lactobacillus casei*-containing milk drink in *Helicobacter pylori*-colonized subjects. Aliment Pharmacol Ther 2003;17(3):429–35.

[17] Sakamoto I, Igarashi M, Kimura K, et al. Suppressive effect of *Lactobacillus gasseri* OLL 2716 (LG21) on *Helicobacter pylori* infection in humans. J Antimicrob Chemother 2001;47(5):709–10.

[18] Shimizu T, Haruna H, Hisada K, et al. Effects of *Lactobacillus gasseri* OLL 2716 (LG21) on *Helicobacter pylori* infection in children. J Antimicrob Chemother 2002;50(4): 617–8.

[19] Canducci F, Armuzzi A, Cremonini F, et al. A lyophilized and inactivated culture of *Lactobacillus acidophilus* increases *Helicobacter pylori* eradication rates. Aliment Pharmacol Ther 2000;14(12):1625–9.

[20] Sheu BS, Wu JJ, Lo CY, et al. Impact of supplement with *Lactobacillus*- and *Bifidobacterium*-containing yogurt on triple therapy for *Helicobacter pylori* eradication. Aliment Pharmacol Ther 2002;16(9):1669–75.

[21] Sykora J, Valeckova K, Amlerova J, et al. Effects of a specially designed fermented milk product containing probiotic *Lactobacillus casei* DN-114 001 and the eradication of *H. pylori* in children: a prospective randomized double-blind study. J Clin Gastroenterol 2005;39(8): 692–8.

[22] Tursi A, Brandimarte G, Giorgetti GM, et al. Effect of *Lactobacillus casei* supplementation on the effectiveness and tolerability of a new second-line 10-day quadruple therapy after failure of a first attempt to cure *Helicobacter pylori* infection. Med Sci Monit 2004;10: CR662–6.

[23] Wendakoon CN, Thomson ABR, Ozimek L. Lack of therapeutic effect of a specially designed yogurt for the eradication of *Helicobacter pylori* infection. Digestion 2002;61(1): 16–20.

[24] Armuzzi A, Cremonini F, Ojetti V, et al. Effect of *Lactobacillus* GG supplementation on antibiotic-associated gastrointestinal side effects during *Helicobacter pylori* eradication therapy: a pilot study. Digestion 2001;63(1):1–7.

[25] Armuzzi A, Cremonini F, Bartolozzi F, et al. The effect of oral administration of *Lactobacillus* GG on antibiotic-associated gastrointestinal side-effects during *Helicobacter pylori* eradication therapy. Aliment Pharmacol Ther 2001;15(2):163–9.

[26] Cremonini F, Di Caro S, Covino M, et al. Effect of different probiotic preparations on anti-*Helicobacter pylori* therapy-related side effects: a parallel group, triple blind, placebo-controlled study. Am J Gastroenterol 2002;97(11):2744–9.

[27] Nista EC, Candelli M, Cremonini F, et al. *Bacillus clausii* therapy to reduce side-effects of anti-*Helicobacter pylori* treatment: randomized, double-blind, placebo controlled trial. Aliment Pharmacol Ther 2004;20(10):1181–8.

[28] Myllyluoma E, Veijola L, Ahlroos T, et al. Probiotic supplementation improves tolerance to *Helicobacter pylori* eradication therapy – a placebo-controlled, double-blind randomized pilot study. Aliment Pharmacol Ther 2005;21(10):1263–72.

[29] Kollaritsch H, Holst H, Grobara P, et al. Prevention of traveler's diarrhea with *Saccharomyces boulardii*. Results of a placebo controlled double-blind study. Fortschr Med 1993;111(9):152–6.

[30] Black FT, Andersen PL, Orskov J, et al. Prophylactic efficacy of lactobacilli on traveler's diarrhea. J Travel Med 1989;7:333–5.

[31] Oksanen PJ, Salminen S, Saxelin M, et al. Prevention of travelers' diarrhoea by *Lactobacillus* GG. Ann Med 1990;22(1):53–6.

[32] Hilton E, Kolakowski P, Singer C, et al. Efficacy of *Lactobacillus GG* as a diarrheal preventive in travelers. J Travel Med 1997;4(1):41–3.

[33] De dios Pozo-Olano J, Warram JH Jr, Gomez RG, et al. Effect of a lactobacilli preparation on traveler's diarrhea. A randomized, double blind clinical trial. Gastroenterology 1978;74(5):829–30.

[34] McFarland LV. Epidemiology, risk factors and treatments for antibiotic associated diarrhea. Dig Dis 1998;16(5):292–307.

[35] D'Souza AL, Rajkumar C, Cooke J, et al. Probiotics in prevention of antibiotic associated diarrhea: meta-analysis. BMJ 2002;324(7350):1361.

[36] Szajewska H, Mrukowicz J. Meta-analysis: non-pathogenic yeast *Saccharomyces boulardii* in the prevention of antibiotic-associated diarrhoea. Aliment Pharmacol Ther 2005;22(5): 365–72.

[37] Siitonen S, Vapaatalo H, Salminen S, et al. Effect of *Lactobacillus* GG yoghurt in prevention of antibiotic associated diarrhea. Ann Med 1990;22(1):57–9.

[38] Arvola T, Laiho K, Torkkeli S, et al. Prophylactic *Lactobacillus* GG reduces antibiotic-associated diarrhea in children with respiratory infections: a randomized study. Pediatrics 1999;104(5):e64.

[39] Vanderhoof JA, Whitney DB, Antonson DL, et al. *Lactobacillus* GG in the prevention of antibiotic-associated diarrhea in children. J Pediatr 1999;135(5):564–8.

[40] Thomas MR, Litin SC, Osman DR, et al. Lack of effect of *Lactobacillus* GG on antibiotic-associated diarrhea: a randomized, placebo-controlled trial. Mayo Clin Proc 2001;76(9):883–9.

[41] Gotz V, Romankiewicz JA, Moss J, et al. Prophylaxis against ampicillin-associated diarrhea with a lactobacillus preparation. Am J Hosp Pharm 1979;36(6):754–7.

[42] Tankanow RM, Ross MB, Ertel IJ, et al. A double-blind, placebo-controlled study of the efficacy of Lactinex in the prophylaxis of amoxicillin-induced diarrhea. DICP 1990;24(4): 382–4.

[43] Clements ML, Levine MM, Ristaino PA, et al. Exogenous lactobacilli fed to man—their fate and ability to prevent diarrheal disease. Prog Food Nutr Sci 1983;7(3–4):29–37.

[44] Adam J, Barret C, Barret-Bellet A, et al. Double blind controlled trial of lyphilized Ultra-Levure. Multicenter study by 26 physicians of 386 cases. Gaz Med Fr 1977;84:2072–81.

[45] Surawicz CM, Elmer GW, Speelman P, et al. Prevention of antibiotic-associated diarrhea by *Saccharomyces boulardii*: a prospective study. Gastroenterology 1989;96(4):981–8.

[46] McFarland LV, Surawicz CM, Greenberg RN, et al. Prevention of beta-lactam-associated diarrhea by *Saccharomyces boulardii* compared with placebo. Am J Gastroenterol 1995;90(3):439–48.

[47] Bleichner G, Blehaut H, Mentec H, et al. *Saccharomyces boulardii* prevents diarrhea in critically ill tube-fed patients. A multicenter, randomized, double-blind placebo-controlled trial. Intensive Care Med 1997;23(5):517–23.

[48] Duman DG, Bor S, Ozutemiz O, et al. Efficacy and safety of *Saccharomyces boulardii* in prevention of antibiotic-associated diarrhoea due to *Helicobacter pylori* eradication. Eur J Gastroenterol Hepatol 2005;17(12):1357–61.

[49] Lewis SJ, Potts LF, Barry RE. The lack of therapeutic effect of *Saccharomyces boulardii* in the prevention of antibiotic-related diarrhea in elderly patients. J Infect 1998;37(3):307–8.

[50] Kotowska M, Albrecht P, Szajewska H. *Saccharomyces boulardii* in the prevention of antibiotic-associated diarrhea in children: a randomized double-blind placebo-controlled trial. Aliment Pharmacol Ther 2005;21(5):583–90.

[51] Wunderlich PF, Braun L, Fumagalli I, et al. Double-blind report on the efficacy of lactic acid-producing *Enterococcus* SF68 in the prevention of antibiotic-associated diarrhea and in the treatment of acute diarrhea. J Int Med Res 1989;17(4):333–8.

[52] Borgia M, Sepe N, Brancato V, et al. A controlled clinical study on *Streptococcus faecium* preparation for the prevention of side reactions during long-term antibiotic treatments. Curr Ther Res 1982;31:266–71.

[53] Orrhage K, Brignar B, Nord CE. Effects of supplements of *Bifidobacterium longum* and *Lactobacillus acidophilus* on the intestinal microbiota during administration of clindamycin. Microb Ecol Health Dis 1994;7:17–25.

[54] Colombel JF, Cortot A, Neut C, et al. Yoghurt with *Bifidobacterium longum* reduces erythromycin-induced gastrointestinal effects. Lancet 1987;2(8549):43.

[55] Elmer GW, McFarland LV. Suppression by *Saccharomyces boulardii* of toxigenic *Clostridium difficile* overgrowth after vancomycin treatment in hamsters. Antimicrob Agents Chemother 1987;31:129–31.

[56] Surawicz CM, McFarland LV, Elmer G, et al. Treatment of recurrent *Clostridium difficile* colitis with vancomycin and *Saccharomyces boulardii*. Am J Gastroenterol 1989;84(10): 1285–7.

[57] Popoola J, Swann A, Warwick G. *Clostridium difficile* in patients with renal failure – management of an outbreak using biotherapy. Nephrol Dial Transplant 2000;15(5):571–4.

[58] McFarland LV, Surawicz CM, Greenberg RN, et al. A randomized placebo-controlled trial of *Saccharomyces boulardii* in combination with standard antibiotics for *Clostridium difficile* disease. JAMA 1994;271(24):1913–8.

[59] Surawicz CM, McFarland LV, Greenberg RN, et al. The search for a better treatment for recurrent *Clostridium difficile* disease: use of high-dose vancomycin combined with *Saccharomyces boulardii*. Clin Infect Dis 2000;31(4):1012–7.

[60] Gorbach SL, Chang TW, Goldin B. Successful treatment of relapsing *Clostridium difficile* colitis with *Lactobacillus* GG. Lancet 1987;2:1519.

[61] Biller JA, Katz AJ, Flores AF, et al. Treatment of recurrent *Clostridium difficile* colitis with *Lactobacillus* GG. J Pediatr Gastroenterol Nutr 1995;21(2):224–6.

[62] Bennett RG, Laughon B, Lindsay J, et al. *Lactobacillus* GG treatment of *Clostridium difficile* infection in nursing home patients. Presented at the 3rd International Conference on Nosocomial Infection. Atlanta, July 31–August 3, 1990.

[63] Pochapin M. The effect of probiotics on *Clostridium difficile* diarrhea. Am J Gastroenterol 2000;95:S11–3.

[64] Wullt M, Hagslatt MJ, Odenholt I. *Lactobacillus plantarum* 299v for the treatment of recurrent *Clostridium difficile*-associated diarrhoea: a double-blind, placebo-controlled trial. Scand J Infect Dis 2003;35:365–7.

[65] Schwan A, Sjölin S, Trottestam U, et al. Relapsing *Clostridium difficile* enterocolitis cured by rectal infusion of normal faeces. Scand J Infect Dis 1984;16:211–5.

[66] Bowden TA, Mansberger AR, Lykins LE. Pseudomembranous enterocolitis: mechanism of restoring floral homeostasis. Am Surg 1981;47:178–83.

[67] Persky SE, Brandt LJ. Treatment of recurrent *Clostridium difficile*–associated diarrhea by administration of donated stool directly through a colonoscope. Am J Gastroenterol 2000;95(11):3283–5.

[68] Aas J, Gessert CE, Bakken JS. Recurrent *Clostridium difficile* colitis: case series involving 18 patients treated with donor stool administered via a nasogastric tube. Clin Infect Dis 2003;36:580–5.

[69] Tvede M, Rask-Madsen J. Bacteriotherapy for chronic relapsing *Clostridium difficile* diarrhoea in six patients. Lancet 1989;1(8648):1156–60.

[70] Seal D, Borriello SP, Barclay F, et al. Treatment of relapsing *Clostridium difficile* diarrhoea by administration of a non-toxigenic strain. Eur J Clin Microbiol 1987;6:51–3.

[71] Mangiante G, Colucci G, Canepari P, et al. *Lactobacillus plantarum* reduces infection of pancreatic necrosis in experimental acute pancreatitis. Dig Surg 2001;18:47–50.

[72] Akyol S, Mas MR, Comert B, et al. The effect of antibiotic and probiotic combination therapy on secondary pancreatic infections and oxidative stress parameters in experimental acute necrotizing pancreatitis. Pancreas 2003;26(4):363–7.

[73] Olah A, Belagyi T, Issekutz A, et al. Randomized clinical trial of specific lactobacillus and fibre supplement to early enteral nutrition in patients with acute pancreatitis. Br J Surg 2002;89(9):1103–7.

[74] Olah A, Belagvi T, Issekutz A, et al. Combination of early nasojejunal feeding with modern symbiotic therapy in the treatment of severe acute pancreatitis (prospective, randomized, double-blind study). Magy Seb 2005;58(3):173–8.

[75] Besselink MGH, Timmerman HM, Buskens E, et al. Probiotic prophylaxis in patients with pre-dicted severe acute pancreatitis (PROPATRIA): design and rationale of a double-blind, pla-cebo-controlled randomized multicenter trial. BMC Surg 2004;4(1):12.
[76] Vanderhoof JA, Young RJ. Pediatric applications of probiotics. Gastroenterol Clin North Am 2005;34:451–63.
[77] Huang JS, Bousvaros A, Lee JW, et al. Efficacy of probiotic use in acute diarrhea in children. A meta-analysis. Dig Dis Sci 2002;47(11):2625–34.

Gastroenterol Clin N Am 35 (2006) 367–391

GASTROENTEROLOGY CLINICS
OF NORTH AMERICA

Diagnosis and Management of Diverticulitis and Appendicitis

Edward P. Dominguez, MD, John F. Sweeney, MD*, Yong U. Choi, MD

Minimally Invasive Surgery, Baylor College of Medicine, 1709 Dryden, Suite 1500, Houston, TX 77030, USA

DIAGNOSIS AND MANAGEMENT OF DIVERTICULITIS

Diverticular disease of the colon is a common problem in the Western world and includes diverticulosis and diverticulitis. Colonic diverticula are outpouchings or pseudodiverticula that occur at the weak points of the colonic wall where small feeding blood vessels enter the circular muscle layer. It seems to be associated with a poor diet with low fiber and high fat [1]. Approximately two thirds of the population greater than 85 years old and one third of the population greater than 45 years old have diverticulosis [2]. The sigmoid colon is the most frequent site of involvement with 65% of patients having the disease at that site. Rarely do patients have disease isolated to other colonic locations without evidence of diverticulosis in the sigmoid colon. For example, diverticulosis isolated to the right colon is uncommon and is seen in less than 5% of patients who have diverticular disease [3–5].

Most patients who have diverticulosis remain asymptomatic; however, 15% to 30% of patients will have complications. Diverticulitis is a complication of diverticulosis that occurs when these outpouchings become infected. Diverticulitis develops in an estimated 15% to 20% of individuals who have diverticulosis [6]. Diverticulitis occurs in a spectrum that ranges from mild to severe. Mild cases of diverticulitis are uncomplicated and consist of mild clinical symptoms or confined pericolonic inflammation. Severe, complicated cases of diverticulitis may be associated with intra-abdominal abscess, generalized purulent peritonitis, fistula formation, perforation, bleeding, or obstruction [6,7]. The ideal therapy for patients who present with diverticulitis varies on the clinical presentation and severity of the disease.

Diagnosis of Diverticulitis
Clinical manifestations
Most patients who have diverticulitis have abdominal pain as their presenting symptom (Table 1). This is associated frequently with fever and a generalized

*Corresponding author. E-mail address: jsweeney@bcm.tmc.edu (J.F. Sweeney).

0889-8553/06/$ – see front matter
doi:10.1016/j.gtc.2006.05.002

Table 1
Diagnostic tests for acute diverticulitis

Tests	Advantages	Disadvantages	Comments
Contrast enema	Low cost Can confirm diagnosis in acute setting	Risk for perforation Cannot grade severity of inflammation or presence of an abscess	Use water-soluble contrast material Barium contraindicated in presence of localized peritonitis
CT	High sensitivity and specificity Can image transmural and extramural disease Patient comfort compared with contrast studies Can classify severity of disease	High cost	Now gold standard for diagnosis of acute diverticulitis Can be used for treatment in conjunction with percutaneous drainage
Ultrasound	Low cost Noninvasive	Operator dependent Difficult to perform with overlying gas-filled loops	Not used readily for diverticulitis
Colonoscopy	Useful in uncomplicated diverticulosis Can evaluate for other diseases (inflammatory bowel disease, ischemic colitis, carcinoma)	Risk for perforation Cannot evaluate extramural disease Can be difficult in setting of acute inflammation	After resolution of acute disease, useful for evaluating the entire colon for other disease processes
Magnetic resonance colonography	Can assess the entire colon accurately Patients not exposed to ionizing radiation	Long time to complete the study Images easily distorted with patient movement/motion artifacts	May increase in use over time but limited use currently

feeling of malaise. The pain typically occurs in the left lower quadrant or suprapubic area. Other less common symptoms that may be seen include diarrhea, constipation, nausea, vomiting, dysuria, and urinary frequency. On physical examination a tender mass in the left lower quadrant is the most common finding. Laboratory examination generally demonstrates a leukocytosis with a left shift. Patients who have severe diverticulitis may present with hypotension, and findings of generalized peritonitis on physical examination [2,7].

Radiologic studies

Radiologic imaging for diverticulitis serves two roles. It allows for diagnosis of diverticulitis in patients who have abdominal pain or other associated clinical symptoms. Also, imaging can be used to assess the severity of diverticulitis and the presence of complications [8]. There are various radiologic options for the evaluation of the colon. These include barium or water-soluble enema, CT scan, ultrasound (US), and MR colonography (MRC).

Colonic contrast studies

Contrast enemas were once considered the gold standard for the diagnosis of diverticulitis; however, because diverticulitis is mostly an extraluminal process, they are now limited in usefulness. A water-soluble enema can confirm the diagnosis of diverticulitis in acute situations but it cannot grade the severity of inflammation or presence of an abscess [8–10]. If a contrast enema is being performed in the setting of acute diverticulitis, water-soluble contrast material should be used with a low-pressure single-contrast study. Barium is contraindicated if there is a presence of localized peritonitis and pericolic abscess, because of a chance of perforation that leads to barium extravasating into the abdominal cavity, which would be highly toxic [8]. With a water-soluble contrast study, the presence of extravasated contrast material outside the colon or into a fistula tract is highly suggestive of diverticulitis [11].

Barium can be used in chronic settings or in demonstrating the distribution of diverticular disease in the absence of diverticulitis. In this setting, the best results are obtained with a proper bowel preparation and using a double-contrast technique. It can be used to confirm the presence of diverticulosis when other differential diagnoses are being entertained [8].

CT scan

CT scanning is considered the imaging modality of choice for the diagnosis of diverticulitis. It has a sensitivity ranging from 85% to 97% [8,9]. It also is the most specific imaging modality for the diagnosis of acute diverticulitis [12]. CT scan is superior to contrast enemas in that it can image transmural and extraluminal disease. It also can image adjacent structures and is more comfortable for the patient. It is significantly less invasive than contrast studies and can be performed in sick patients [8,9].

Another advantage of CT scans is the ability to classify diverticulitis by the severity of the disease. Buckley and colleagues [12] classified diverticulitis as mild, moderate, and severe. Mild diverticulitis was evidenced by bowel wall thickening and pericolic fat stranding. Moderate diverticulitis consists of bowel wall thickening greater than 3 mm with phlegmon or small abscess. Severe diverticulitis is defined as bowel wall thickening greater than 5 mm, localized perforation or subdiaphragmatic free air, and abscess greater than 5 cm [12]. Hinchey and colleagues [13] developed a classification for perforated diverticular disease in relation to CT scan findings. Hinchey stage I consists of pericolic abscess or phlegmon. Stage II is abscess in the pelvis, intra-abdominal cavity, or retroperitoneal space. Hinchey stage III is represented by generalized purulent peritonitis. Stage IV is generalized fecal peritonitis [14]. With these stages in mind, the approach to the management of diverticulitis can be formulated.

CT scans also can be used as a form of treatment when combined with CT-guided drainage.

Ultrasound

Another radiologic approach in the diagnosis of diverticulitis is abdominal US. This is a low cost, noninvasive imaging study; however, it is operator dependent and diverticulitis may be difficult to evaluate. Common criteria that are used for US diagnosis of diverticulitis are colonic mural thickening, pericolic inflammation, and the visualization of the diverticula. With these criteria, other etiologies, such as Crohn's disease, penetrating colonic cancer, ischemic colitis, or other inflammatory conditions, must be ruled out [15].

Hollerweger and colleagues [15] reported findings using an inflamed diverticulum as a sign of diverticulitis. The overall sensitivity was 77% and the specificity was 99%. In uncomplicated disease, the sensitivity was 96%. In patients who had complicated diverticulitis, it was difficult to visualize the diverticulum. Another sonographic finding for acute colonic diverticulitis, as reported by Kori and colleagues [16], is the "dome sign"—a hypoechoic mass protruding at the outer surface of the intestinal wall. In patients with right-sided abdominal pain, 100% of those with a dome sign had diverticulitis as the etiology of the pain. This allowed differentiation from acute appendicitis [16].

Endoscopic procedures

Colonoscopy is useful in diagnosing patients who have uncomplicated diverticulosis; however, it generally is contraindicated in patients who have acute diverticulitis because of the increased risk for perforation. It only should be considered when inflammatory bowel disease, ischemic colitis, or carcinoma are suspected highly [9,17,18]. It is a useful tool in patients who have been treated for diverticulitis. A colonoscopy is indicated in these patients to evaluate for underlying neoplastic disease [18]. When performing a colonoscopy after an episode of diverticulitis, a pediatric colonoscope may improve success if a standard adult colonoscope is difficult to pass through a fixed sigmoid because of a history of inflammation [19].

MR colonography

MRC is a new imaging technique that has been applied to patients who have diverticulitis. At times, colonoscopy can be difficult to complete all the way to the cecum. Patients with a history of severe diverticulitis may have stenosis or fixation of the sigmoid colon. Because it is important to evaluate patients who have diverticular disease for other pathology, MRC can be used to assess the remaining colon accurately. To perform an MRC, a patient undergoes the same bowel preparation as for a colonoscopy. Then, a rectal tube is passed and the colon is filled with 2000 to 2500 mL of water. The patient undergoes MRI, and three-dimensional images are obtained before and after injection of gadolinium-based contrast agents [20,21]. Hartmann and colleagues [22] reported sensitivity of 100% by MRC for detection of polyps at least 10 mm in diameter and 84.2% for polyps between 6 mm and 9 mm in diameter.

MRC also can be used for detection of diverticulitis. Heverhagen and colleagues [23] reported using MRC without any injection of contrast material. In 20 patients who had documented acute diverticulitis, MRC accurately diagnosed 19 patients. Schreyer and colleagues [24] reported correctly diagnosing diverticulitis in 14 patients when MRC results were compared with the gold standard of CT scan. More recently, Ajaj and colleagues [21] reported a sensitivity and specificity of 86% and 92% for detection of sigmoid diverticulitis with dark-lumen MRC. The advantage of MRC over CT scan or barium enema is that patients are not exposed to ionizing radiation. MRC also provides the ability to evaluate the entire colon completely in patients who are unable to tolerate colonoscopy; however, this enthusiasm must be tempered by the fact that MRC takes longer than CT scan to complete. Also, patients who have lower abdominal pain may not be able to be still for a prolonged period of time and motion artifacts could distort the images [24].

Management of Diverticulitis
Medical treatment

In general, the initial treatment for uncomplicated diverticulitis should be nonoperative unless an absolute indication for surgery (eg, peritonitis) exists (Table 2). Patients who have mild diverticulitis can be treated as an outpatient with broad-spectrum oral antibiotics that target aerobic and anaerobic gram-negative rods. These include clinically stable patients with mild symptoms and no peritoneal signs on abdominal examination, who are able to tolerate oral intake. Clear liquids should be initiated until the symptoms resolve at which time diet can be advanced slowly [11,18]. When treating a patient who has diverticulitis as an outpatient, close follow-up is important. Symptomatic improvement should be seen in 2 to 3 days. Antibiotics should be continued for 7 to 10 days. If a patient has increasing pain, fever, or the inability to tolerate oral intake, hospitalization may be necessary [11,18].

If a patient needs to be hospitalized for diverticulitis, he/she should not be allowed to have anything by mouth. Intravenous (IV) fluids and IV broad-spectrum antibiotics that target aerobic and anaerobic gram-negative rods should be instituted. Once again, symptoms should improve in 2 to 3 days. If patients respond to IV antibiotics, diet can be advanced slowly. Antibiotics can be switched to an oral agent with good bioavailability, and the patient discharged, to complete the 7- to 10-day antibiotic course. If patients do not improve, then a surgical consultation is warranted [11,18].

Patients respond well to nonoperative treatment. For first episodes of diverticulitis, 50% to 85% of patients respond to antibiotics and do not require surgery. Only 15% to 30% of patients who are admitted after their first diverticulitis episode require surgery during the same hospitalization [4,11,18,25]. The question about patients who respond to medical management is "Who will recur and who will benefit from elective surgery?".

Table 2
Controversies in the management of acute diverticulitis

Topic	Recommended	Alternative	Comments
Abscess management	CT-guided percutaneous drainage	Resection with diverting ostomy and Hartman's Pouch Resection with primary anastomosis	Primary anastomosis is controversial but some studies report good success
Indications for early surgery	After first episode of severe diverticulitis in young patients Patients who have complications from diverticulitis after the first episode Patients who require chronic immunosuppression	Use same criteria for young patients as for older patients	Indications for early surgery is controversial and there are no universally accepted criteria
Indications for elective surgery	After the second episode of diverticulitis	No surgery unless patients develop complications	Criteria for elective surgery not defined clearly Must evaluate risk and benefits for each individual
Method of surgery (open versus laparoscopic)			No definite criteria for recommendation of laparoscopic versus open surgery. Depends on patient and the experience and comfort level of the surgeon.

CT-guided drainage

When perforation of a diverticulum occurs, an intra-abdominal abscess may form. A CT scan will identify the size and location of the abscess. A small localized abscess may be treated with antibiotics [4,9,11]; however, if there is a large abscess or patients do not respond to antibiotics, a CT scan–guided drainage can be performed [4,6,9,11,18]. Percutaneous drainage has a great advantage in that it can control sepsis immediately without the need for general anesthesia. It also can eliminate the need for a two-stage procedure with an interval colostomy, and allow a patient to be prepared properly for a single-stage procedure [4,6,11]. CT-guided drainage is successful. The success rates for stabilizing patients and allowing for a subsequent one-stage procedure ranges from 74% to 93.7% [4,6,9]. Percutaneous drainage is a palliative procedure and should not be considered a definitive treatment. Patients should have an elective resection performed in approximately 3 to 4 weeks.

Surgical treatment

If patients do not respond to medical management or cannot be controlled with percutaneous drainage, surgery should be considered. There are various discussions on the type of surgical resection for a patient who does not respond to nonoperative management. The consensus development conference from 1999 stated that there was no valid data regarding the best treatment for purulent peritonitis. The options include resection of the diseased segment with a Hartmann's pouch and end-colostomy or resection with primary anastomosis with or without a diverting stoma [25]. A review of other articles gives the same type of options without a definitive choice of surgery. It reports a feasibility of resection with primary anastomosis without diversion. Wasvary and colleagues [26] reported no need for a proximal diversion after primary anastomosis in patients who had pericolic or pelvic abscess. This one-stage approach results in a shorter hospital stay and does not require a second operation; however, a two-stage procedure with an initial resection and proximal diversion is indicated in patients who have severe inflammation and substantial fecal contamination [27,28].

The timing for an elective operation to treat diverticulitis is not defined clearly. Of those patients who respond to antibiotics, 7% to 62% have a recurrence of acute diverticulitis [1,4,11]. After the second episode of diverticulitis, the probability of a third episode is greater than 50% [18]. Recurrent attacks of diverticulitis are less likely to respond to medical management. Therefore, elective surgery is recommended by many surgeons after the second episode of diverticulitis [4,9,11,25,28]. Patients who have complicated diverticulitis may benefit from resection after the first episode [28]; however, this is not a hard and fast rule and the risks and benefits for each individual patient must be evaluated. A patient who requires chronic immunosuppression may benefit from elective surgery after the first episode of diverticulitis. There also is controversy about whether younger patients should have an elective resection after the first episode [4,11,25]. Broderick-Villa and colleagues [29] and Lorimer [30] reported low recurrence rates after initial response to medical management, and elective resection did not prevent late major complications of diverticular disease. Therefore, elective resection was not recommended.

Young patients

The prevalence of diverticulitis in patients who are younger than 50 years old ranges from 5% to 10% [31–33]. Controversy exists on how to treat these patients. Some investigators describe younger patients as having more virulent disease with more complications than do older patients, whereas others do not report a particularly aggressive course [31,33]. There is no agreement on the timing for elective surgical resection. There are reports in the literature that support early resection after the first episode of diverticulitis in younger patients [32,34]. Other reports indicate that there is no absolute need for surgical resection after the first episode, and similar factors should be considered before elective surgery as for older patients [31,33,35]. Chautems and colleagues [36] recommended elective surgical resection for patients less than 50 years old after the first acute episode only if they had severe diverticulitis on CT scan.

Laparoscopic surgery

There has been an increasing volume of data for laparoscopic resection for diverticular disease. It has shown a low complication rate (<10%), shortened hospital stay (2–5 days), and a decrease in length of ileus (1–3 days) [37]. When performed by experienced laparoscopic surgeons, there was no increase in morbidity for laparoscopic surgery for diverticulitis compared with laparoscopic surgery for other diseases [38]. Higher conversion rates seem to be limited to patients who have complicated diverticulitis to include severe inflammation, abscess, and fistulas. For uncomplicated diverticulitis, the conversion rate is acceptable and the laparoscopic approach is a great option [38,39]. Recently, there are reports that even in the presence of abscesses or fistulas, laparoscopic colon resection is feasible with good results when performed by experienced surgeons [40,41].

Complications

Diverticulitis can lead to various complications. These include intra-abdominal abscess, fistula, obstruction, and hemorrhage. Patients with an abscess can be managed with antibiotics for a small abscess or CT-guided drainage for a larger abscess. If the patient continues to deteriorate, emergent surgery is needed with a single-stage or two-stage surgical resection. Fistulas are managed surgically during resection of the diseased segment. If a patient has bowel obstruction, he/she usually can be managed with nonoperative therapy—bowel rest and treatment of diverticulitis with antibiotics. Complete obstruction is unusual. Recurrent attacks of diverticulitis can lead to strictures that are diagnosed by a barium enema. A colonoscopy should be performed to rule out stricture that is due to a neoplasm. If the bowel obstruction does not resolve with bowel rest and nasogastric decompression, surgical intervention is necessary [4,9,28]. Finally, patients may experience hemorrhage from diverticular disease. For most patients, diverticular bleeding is self-limited. The first step is to resuscitate and stabilize the patient. Then, the bleeding source needs to be identified. This can be done with a nuclear medicine scan, angiography, or colonoscopy. Although most diverticular disease occurs in the left colon, bleeding occurs more from right-sided diverticular disease. Angiographic embolization can be used to stop the bleeding. Colonoscopy also can be therapeutic in conjunction with injection, heater probe, or fibrin sealant. If bleeding continues, surgical intervention with segmental resection is performed. If patients have persistent bleeding and no definite bleeding site is identified, a subtotal colectomy may be required [4,9].

Conclusion

Diverticulitis is a disease of the elderly but more young people are being diagnosed in recent years. There are many diagnostic tools available. This is a disease that can be treated successfully by medical treatment or surgery. There are many controversies on the proper timing for elective surgical intervention. Successful diagnosis and treatment of diverticulitis requires a multidisciplinary approach among the gastroenterologists, surgeons, and radiologists.

DIAGNOSIS AND MANAGEMENT OF APPENDICITIS

The term "appendicitis" and the recognition that the definitive therapy for appendicitis is removal of the inflamed appendix date back to the 1890s. The appendectomy is the most commonly performed emergent operation in the world. More than 250,000 appendicitis-related admissions occur annually in the United States, totaling nearly three billion dollars in hospital charges [42]. The current incidence of appendicitis is 86 per 100,000 patients per year with a lifetime risk of 6.7% for women and 8.6% for men [43,44].

Appendicitis occurs when the appendiceal lumen becomes obstructed by fecaliths, hypertrophied lymphatic tissue, tumor, or foreign bodies. The appendix becomes distended as mucosal secretion and bacterial proliferation continue in the face of the obstructed appendiceal lumen. The distension of the appendix initially causes a vague dull pain in the periumbilical area, secondary to stimulation of visceral afferent nerves. As the serosal covering of the appendix becomes inflamed, the parietal localization in the right lower quadrant begins. If the process continues without relief, perforation of the appendix occurs. The organisms that are involved in appendicitis typically are *Bacteroides fragilis* and *Escherichia coli*, but polymicrobial isolates are common.

A timely and accurate diagnosis of appendicitis is important to prevent appendiceal perforation. Therefore, surgeons will accept a certain number of normal or negative appendectomies to minimize the incidence of perforated appendicitis. Negative appendectomy rates are acceptable because perforated appendicitis is associated with a fourfold increase in morbidity and an 11-fold increase in mortality compared with acute appendicitis [45]. There is an inverse relationship between the negative appendectomy rate and the perforation rate [46,47]. In the United States, a 15% negative appendectomy rate has been reported and is more common in women than in men (22% versus 9%, respectively) [44,49]. In cases where the diagnosis of appendicitis has been missed and litigation has been pursued, the perforation rate approached 95% [50]. Patients who have perforated appendicitis have been reported to wait up to 2.5 times longer to seek medical care than those who have acute appendicitis [46,51]. Patients in whom the diagnosis of appendicitis has been missed are less likely to appear in distress, have right lower quadrant pain, or complain of nausea [50]. These atypical presentations prompt less surgical evaluations and more misdiagnoses of gastroenteritis.

Diagnosis of Appendicitis

Clinical diagnosis

Despite advances in diagnostics, the clinical history and physical examination remain paramount to the diagnosis of appendicitis (Table 3). Although a variety of presentations may be noted, the classic order of events, as described by Sir

Table 3
Diagnostic tests for suspected acute appendicitis

Tests	Advantages	Disadvantages	Comments
Blood studies alone without imaging	Cheap, readily available	Not specific enough to be used alone	Usually coupled with imaging unless high clinical suspicion
CT	Identifies other intra-abdominal pathology; diagnostic accuracy increasing	Expensive, must have timely reading from radiologist; reluctance of use in pregnancy	Most commonly ordered imaging test; no consensus on contrast route
CT with oral contrast	Visualizes the bowel and surrounding structures	Aspiration risk, not tolerated well by ill patients	Used routinely in many centers; controversial
CT with IV contrast	Visualizes the bowel wall and mesenteric vessels	Extravasation, skin reaction, potential renal damage	Used routinely in some centers; controversial
Ultrasound	Noninvasive, no contrast required; safe in pregnancy	Highly operator dependent	Based on an individual center's experience; typically first test in pregnancy
Tagged leukocyte study	Helpful in intermediate cases	Expensive, time consuming; false positives, not widely available	Not used widely
Colonoscopy	Highly sensitive; evaluates entire colon for other pathology	Risk for perforation; requires bowel preparation	Helpful in nonacute setting where diagnosis is in question

Zachary Cope [52], of pain, followed by nausea and vomiting, local iliac tenderness, fever, and leukocytosis still apply. Classically, the pain is recognized initially in the periumbilical or epigastric regions and subsequently localizes to the right lower quadrant over several hours; however, pain descriptions may differ based on the position of the appendix. For example, when the appendix is retrocecal, the initial pain manifestation may be in the right iliac or flank region. Additionally, a long appendix that crosses the midline may cause left lower quadrant pain. Nausea and anorexia are present nearly always and typically occur after the onset of pain. Vomiting may accompany the nausea, but rarely occurs before the onset of pain if appendicitis is present.

Perhaps no other pathologic process in the abdomen has better known physical examination findings than does appendicitis. An examiner often finds the subjects laying flat and motionless with their right leg drawn up to relieve the pressure of the right lower quadrant inflammatory mass. It should be emphasized that, as with pain location, physical examination findings are widely dependent on the position of the appendix. Most patients, at some time in their course, exhibit tenderness in the right lower quadrant. Direct rebound tenderness in this area is a response to the inflamed appendix and its proximity to the peritoneal surface. This localized peritoneal irritation also may be demonstrated by indirect referred tenderness in the right lower quadrant that is elicited with left lower quadrant pressure (ie, Rovsing's sign). Involuntary guarding refers to muscle contraction in response to the inflamed parietal peritoneum. This finding, along with rebound tenderness, is an independent predictor of appendicitis [53]. Cutaneous hyperesthesias on the right at the levels of T10, T11, and T12 dermatomes may be present, but are assessed rarely. A positive "psoas sign" occurs when a patient experiences pain while on their left side and an examiner slowly extends the right thigh. Pain occurs as the iliopsoas is irritated by the inflamed appendix. In turn, the obturator sign may be elicited by an examiner internally rotating the flexed right thigh while the patient is supine. This brings the obturator internus in contact with an irritated pelvis, which produces hypogastric pain. Finally, the patient's temperature is a poor predictor of appendicitis [54], but when high and accompanied by tachycardia, a ruptured appendicitis with intra-abdominal abscess should be suspected.

Often, the patient has been premedicated with narcotics before surgical evaluation. This remains a controversial practice that is promoted by emergency physicians and discouraged by surgeons. Keeping with classic surgical dogma, surgeons worry that adequate analgesic relief may alter the accuracy of diagnosis and the ability to obtain informed consent [52,55]. The logistical difficulties that are inherent to this problem, including patient randomization, adequate sample sizes, blinding of patient and examiner, actual disease process causing the pain, and varied availability of operating rooms, have made multicenter studies and evidence-based approaches unobtainable [56]. In the small studies that exist, judicious and appropriate doses of narcotic analgesia seem to provide significant pain relief without altering physical examination findings or the diagnostic process in patients who truly have appendicitis [56–58]. LoVecchio and colleagues [59] reported that 5 mg or 10 mg of morphine, given to patients who have acute abdominal pain, significantly alters their physical examination findings (tenderness and localization) without altering their diagnosis or management when compared with placebo. In one retrospective review, up to 50% of patients with a misdiagnosis of appendicitis required narcotic pain medicine before discharge from the emergency room, which emphasizes the need for observation and experienced surgical evaluation if narcotics are given [50].

Laboratory diagnosis

As radiographic diagnostic modalities have improved, less emphasis has been placed on laboratory diagnosis in patients who present with suspected appendicitis. Although laboratory evaluation is cheap, rapid, and readily available, elevated values are weak predictors of appendicitis when viewed alone. Several studies have demonstrated the proportion of polymorphonuclear cells and the white blood cell (WBC) count are important diagnostic predictors of appendicitis [46,53,60–62]. One such study suggested that a WBC count of greater than 12,300/mL is associated with a twofold increase in appendicitis in patients who had suspected appendicitis [63]; however, several studies have reported that WBC counts of greater than 10,000/mL was only 76% to 93% sensitive and 38% to 63% specific for appendicitis [54,64]. This lack of specificity precludes surgeons from taking a patient to surgery based on WBC count alone.

Although there is no single laboratory value that is particularly accurate by itself, a combination of values may be promising. Dueholm and colleagues [64] reported that when WBC count, neutrophil differential, and C-reactive protein levels are within the normal reference ranges, the negative predictive value is 100%. When the diagnosis is otherwise in doubt, this "triple test" may identify patients who warrant further observation rather than undergoing a likely negative laparotomy. Similar findings have been reported when combining WBC and C-reactive protein with and without phospholipase A2 [65,66]. If the patient has a WBC count of greater than 18,000/mL perforation or another diagnosis should be entertained. A urine analysis sample may have red blood cells or WBCs, but typically not bacteria.

Role of imaging in diagnosis

Advances in the diagnostic accuracy of imaging have altered the approach to patients who have suspected appendicitis. Adjunctive diagnostic tests may be used in cases where the presentation is atypical or other tests are equivocal. This is especially applicable in the pediatric population and in women of child-bearing age in whom the correct diagnosis may be elusive. Plain films are not performed routinely or considered mandatory but may reveal an appendicolith, a localized ileus, or a unsuspected pneumonia. Barium enema is used rarely as a diagnostic modality in this disease. Some of the more commonly recommended diagnostic images include leukocyte-tagged studies, US, and computed tomography.

Leukocyte-tagged studies

Technetium-labeled WBC scans have been used in atypical presentations with sensitivities of 85% to 98%, accuracies of 89% to 97%, and a reduction in negative appendectomy rates [67–69]. These tests are expensive, time consuming, not universally available, and susceptible to false positives because any inflammation may cause WBC accumulation. For these reasons, leukoscintingraphy is not used widely as an aid in the diagnosis of appendicitis.

Ultrasound

Much has been written in the surgical, radiology, and gastroenterology literature about the efficacy of US in the setting of appendicitis. US is an attractive diagnostic imaging option because it is inexpensive, rapid, noninvasive, safe in pregnancy, and does not require contrast; however, US can be considered useful in the evaluation for appendicitis only if it improves upon the most commonly used diagnostic tool: clinical impression. Findings that are suggestive of appendicitis include a thickened, noncompressible, blind-ended wall that is greater than 6 mm in diameter. Other findings include the absence of gas in the appendiceal lumen, the presence of blood flow in the appendiceal wall, and appendicoliths [70,71]. If the diameter of the outer appendiceal wall is greater than 6 mm in the anterior–posterior direction, sensitivities and negative predictive values up to 98% to 100% have been reported, but with a specificity of only 68% [72,73]. Franke and colleagues [70] reported the presence of a target sign as the most clinically diagnostic finding. Other potentially important findings that are identified by US include right-sided diverticulitis, colitis, terminal ileitis, mesenteric lymphadenitis, ovarian cysts, tubo-ovarian abscesses, and ectopic pregnancies [74,75]. If the symptoms suggest a gynecologic origin, an endovaginal US should be considered. The accuracy of using US findings to diagnose appendicitis is operator dependent [74,76,77].

CT

Findings on CT that are suggestive of appendicitis include abnormalities of the appendix, such as an enlarged appendix greater than 6 mm, wall thickening, and appendicoliths, as well as right lower quadrant inflammatory changes (eg, fat stranding, fluid, phlegmon, abscess, free air, adenopathy, adjacent bowel thickening) [78]. Rao and colleagues [78] reported finding an enlarged appendix greater than 6 mm and right lower quadrant fatty stranding in 93% of patients who had appendicitis. Using focused, helical imaging after administration of rectal contrast, the same group reported an accuracy, sensitivity, and specificity of 98% [79]. This technique resulted in a change in management in more than 50% of patients in whom appendicitis was suspected, which prevented unnecessary appendectomies and admissions and identified other diagnoses [79]. The same group increased the sensitivity to 100% when adding oral contrast while limiting the overall radiation exposure to one third of a standard CT of the abdomen and pelvis [80].

During this same time period, this group also convincingly described a significant reduction in cost when CT was used routinely in the evaluation by preventing unnecessary appendectomies, observations before necessary appendectomies, and admissions when appendicitis was not present [79,81]. Five years later, using various contrast regimens and thin, focused cuts, this group reported a negative appendectomy rate of 3% [82]. In this latest series, only 12% of patients went to surgery without CT evaluation and equivocal readings were reported in only 1.9% of adult cases. These results indicate that the diagnostic value of CT improves as a center's experience increases.

Compare and "contrast"

Controversy abounds as to the best CT technique to use with arguments for and against oral contrast, rectal contrast, IV contrast, triple contrast, and no contrast at all. The use of IV contrast aids in visualization of the bowel wall and may increase visualization of an inflamed appendix without the delay or burden of oral or rectal contrast administration. Studies that evaluated IV contrast have reported only adequate sensitivities of 92% and accuracies from 91% to 98% [83,84]. Jacobs and colleagues [85] compared a focused approach using oral contrast with an unfocused approach with IV contrast added; IV contrast significantly improved the reader's ability to identify appendicitis as well as alternative diagnoses.

Evaluation of the abdomen without any contrast enhancement avoids the administration of IV contrast and the potential for injection site extravasation, renal damage, contrast allergy, skin rash, respiratory compromise, and death [86]. Additionally, the routine administration of oral contrast, which may not be tolerated well by a patient who is nauseated, presents an additional risk of aspiration if general anesthesia is required and commonly delays study completion for several hours [87]. Additionally, unenhanced CT is generally less expensive, does not require the presence of a radiologist, and avoids the discomfort and theoretic perforation risk of rectal contrast administration [88]. Unenhanced CT evaluation has sensitivities reported from 96%, specificities of 99%, and accuracy of 97% [89]. Peck and colleagues [88], in a large rural setting, described reducing their negative appendectomy rates to 5% while maintaining an accuracy of 97% with unenhanced CT scans. Without any contrast a normal appendix was reported to be visualized in 79% of cases with adequate interobserver agreement [90].

Recently, Anderson and colleagues [91] systematically reviewed 23 mostly prospective reports and compared the diagnostic value of CT with rectal, oral, rectal and oral, oral and IV, and no contrast. Overall, sensitivities ranged from 83% to 97%, specificities ranged from 93% to 98%, and accuracies ranged from 92% to 97%. Unenhanced studies exhibited higher specificity, positive predictive value, and accuracy, while maintaining similar sensitivity and negative predictive value as compared with contrast studies [91]. The explanation for this is unclear and may be due, in part, to publication bias. Regardless, a limited number of prospective, randomized studies have led to a lack of a national standard.

CT controversies

Not all reports have been supportive of routine CT usage. Lee and colleagues [92] found that rather than increasing diagnostic accuracy, CT delayed management and provided less benefit than did diagnostic laparoscopy. Recently, Garfield and colleagues [93] reported that the routine use of CT increased time in the emergency room by an average of 9 hours without increasing diagnostic accuracy. Perez and colleagues [94], however, reported that their negative appendectomy rate increased from 12% to 17% after CT was introduced in their series, while significantly increasing the length of stay in the emergency room. A recent prospective, randomized comparison of clinical assessment versus CT with IV and oral contrast revealed similar accuracies (90% versus 92%) and a higher sensitivity for clinical assessment (100% versus 91%) [95]. Length of stay and total costs were similar, but time to operating room was increased when CT was used. These studies call to light the legitimate concerns about institutional variability between who orders the CT and who interprets it, which ultimately may lead to discrepancies [96]. Recently, Flum and colleagues

[48] analyzed the records of patients who had appendicitis in a large health care system and found no increase in the accuracy of diagnosis, despite the increasing use of CT and US.

These studies fuel the skepticism that some surgeons have over relying on imaging to diagnose a clinical disease. In a recent survey of practicing surgeons, 62% believed that CT scan was overused and 74% believed its accuracy to be less than the stated 98% [97]. As a result, most of these respondents order CT scans in the evaluation of appendicitis less than 50% of the time. In most cases (63%), the CT is ordered by an emergency medicine physician, and, alarmingly, in more than 30% of cases the scan may be interpreted by someone other than an attending radiologist [97].

Less than 1% of all appendectomies turn out to be for neoplasms, and up to 40% of these may present clinically as appendicitis [98]. CT evaluation may suggest an appendiceal neoplasm in some cases, which could alter the operative approach. Pickhardt and colleagues [98] reported that 95% of primary appendiceal neoplasms were larger than 15 mm on CT or had concerning morphologic abnormalities.

Role of colonoscopy in diagnosis of appendicitis

Gastroenterologists are not asked to perform colonoscopies infrequently in patients who present with right lower quadrant pain when symptoms are not specific, when imaging studies are nondiagnostic, when appendectomy has been performed, or when the symptoms are chronic [99]. These patients often have CT scans that suggest diagnoses other than appendicitis, including inflammatory bowel disease, diverticulitis, colitis, or cecal cancer. Findings that are suggestive of appendicitis include mucosal hyperemia, bulging at the area of the orifice, spontaneous discharge of pus, and discharge of pus following forceps biopsy [100,101]. Uehara and colleagues [100] reported these findings during a routine colonoscopy in an asymptomatic patient who underwent immediate appendectomy with pathologically confirmed appendicitis. Inflammation in the remainder of the appendix following appendectomy, referred to as stump appendicitis, also has been diagnosed in this fashion [102]. Although determining the exact diagnostic accuracy of colonoscopy for appendicitis is challenging, Chang and colleagues [101], in their retrospective review, estimated a sensitivity of 100% and a specificity of 99%. Ohtaka and colleagues [103] reported the diagnosis of a suspected periappendiceal abscess found by chance during a colonoscopic biopsy near a cecal lesion leading to successful endoscopic drainage of pus. Colonoscopy does present the theoretic risk for furthering or creating abscess formation with insufflation and bowel preparation as well as aggravating symptoms.

Management of Appendicitis

Except in areas of remote medical care, appendectomy has been the treatment of appendicitis since the entity was described first. A decade ago, Erickson and Granstrom [104] randomized patients who had appendicitis to antibiotic therapy for 10 days or appendectomy. The nonoperative group was treated successfully in 95% of cases; however, 35% of cases recurred with rupture or phlegmon within an average of 7 months.

Patients who are diagnosed with appendicitis should be hydrated adequately and started on antibiotics. In the case of uncomplicated appendicitis, a third-generation cephalosporin is administered for 24 hours or less. For more complicated infections, broader antibiotic coverage with carbapenems or triple coverage with a cephalosporin, metronidazole, and an aminoglycoside is instituted before appendectomy (Table 4).

Open appendectomy

The incision of choice for an open appendectomy (OA; McBurney's, Rocky-Davis, midline) is based on the point of maximal tenderness or image findings that facilitate localizing the appendix and the ligating appendiceal artery. The inflamed appendix is removed by simple ligation, purse string ligation, or gastrointestinal stapler, and the peritoneal cavity is irrigated. The remaining wound is closed in layers, except in the case of perforation whereby the skin and subcutaneous tissue are packed open to minimize the risk for wound infection. If, upon evaluation, the appendix is normal, a methodical search is performed to find the source of pathology with special attention to the small bowel and, in the female patient, pelvic structures.

Laparoscopic appendectomy

To perform a laparoscopic appendectomy (LA), access to the abdominal cavity is gained in the periumbilical region and a laparoscope is inserted. This allows for visualization of the entire abdominal cavity. Two or three additional

Table 4
Controversies in the management of suspected acute appendicitis

Topic	Recommended	Alternative	Comments
Pain management	Judicious use for patient comfort during work-up	Withhold all pain medicines before evaluation by surgical team	Most recent studies show small incremental doses of narcotics do not alter diagnostic accuracy
Prophylactic antibiotics	Acute: perioperative abx only Ruptured: IV abx until hospital discharge followed by po abx for 7–10 days	Ruptured: IV abx while in hospital and no abx at discharge	No consensus but most surgeons continue oral abx after discharge when appendix was ruptured
Open versus laparoscopic	Laparoscopic	Open	Should be based on surgeon's experience and preference
Abscess management	CT-guided percutaneous drainage, IV abx, interval appendectomy	Open exploration, appendectomy, drainage	Excellent results reported with initial percutaneous drainage

Abbreviations: abx, antibiotics; po, by mouth.

operating trocars are placed to facilitate exposure and dissection of the appendix. The base of the appendix and the appendiceal mesentery are transected using an endoscopic stapling device. The specimen is removed from the abdomen using a small specimen bag and the small incisions are closed. As with an OA, if the appendix appears grossly normal an extensive search for other pathology is undertaken.

Laparoscopic versus open appendectomy: which approach is better?

The advantages of an LA compared with a conventional OA are debatable. A recent review of a nationwide database and several meta-analyses have reported less wound infections, less pain, less complications, and faster recovery following LA [105–107]; however, there is no consensus among the most recent prospective randomized trials over the last 10 years [108–124]. Some studies have revealed that LA is associated with less pain medication and shorter hospital stay [109–111,118–120], whereas others reported fewer wound infections [109,111,113,119,120]. Others demonstrate no difference between LA and OA in wound infection rates, complications [108,110,112–118,121,124], or hospital stay [108,112–115,117,121,124]. A recent, well-designed, prospective, randomized, double-blinded study revealed no differences in complications, pain, activity, hospital discharge, or resumption of diet [123].

LA, on average, takes 18 minutes longer than does OA, and conversion rates from LA to OA range from 5% to 23% [108–124]. Longer operating room times result in higher costs unless patients are sent home earlier. LA may be associated with less cost when indirect costs are considered, such as return to work, in otherwise healthy patients [116,118]. Several of the prospective, randomized studies suggest this advantage by demonstrating quicker time to full recovery and activity [109–111,114,116–119,121,124], whereas others have refuted this advantage [115,122,123]. Laine and colleagues [114] randomized young women who had presumed appendicitis to open exploration or laparoscopy, and revealed the added benefit of laparoscopy by establishing the diagnosis in 96% versus 72% for open surgery, which resulted in a lower negative appendectomy rate (44% to 4%). In a similarly designed trial, Larsson and colleagues [125] reduced the negative appendectomy rate from 34% to 7%, and identified gynecologic pathology when the appendix was normal that was not picked up during OA. In men, the advantages are less clear [110,112,122]. When the appendix is found to be ruptured during laparoscopy, appendectomy can be performed safely, but open conversion rates are higher [126–128]. We advocate LA at Baylor College of Medicine for two reasons. The laparoscopic approach provides superior visualization of the abdominal cavity and allows for a more thorough exploration of the abdominal cavity should the appendix appear normal. Additionally, it is an advanced laparoscopic procedure that gives surgeons experience with manipulating the bowel laparoscopically; this makes them more comfortable with laparoscopic techniques that are essential for small and large intestinal resections.

Abscess

In up to 25% of cases the appendix is ruptured or a periappendiceal abscess is present [49]. If ruptured appendicitis or abscess is noted, the appendix is removed, the peritoneum is irrigated, and the wound is allowed to heal by secondary intention or delayed primary closer to avoid infection. If broad-spectrum antibiotics are initiated, sampling of peritoneal fluid for culture seems to be unnecessary, except in immunocompromised patients [129]. With the increasing use of preoperative imaging, patients who have periappendiceal abscesses often are diagnosed preoperatively. These patients are treated best with nonoperative management and selective image-guided percutaneous drainage. Immediate operation in these patients results in higher complication rates and longer hospital stays [130,131]. After drainage and antibiotic therapy, these patients should be encouraged to return for interval appendectomy. A significant number of these patients has recurrent appendicitis, but it often is difficult to convince a patient to return for surgery when they are asymptomatic.

Postoperative care

Postoperative complications include wound infections, intra-abdominal abscess, bowel obstruction, and rarely, hernia. These are more likely to occur in patients who have had ruptured appendicitis. Following successful appendectomy for acute, nonruptured appendicitis, antibiotics are discontinued and a diet is resumed. Typically, patients are discharged the next day. In the case of ruptured appendicitis, broad-spectrum IV antibiotics are continued postoperatively. Recently, Taylor and colleagues [132] randomized patients who had acute and perforated appendicitis to placebo or oral antibiotics following IV antibiotics. They reported no significant difference in postoperative infections between groups, which suggests that hospital discharge with oral antibiotics may be unnecessary; however, it is common clinical practice to discharge patients who had ruptured appendicitis with oral antibiotics for 7 to 10 days.

Appendicitis in Pregnancy

Appendicitis complicates 1 in 1500 pregnancies, and is the most frequent reason for nonobstetric surgery during pregnancy [133]. The diagnosis of appendicitis in pregnancy is challenging secondary to the altered location of the appendix, the overlap of signs and symptoms, and the reluctance to perform unnecessary surgery in a pregnant patient. The danger of a missed diagnosis of appendicitis is associated with an increase risk for ruptured appendicitis and peritonitis, which are associated with 10% fetal loss rates [134]. Perforation rates were reported to range from 12% to 55% [133,135].

Because of the limitations of imaging modalities in these patients, physical examination and history are the most important parts of the evaluation. Often, US is the first image obtained, but operator experience and the inconsistent location of the appendix in this population hampers the accuracy, especially in the third trimester. CT is beneficial in diagnosis when used with limited helical scanning at less than 0.003 Gy [136]. Because of potential teratogenesis, emphasis is placed on balancing the image quality and the radiation dose [137]. Several small studies demonstrated the successful use of MRI in this group citing the avoidance of contrast and the lack of biologic risk [138,139]. When appendicitis is suspected, a laparoscopic approach is a safe and effective surgical option [140].

Appendicitis in the Elderly

As life expectancy increases, the frequency of appendicitis in the elderly is more common. Up to 74% may have atypical presentations and often delay seeking medical evaluation, which contributes to the difficulty in making an accurate diagnosis [141]. Even after presentation, these patients often are misdiagnosed by physicians who assume other diagnoses or are more concerned with the co-morbidities. These patients often end up being admitted with presumed diverticulitis or partial small bowel obstruction. Not surprisingly, this population has perforation rates that range from 51% to 72% [43,141,142] and higher morbidity and mortality [142]. Storm-Dickerson and Horattas [141] reported a decrease in ruptured appendicitis in this population from 72% to 51% with the earlier use of CT. Additionally, a recent, large observational study revealed that a laparoscopic approach in this population was safe and resulted in shorter hospital stays and fewer complications [143]. Whatever the operative approach, the best outcomes in this population result from a high index of suspicion for appendicitis and abdominal imaging when necessary.

SUMMARY

Diverticulitis and appendicitis are common infections of the gastrointestinal tract that require urgent medical and surgical attention. Successful management of these conditions requires a multidisciplinary approach among primary care providers, gastroenterologists, surgeons, and radiologists. The diagnosis of appendicitis, in particular, can be difficult. Advances in radiographic imaging have improved the diagnostic accuracy in these infections. Minimally invasive surgical techniques have improved the patient's postoperative recovery when surgery is necessary in the management of these conditions.

References

[1] Mueller MH, Glatzle J, Kasparek MS, et al. Long-term outcome of conservative treatment in patients with diverticulitis of the sigmoid colon. Eur J Gastroenterol Hepatol 2005;17: 649–54.

[2] Chandra V, Nelson H, Russell D, et al. Impact of primary resection on the outcome of patients with perforated diverticulitis. Arch Surg 2004;139:1221–4.

[3] Martinez SA, Cheanvechai V, Alasfar FS, et al. staged laparoscopic resection for complicated sigmoid diverticulitis. Surg Laparosc Endosc Percutan Tech 1999;9(2):99–105.

[4] Stollman NH, Raskin JB. Diagnosis and management of diverticular disease of the colon in adults. Am J Gastroenterol 1999;94(11):3110–21.

[5] Otterson MF, Korus GB. Diverticular disease. In: Mulholland MW, Lillemoe KD, Doherty GM, et al, editors. Greenfield's surgery. Scientific principles and practice. 4th edition. Philadelphia: Lippincott Williams & Wilkins; 2006. p. 1130–7.

[6] Kaiser AM, Jiang JK, Lake JP, et al. The management of complicated diverticulitis and the role of computed tomography. Am J Gastroenterol 2002;100:910–7.

[7] Chapman J, Davies M, Wolff B, et al. Complicated diverticulitis. Is it time to rethink the rules? Ann Surg 2005;242:576–81.

[8] Halligan S, Saunders B. Imaging diverticular disease. Best Pract Res Clin Gastroenterol 2002;16(4):595–610.

[9] Farrell RJ, Farrell JJ, Morrin MM. Diverticular disease in the elderly. Gastroenterol Clin North Am 2001;30(2):485–96.

[10] Whetsone D, Hazey J, Pofahl WE, et al. Current management of diverticulitis. Curr Surg 2004;61(4):361–5.

[11] Stollman NH, Raskin JB. Diverticular disease of the colon. Lancet 2004;363:631–9.

[12] Buckley O, Geoghegan T, O'Riordain DS, et al. Computed tomography in the imaging of colonic diverticulitis. Clin Radiol 2004;59:977–83.

[13] Hinchey EJ, Schaal PG, Richards GK. Treatment of perforated diverticular disease of the colon. Adv Surg 1978;12:85–109.

[14] Lohrmann C, Ghanem N, Pache G, et al. CT in acute perforated sigmoid diverticulitis. Eur J Radiol 2005;56:78–83.

[15] Hollerweger A, Macheiner P, Rettenbacher T. Colonic diverticulitis: diagnostic value and appearance of inflamed diverticula—sonographic evaluation. Eur Radiol 2002;11: 1956–63.

[16] Kori T, Nemoto M, Maeda M, et al. Sonographic features of acute colonic diverticulitis: the "dome sign". J Clin Ultrasound 2000;28:340–6.

[17] Lee JG, Leung JW. Colonoscopic diagnosis of unsuspected diverticulosis. Gastrointest Endosc 2002;55(6):746–8.

[18] Salzman H, Lillie D. Diverticular disease: diagnosis and treatment. Am Fam Physician 2005;72:1229–34.

[19] Marshall JB. Use of pediatric colonoscope improves the success of total colonoscopy in selected adult patients. Gastrointest Endosc 1996;44(6):675–8.

[20] Hartmann D, Bassler B, Schilling D, et al. Incomplete conventional colonoscopy: magnetic resonance colonography in the evaluation of the proximal colon. Endoscopy 2005;37: 816–20.

[21] Ajaj W, Ruehm SG, Lauenstein T, et al. Dark-lumen magnetic resonance colonography in patients with suspected sigmoid diverticulitis: a feasibility study. Eur Radiol 2005;15: 2316–22.

[22] Hartmann D, Bassler B, Schilling D, et al. Colorectal polyps: detection with dark-lumen MR colonography versus conventional colonoscopy. Radiology 2006;238(1):143–9.

[23] Heverhagen JT, Zielke A, Ishaque N, et al. Acute colonic diverticulitis: visualization in magnetic resonance imaging. Magn Reson Imaging 2001;19:1257–77.

[24] Schreyer AG, Furst A, Agha A, et al. Magnetic resonance imaging based colonography for diagnosis and assessment of diverticulosis and diverticulitis. Int J Colorectal Dis 2004;19:474–80.

[25] Kohler L, Sauerland S, Neugebauer E, et al. Diagnosis and treatment of diverticular disease: results of a Consensus Development Conference. Surg Endosc 1999;13: 430–6.

[26] Wasvary H, Turfah F, Kadro O, et al. Same hospitalization resection for acute diverticulitis. Am Surg 1999;65:632–6.

[27] Wolff BG, Devine RM. Surgical management of diverticulitis. Am Surg 2000;66: 153–6.

[28] Wong WD, Wexner SD, Lowry A, et al. practice parameters for the treatment of sigmoid diverticulitis-supporting documentation. The Standards Task Force of The American Society of Colon and Rectal Surgeons. Dis Colon Rectum 2000;43(3):290–7.

[29] Broderick-Villa G, Burchette RJ, Collins C, et al. Hospitalization for acute diverticulitis does not mandate routine elective colectomy. Arch Surg 2005;140:576–83.

[30] Lorimer JW. Is prophylactic resection valid as an indication for elective surgery in diverticular disease? Can J Surg 1997;40(6):445–8.

[31] Biondo S, Pares D, Rague JM, et al. Acute colonic diverticulitis in patients under 50 years of age. Br J Surg 2002;89:1137–41.
[32] Konvolinka CW. Acute diverticulitis under age forty. Am J Surg 1994;167:562–5.
[33] West SD, Robinson EK, Delu AN, et al. Diverticulitis in the younger patient. Am J Surg 2003;186:743–6.
[34] Cunningham MA, Davis JW, Kaups KL. Medical versus surgical management of diverticulitis in patients under age 40. Am J Surg 1997;174:733–6.
[35] Guzzo J, Hyman N. Diverticulitis in young patients: is resection after a single attack always warranted? Dis Colon Rectum 2004;47(7):1187–91.
[36] Chautems RC, Ambrosetti P, Ludwig A, et al. Long-term follow-up after first acute episode of sigmoid diverticulitis: is surgery mandatory? A prospective study of 118 patients. Dis Colon Rectum 2002;45(7):962–6.
[37] Senagore AJ. Laparoscopic sigmoid colectomy for diverticular disease. Surg Clin North Am 2005;85:19–24.
[38] Schwandner O, Farke S, Bruch HP. Laparoscopic colectomy for diverticulitis is not associated with increased morbidity when compared with non-diverticular disease. Int J Colorectal Dis 2005;20:165–72.
[39] Vargas HD, Ramirez RT, Hoffman GC, et al. Defining the role of laparoscopic-assisted sigmoid colectomy for diverticulitis. Dis Colon Rectum 2000;43(12):1726–31.
[40] Pugliese R, Lernia SD, Scandroglio I, et al. Laparoscopic treatment of sigmoid diverticulitis. A retrospective review of 103 cases. Surg Endosc 2004;18:1344–8.
[41] Laurent SR, Detroz B, Detry O, et al. Laparoscopic sigmoidectomy for fistulized diverticulitis. Dis Colon Rectum 2005;48(1):148–52.
[42] Davies GM, Dasbach EJ, Teutsch S. The burden of appendicitis-related hospitalizations in the United States in 1997. Surg Infect (Larchmt) 2004;5:160–5.
[43] Korner H, Sondenaa K, Soreide JA, et al. Incidence of acute nonperforated and perforated appendicitis: age-specific and sex-specific analysis. World J Surg 1997;21:313–7.
[44] Addiss DG, Shaffer N, Fowler BS, et al. The epidemiology of appendicitis and appendectomy in the Unites States. Am J Epidemiol 1990;132:910–25.
[45] Velanovich V, Satava R. Balancing the normal appendectomy rate with the perforated appendicitis rate. Am Surg 1992;52:264–9.
[46] Colson M, Skinner KA, Dunnington G. High negative appendectomy rates are no longer acceptable. Am J Surg 1997;174:723–7.
[47] Korner H, Sondenaa K, Soreide A, et al. Structured data collection improves the diagnosis of acute appendicitis. Br J Surg 1998;85:341–4.
[48] Flum DR, McClure TD, Morris A, et al. Misdiagnosis of appendicitis and the use of diagnostic imaging. J Am Coll Surg 2005;201:933–9.
[49] Flum DR, Morris A, Koepsell T, et al. Has misdiagnosis of appendicitis decreased over time? JAMA 2001;286:1748–53.
[50] Rusnak RA, Borer JM, Fastow JS. Misdiagnosis of acute appendicitis: common features discovered in cases after litigation. Am J Emerg Med 1994;12:397–402.
[51] Temple CL, Huchcroft SA, Temple WJ. The natural history of appendicitis in adults. Ann Surg 1995;221:278–81.
[52] Cope Z. Appendicitis. London: Oxford; 1972.
[53] Andersson RE, Hugander AP, Ghazi SH, et al. Diagnostic value of disease history, clinical presentation, and inflammatory parameters of appendicitis. World J Surg 1999;23:133–40.
[54] Cordall T, Glasser J, Guss DA. Clinical value of the total white blood cell count and temperature in the evaluation of patients with suspected appendicitis. Acad Med 2004;11:1021–7.
[55] Graber M, Ely J, Clarke S, et al. Informed consent and general surgeons' attitudes toward the use of pain medication in the acute abdomen. Am J Emerg Med 1999;17:113–6.
[56] Wolfe JM, Smithline HA, Phipen S, et al. Does morphine change the physical examination in patients with acute appendicitis? Am J Emerg Med 2004;22:280–5.

[57] Vermeulen B, Morabia A, Unger P, et al. Acute appendicitis: influence of early pain relief on the accuracy of clinical and US findings in the decision to operate- a randomized trial. Radiology 1999;210:639–43.

[58] Mahadevan M, Graff L. Prospective randomized study of analgesic use for ED patients with right lower quadrant abdominal pain. Am J Emerg Med 2000;18:753–6.

[59] LoVecchio F, Oster N, Sturmann K, et al. The use of analgesics in patients with acute abdominal pain. J Emerg Med 1997;15:775–9.

[60] Andersson RE. Meta-analysis of the clinical and laboratory diagnosis of appendicitis. Br J Surg 2004;91:28–37.

[61] Landau O, Watemberg S, Arber N, et al. Retrospective analysis of the benefit of various acute-phase reactants for the diagnosis of acute appendicitis. Dig Surg 1996;13: 457–9.

[62] Hallan S, Asberg A, Edna T. Additional value of biochemical tests in suspected acute appendicitis. Eur J Surg 1997;163:533–8.

[63] Korner H, Soreide JA, Sondenaa K. Diagnostic accuracy of inflammatory markers in patients operated on for suspected acute appendicitis: a receiver operating characteristic curve analysis. Eur J Surg 1999;165:679–85.

[64] Dueholm S, Bagi P, Bud M. Laboratory aid in the diagnosis of acute appendicitis. Dis Col Rectum 1989;32:855–9.

[65] Gronroos JM, Forsstrom JJ, Irjala K, et al. Phospholipase A2, C-reactive protein, and white blood cell count in the diagnosis of acute appendicitis. Clin Chem 1994;40:1757–60.

[66] Gronroos JM, Gronroos P. Leukocyte count and C-reactive protein in the diagnosis of acute appendicitis. Br J Surg 1999;86:501–4.

[67] Evetts BK, Foley CR, Latimer RG, et al. Tc-99m hexamethylpropyleneamineoxide scanning for the detection of acute appendicitis. J Am Coll Surg 1994;179:197–201.

[68] Rypins EB, Evans DG, Hinrichs W, et al. Tc-99-m-HMPAO white blood cell scan for diagnosis of acute appendicitis in patients with equivocal clinical presentation. Ann Surg 1997;226:58–65.

[69] Yan D-C, Shiau Y-C, Wang J-J, et al. Improving the diagnosis of acute appendicitis in children with atypical clinical findings using the technetium-99m hexamethylpropylene amine oxime-labeled white-blood-cell abdomen scan. Pediatr Radiol 2002;32:663–6.

[70] Franke C, Bohner H, Yang Q, et al. Ultrasonography for diagnosis of acute appendicitis: results of a prospective multicenter trial. World J Surg 1999;23:141–6.

[71] Rettenbacher T, Hollerweger A, Gritzmann N, et al. Appendicitis: should diagnostic imaging be performed if the clinical presentation is highly suggestive of the disease? Gastroenterology 2002;123:992–8.

[72] Rettenbacher T, Hollerweger A, Macheiner P, et al. Outer diameter of the veriform appendix as a sign of acute appendicitis: evaluation at US. Radiology 2001;218:757–62.

[73] Kessler N, Cyteval C, Gallix B, et al. Appendicitis: evaluation of sensitivity, specificity, and predictive values of US, Doppler US and laboratory findings. Radiology 2004;203: 472–8.

[74] Lee J, Jeong YK, Hwang JC, et al. Graded compression sonography with adjuvant use of a posterior manual compression technique in the sonographic diagnosis of acute appendicitis. AJR Am J Roentgenol 2002;178:863–8.

[75] Kaneko K, Tsuda M. Ultrasound-based decision making in the treatment of acute appendicitis in children. J Ped Surg 2004;39:1316–20.

[76] Zielke A, Sitter H, Rampp T, et al. Clinical decision-making, ultrasonography and scores for evaluation of suspected acute appendicitis. World J Surg 2001;25:578–84.

[77] Chen S, Chen K, Wang S. Abdominal sonography screening of clinically diagnosed or suspected appendicitis before surgery. World J Surg 1998;22:449–52.

[78] Rao PM, Rhea JT, Novelline RA, et al. Sensitivity and specificity of the individual CT signs of appendicitis: experience with 200 helical appendiceal CT examinations. J Comput Assist Tomogr 1997;21(5):686–92.

[79] Rao PM, Rhea JT, Novelline RA, et al. Effect of computed tomography of the appendix on treatment of patients and use of hospital resources. N Engl J Med 1998;338(3): 141–6.

[80] Rao PM, Rhea JT, Novelline RA, et al. Helical CT technique for the diagnosis of appendicitis: prospective evaluation of a focused appendix CT examination. Radiology 1997;202:139–44.

[81] Rhea JT, Rao PM, Novelline RA, et al. A focused appendiceal CT technique to reduce the cost of caring for patients with clinically suspected appendicitis. AJR Am J Roentgenol 1997;169:113–8.

[82] Rhea JT, Halpern EF, Ptak T. The status of appendiceal CT in an urban medical center 5 years after its introduction: experience with 753 patients. AJR Am J Roentgenol 2005;184: 1802–8.

[83] Iwahashi N, Kitagawa Y, Mayumi T, et al. Intravenous contrast-enhanced computed tomography in the diagnosis of acute appendicitis. World J Surg 2005;29:83–7.

[84] Choi YH, Fischer E, Hoda SA. Appendiceal CT in 140 cases diagnostic criteria for acute and necrotizing appendicitis. Clin Imaging 1998;22:252–71.

[85] Jacobs JE, Birnbaum BA, Macari M, et al. Acute appendicitis: comparison of helical CT diagnosis-focused technique with oral contrast material versus nonfocused technique with oral and intravenous contrast material. Radiology 2001;220:683–90.

[86] Rao PM, Rhea JT, Rattner DW, et al. Introduction of appendiceal CT: impact on negative appendectomy and appendiceal perforation rates. Ann Surg 1999;229(3):344–9.

[87] Wijetunga R, Tan BS, Rouse JC. Diagnostic accuracy of focused appendiceal CT in clinically equivocal cases of acute appendicitis. Radiology 2001;221:747–53.

[88] Peck J, Peck A, Peck C, et al. The clinical role of noncontrast helical computed tomography in the diagnosis of acute appendicitis. Am J Surg 2000;180:133–6.

[89] Lane MJ, Liu DM, Huynh MD. Suspected acute appendicitis: nonenhanced helical CT in 300 consecutive patients. Radiology 1999;213:341–6.

[90] Benjaminov O, Atri M, Hamilton P, et al. Frequency of visualization and thickness of normal appendix at nonenhanced helical CT. Radiology 2002;225:400–6.

[91] Anderson BA, Salem L, Flum DR. A systematic review of whether oral contrast is necessary for the diagnosis of appendicitis in adults. Am J Surg 2005;190:474–8.

[92] Lee SL, Walsh AJ, Ho HS. Computed tomography and ultrasonography do not improve and may delay the diagnosis and treatment of acute appendicitis. Arch Surg 2001;136: 556–62.

[93] Garfield JL, Birkhahn RH, Gaeta TJ. Diagnostic pathways and delays on route to operative intervention in acute appendicitis. Am Surg 2004;70:1010–3.

[94] Perez J, Barone JE, Wilbanks TO, et al. Liberal use of computed tomography scanning does not improve diagnostic accuracy in appendicitis. Am J Surg 2003;185:194–7.

[95] Hong JJ, Cohn SM, Ekeh P, et al. A prospective study of clinical assessment versus computed tomography for the diagnosis of acute appendicitis. Surg Infect 2003;4(3): 231–9.

[96] Maluccio MA, Covey AM, Weyant MJ. A prospective evaluation of the use of emergency department computed tomography for suspected acute appendicitis. Surg Infect (Larchmt) 2001;2(3):205–14.

[97] Sarkaria IS, Eachempati SR, Weyant MJ, et al. Current surgical opinion of computed tomography for acute appendicitis. Surg Infect (Larchmt) 2004;5(3):243–52.

[98] Pickhardt PJ, Levy AD, Rohrmann CA, et al. Primary neoplasms of the appendix manifesting as acute appendicitis: CT findings with pathologic comparison. Radiology 2002;224: 775–81.

[99] Johnson TR, DeCosse JJ. Colonoscopic diagnosis of grumbling appendicitis. Lancet 1998;351:495.

[100] Uehara A, Ohta H, Nagamine M, et al. Colonoscopic diagnosis of asymptomatic acute appendicitis. Am J Gastroenterol 2000;95:3010–1.

[101] Chang H, Yang S, Myung S, et al. The role of colonoscopy in the diagnosis of appendicitis in patients with atypical presentations. Gastrointest Endosc 2002;56:343–8.

[102] Nahon P, Nahon S, Hoang J, et al. Stump appendicitis diagnosed by colonoscopy. Am J Gastroenterol 2002;97:1564–5.

[103] Ohtaka M, Asakawa A, Kashiwagi A, et al. Pericecal appendiceal abscess with drainage during colonoscopy. Gastrointest Endosc 1999;49:107–9.

[104] Erickson S, Granstrom L. Randomized controlled trial of appendectomy versus antibiotic therapy for acute appendicitis. Br J Surg 1995;82:166–9.

[105] Golub R, Siddiqui F, Pohl D. Laparoscopic versus open appendectomy: a meta- analysis. J Am Coll Surg 1998;186:545–53.

[106] Chung RS, Rowland DY, Li P, et al. A meta-analysis of randomized controlled trials of laparoscopic versus conventional appendectomy. Am J Surg 1999;177:250–6.

[107] Guller U, Hervey S, Purves H, et al. Laparoscopic versus open appendectomy. Outcomes comparison based on a large administrative database. Ann Surg 2004;239: 43–52.

[108] Martin LC, Puente I, Sosa JL, et al. Open vs laparoscopic appendectomy. A prospective randomized comparison. Ann Surg 1995;222:256–62.

[109] Ortega AE, Hunter JG, Peters JH, et al. A prospective, randomized comparison of laparoscopic appendectomy with open appendectomy. Am J Surg 1995;169:208–13.

[110] Cox MR, McCall JL, Toouli J, et al. Prospective randomized comparison of open versus laparoscopic appendectomy in men. World J Surg 1996;20:263–6.

[111] Hansen JB, Smithers BM, Schache D, et al. Laparoscopic versus open appendectomy: prospective randomized trial. World J Surg 1996;20:17–21.

[112] Mutter D, Vix M, Bui A, et al. Laparoscopy not recommended for routine appendectomy in men: results of a prospective randomized study. Surgery 1996;120:71–4.

[113] Kazemier G, de Zeeuw GR, Lange JF, et al. Laparoscopic vs open appendectomy. A randomized clinical trial. Surg Endosc 1997;11:336–40.

[114] Laine S, Rantala A, Gullichsen R, et al. Laparoscopic appendectomy—is it worthwhile? A prospective, randomized study in young women. Surg Endosc 1997;11:95–7.

[115] Minne L, Varner D, Burnell A, et al. Laparoscopic vs open appendectomy. Prospective randomized study of outcomes. Arch Surg 1997;132:708–12.

[116] Heikkinen TJ, Haukipuro K, Hulkko A. Cost-effective appendectomy. Open or laparoscopic? A prospective randomized study. Surg Endosc 1998;12:1204–8.

[117] Hellberg A, Rudberg C, Kullman E, et al. Prospective randomized multicenter study of laparoscopic versus open appendectomy. Br J Surg 1999;86:48–53.

[118] Long KH, Bannon MP, Zietlow SP, et al. A prospective comparison of laparoscopic appendectomy with open appendectomy: clinical and economic analyses. Surgery 2001;129: 390–400.

[119] Pedersen AG, Petersen OB, Wara P, et al. Randomized clinical trial of laparoscopic versus open appendectomy. Br J Surg 2001;88:200–5.

[120] Marzouk M, Khater M, Elsadek M, et al. Laparoscopic vs open appendectomy. A prospective comparative study of 227 patients. Surg Endosc 2003;17:721–4.

[121] Milewczyk M, Michalik M, Ciesielski M. A prospective, randomized, unicenter study comparing laparoscopic and open treatments of acute appendicitis. Surg Endosc 2003;17: 1023–8.

[122] Ignacio RC, Burke R, Spencer D, et al. Laparoscopic vs open appendectomy. What is the real difference? Surg Endosc 2004;18:334–7.

[123] Katkhouda N, Mason RJ, Towfigh S, et al. Laparoscopic versus open appendectomy. A prospective randomized double-blind study. Ann Surg 2005;242:439–50.

[124] Moberg AC, Berndsen F, Palmquist I, et al. Randomized clinical trial of laparoscopic versus open appendectomy for confirmed appendicitis. Br J Surg 2005;92:298–304.

[125] Larsson P, Henriksson G, Olsson M, et al. Laparoscopy reduces unnecessary appendectomies and improves diagnosis in fertile women. Surg Endosc 2001;15:200–2.

[126] Wullstein C, Barkhausen S, Gross E. Results of laparoscopic vs conventional appendectomy in complicated appendicitis. Dis Colon Rectum 2001;44:1700–5.

[127] So J, Chiong E, Chiong E, et al. Laparoscopic appendectomy for perforated appendicitis. World J Surg 2002;26:1485–8.

[128] Ball CG, Kortbeek JB, Kirkpatrick AW, et al. Laparoscopic appendectomy for complicated appendicitis. Surg Endosc 2004;18:969–73.

[129] Soffer D, Zait S, Klausner J, et al. Peritoneal cultures and antibiotic treatment in patients with perforated appendicitis. Eur J Surg 2001;167:214–6.

[130] Oliak D, Yamini D, Udani VM, et al. Initial nonoperative management for periappendiceal abscess. Dis Colon Rectum 2001;44:936–41.

[131] Brown C, Abrishami M, Muller M, et al. Appendiceal abscess: immediate operation or percutaneous drainage? Am Surg 2003;69:829–33.

[132] Taylor E, Berjis A, Bosch T, et al. The efficacy of postoperative oral antibiotics in appendicitis: a randomized prospective double-blinded study. Am Surg 2004;70:858–62.

[133] Mourad J, Elliot JP, Erickson L, et al. Appendicitis in pregnancy: new information that contradicts long-held beliefs. Am J Obstet Gynecol 2000;182:1027–9.

[134] Cohen-Kerem R, Railton C, Oren D, et al. Pregnancy outcome following non-obstetric surgical intervention. Am J Surg 2005;190:467–73.

[135] Tracey M, Fletcher HS. Appendicitis in pregnancy. Am Surg 2000;66:555–60.

[136] Castro MA, Shipp TD, Castro EE, et al. The use of computed tomography in pregnancy for the diagnosis of acute appendicitis. Am J Obstet Gynecol 2001;184:954–7.

[137] Wagner LK, Huda W. When a pregnant woman with suspected appendicitis is referred for a CT scan, what should a radiologist do to minimize potential radiation risks? Pediatr Radiol 2004;34:589–90.

[138] Oto A, Ernst RD, Shah R, et al. Right-lower-quadrant pain and suspected appendicitis in pregnant women: evaluation with MR imaging-initial experience. Radiology 2005;234:445–51.

[139] Cobben LP, Groot I, Haans L, et al. MRI for clinically suspected appendicitis during pregnancy. AJR Am J Roentgenol 2004;183:671–5.

[140] Rollins MD, Chan KJ, Price RR. Laparoscopy for appendicitis and cholelithiasis during pregnancy. Surg Endosc 2004;18:237–41.

[141] Storm-Dickerson TL, Horattas MC. What have we learned over the past 20 years about appendicitis in the elderly. Am J Surg 2003;185:198–201.

[142] Hiu TT, Major KM, Avital I, et al. Outcome of elderly patients with appendicitis. Arch Surg 2002;137:995–1000.

[143] Guller U, Jain N, Peterson ED, et al. Laparoscopic appendectomy in the elderly. Surgery 2004;135:479–88.

Gastroenterol Clin N Am 35 (2006) 393–407

GASTROENTEROLOGY CLINICS
OF NORTH AMERICA

The Management of Suspected Pancreatic Sepsis

Tyler M. Berzin, MD, Koenraad J. Mortele, MD,
Peter A. Banks, MD*

Department of Medicine, Division of Gastroenterology, Department of Radiology,
and Center for Pancreatic Disease, Brigham and Women's Hospital, 75 Francis Street,
Boston, MA 02115, USA

According to the Atlanta Symposium of 1992, severe acute pancreatitis is defined as pancreatitis associated with organ failure or local complications (necrosis, pseudocyst, or abscess) [1]. The Atlanta criteria for organ failure are (1) $PaO_2 \leq 60$ mm Hg; (2) shock (systolic blood pressure ≤ 90 mm Hg); (3) creatinine > 2.0 mg/dL after rehydration; and (4) gastrointestinal bleeding (>500 mL/24 h). Among these criteria, most clinicians agree that respiratory failure, renal failure, and shock are the three major components.

Pancreatic necrosis is defined as areas of devitalized parenchyma usually associated with peripancreatic fat necrosis. Approximately 15% of cases of acute pancreatitis are necrotizing and the remaining 85% are interstitial. The distinction between necrotizing pancreatitis and interstitial pancreatitis can be made reliably with the use of contrast-enhanced CT. CT diagnosis of pancreatic necrosis requires the identification of distinct areas of nonenhanced pancreatic parenchyma of at least 3 cm in size or involving more than 33% of the pancreas (Figs. 1–3) [2]. After several weeks, the peripancreatic inflammation that is associated frequently with pancreatic necrosis subsides. The process may coalesce as an encapsulated region of necrotic tissue and fluid (see Figs. 2 and 3). The resulting collection is still termed a pseudocyst by many clinicians. More recently, the term "organized necrosis" was introduced in recognition of the fact that the encapsulated structure is composed of necrotic pancreatic tissue as well as fluid.

Extrapancreatic fluid collections, which may form during interstitial and necrotizing pancreatitis, are defined by the Atlanta Symposium as collections of pancreatic fluid that have extravasated out of the pancreas into the anterior pararenal space, and at times, elsewhere (see Fig. 1). Most extrapancreatic fluid

*Corresponding author. *E-mail address:* pabanks@partners.org (P.A. Banks).

0889-8553/06/$ – see front matter
doi:10.1016/j.gtc.2006.03.007

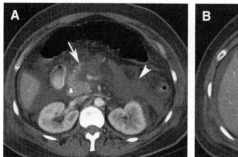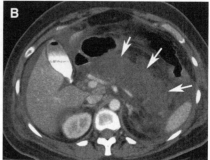

Fig. 1. 60-year-old man who has necrotizing pancreatitis secondary to gallstones. (A) Axial intravenous contrast-enhanced CT image through the pancreatic head shows necrosis of the pancreatic gland with clear demarcation (*arrow*) between necrotic and viable enhancing tissue. Note presence of a biliary stent, ascites, and an acute fluid collection (*arrowhead*) in the anterior pararenal space. (B) Axial intravenous contrast-enhanced CT image through the body and tail shows subtotal necrosis of the pancreatic gland (*arrows*). Contrast material is identified in the gallbladder from the previous endoscopic retrograde cholangiopancreatography procedure (with biliary stent placement).

collections resolve spontaneously, but some may encapsulate and evolve into pseudocysts.

A pancreatic pseudocyst is a local collection of extrapancreatic fluid that is encapsulated by a nonepithelialized wall. A pseudocyst typically matures approximately 4 to 6 weeks after the onset of acute pancreatitis. In contrast to organized necrosis, pseudocysts are located most frequently adjacent to the pancreas and contain little, if any, pancreatic tissue. A pancreatic abscess is a late phenomenon that usually develops more than 5 weeks after the initial episode of pancreatitis. An abscess is a focal collection of pus that develops within an area of minimal pancreatic necrosis. Incomplete debridement of necrosis also may lead to development of a pancreatic abscess.

SEVERE ACUTE PANCREATITIS
Severe acute pancreatitis develops in two phases. The initial phase is dominated by the systemic inflammatory response syndrome (SIRS) that usually occurs during the first week of the disease and resolves spontaneously or culminates in organ failure. The criteria for SIRS are (1) temperature $\leq 36°C$ or $\geq 38°C$; (2) heart rate ≥ 90 beats/min; (3) respiratory rate ≥ 20 breaths/min; and (4) white blood cell count ≤ 4000 cells/mm^3 or $\geq 12,000$ cells/mm^3 or $> 10\%$ bands. The second phase of severe acute pancreatitis is dominated by the late effects of necrotizing pancreatitis, the most significant of which is infected necrosis associated with organ failure. Approximately half of infections occur during the first 10 to 21 days of illness, and the rest occur after this interval [3,4]. Among patients who have necrotizing pancreatitis, estimates of the

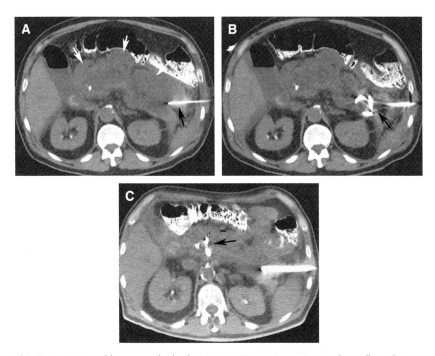

Fig. 2. A 45-year-old woman who had necrotizing pancreatitis improved initially and was re-admitted for fever and leukocytosis 3 weeks after clinical onset. Infected necrosis was diagnosed by CT-guided fine needle aspiration. (A) Axial contrast-enhanced CT image shows organized necrosis of the pancreas (*white arrows*). Infected necrosis was documented by percutaneous CT-guided aspiration using a 20-gauge Chiba needle (*black arrow*). (B) Initially, the patient was managed with aggressive percutaneous CT-guided catheter drainage (4 12F catheters). Unenhanced CT image shows location of a catheter (*black arrow*) in the tail. (C) Unenhanced CT image shows location of a catheter (*black arrow*) in the head with near complete drainage of the organized necrosis. Percutaneous drainage did not eliminate the infected necrosis completely; the patient underwent surgical debridement.

prevalence of infected necrosis have ranged from as high as 70% to as low as 16% to 37% in more recent studies [5–7].

PANCREATIC INFECTION, ORGAN FAILURE, AND MORTALITY

Pancreatic infection as a complication of acute pancreatitis occurs typically in the setting of pancreatic necrosis and rarely in association with extrapancreatic fluid collections and pancreatic pseudocysts. Pancreatic abscesses also are rare [1]. The mortality of infected necrosis is approximately 30%, compared with 12% for sterile necrosis [2]. Approximately one half of deaths in acute pancreatitis occur during the first 2 weeks as a direct result of persistent organ failure, whereas the remaining deaths occur after 2 weeks and primarily are attributable to infected necrosis and organ failure [5,7,8].

Approximately 50% of patients who have necrotizing pancreatitis develop organ failure, compared with less than 10% of patients who have interstitial

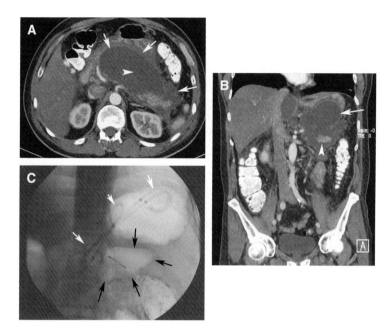

Fig. 3. 55-year-old patient who had necrotizing pancreatitis was readmitted for abdominal pain and malaise 3 weeks after the initial episode of acute pancreatitis. Because of intractable pain, the patient required debridement, whether the necrosis was sterile or infected. Axial (A) and coronal (B) contrast-enhanced CT images through the pancreatic bed show organized necrosis (*arrows*) in the pancreatic bed. Note areas of nonliquefied fat (*arrowhead*) in the collection (A) and remnant pancreatic tail (*arrowhead; B*). (C) The patient underwent endoscopic cyst gastrostomy with debridement of infected pancreatic necrosis (*black arrows outline the collection*). Continuity between the stomach and the cavity was maintained using three double-looped pigtail catheters (*white arrows*).

pancreatitis [2,5]. The prevalence of organ failure is higher in patients who have infected necrosis than in those who have sterile necrosis [5,7,9]. Organ failure occurs less commonly in association with infected extrapancreatic fluid collections, infected pseudocysts, and pancreatic abscesses than in association with infected pancreatic necrosis; mortality also is much lower for these conditions.

MICROBIOLOGY OF PANCREATIC INFECTIONS

There seem to be multiple pathways by which microorganisms may enter pancreatic tissue, including biliary and duodenal-pancreatic reflux, hematogenous and lymphatic dissemination, and local bacterial translocation from the gut [6,10–12]. Clinical studies and evidence from animal models point toward a key role for bacterial translocation across the colonic mucosa in acute illnesses [13–15].

Gut-derived gram-negative bacteria, including *Escherichia coli*, *Klebsiella*, and *Pseudomonas*, are the most common pathogens that are identified in pancreatic infections; this suggests that the colonic mucosal barrier may be compromised in severe acute pancreatitis, which encourages the translocation of enteric organisms [16–18]. Gram-positive organisms, including *Staphylococcus aureus* and *S enterococcus* species, also are found in infected necrosis. Resistant gram-positive cocci, along with fungi, are of increasing concern in patients who have necrotizing pancreatitis and are exposed to broad-spectrum antibiotics [6,19,20]. Cultures reveal monomicrobial infections in approximately 66% to 88% of patients who have infected necrosis [6,18]. Necrotic, devitalized pancreatic tissue lacks the immunologic mechanisms to prevent the proliferation of bacteria and fungi. Antibiotic penetration also is limited in necrotic tissue.

DIAGNOSIS OF INFECTED PANCREATIC NECROSIS
Clinical Evaluation

There are no reliable clinical parameters to distinguish sterile from infected pancreatic necrosis. Markers of systemic inflammation, such as fever and leukocytosis, usually are increased in infected necrosis, but may be increased to the same extent in severe sterile necrosis [3]. Plasma C-reactive protein (CRP) levels that exceed 150 mg/L suggest pancreatic necrosis, but CRP levels seem to be equivalent in patients who do or do not have infected necrosis [21,22]. Procalcitonin, which is released from the thyroid gland in the setting of bacterial infection and sepsis, has been proposed as a potential marker for infection in a broad array of medical conditions [22–24]. An increased procalcitonin level seems to be promising as a marker for infection in necrotizing pancreatitis, with several small studies reporting a 75% to 94% sensitivity and 83% to 91% specificity for infected pancreatic necrosis [25,26]. Additional study is necessary to confirm its accuracy in helping to distinguish sterile from infected pancreatic necrosis. Interleukin-6, phospholipase A2, and other serum markers also are under investigation for their role in assessing the likelihood of necrosis and infection in pancreatitis, but available data are more limited.

Clinical scoring systems, such as Ranson's criteria and Acute Physiology and Chronic Health Evaluation II, can be of use in distinguishing mild from severe pancreatitis, but are not useful in identifying infection among patients who have pancreatic necrosis [5,9,27]. Organ failure is more common in infected necrosis than in sterile necrosis, but it has not been validated in predicting the likelihood of infection [5,7,9].

In summary, pancreatic infection should be suspected in patients who have necrotizing pancreatitis and leukocytosis, fever, or organ failure that persists for at least 7 to 10 days after initial presentation. Infected necrosis also should be considered strongly in patients who develop leukocytosis, fever, or organ failure after several weeks of apparent clinical improvement or who continue to experience abdominal pain, anorexia, or malaise after several weeks of illness (see Fig. 3).

Radiographic Findings

Contrast-enhanced CT scan is the primary imaging modality that is used to identify pancreatic necrosis, and a CT severity index can be useful in quantifying the extent of necrosis [28]. In some studies [9,29,30], but not in others [5,31,32], the extent of pancreatic necrosis is correlated with the likelihood of infection, but it has not been validated as a predictor of infection. Therefore, there are no specific radiologic features that identify pancreatic infection except the rare presence of air bubbles within the necrotic pancreas on CT scan [33].

Fine Needle Aspiration

Image-guided percutaneous fine needle aspiration has become a valuable tool in the diagnosis of infected pancreatic necrosis (see Fig. 2). When performed by a trained interventional radiologist in an experienced radiologic unit, the procedure can be performed safely and accurately, even on patients who have multisystem organ failure [3,18]. The specimen should be carried immediately to the microbiology lab for gram stain and culture. Antibiotics should be initiated in response to a positive gram stain while culture results are pending. It has been the authors' experience that a Gram stain reveals organisms in almost all cases of bacterial infection of pancreatic necrosis, although on rare occasions a gram stain is negative and the culture is positive [3]. A positive culture from fine needle aspiration is the gold standard for confirming infected necrosis. CT-guided fine needle aspiration has been reported to have a sensitivity and specificity for infected necrosis that exceed 95% [18], and ultrasound guidance achieves a sensitivity and specificity of 88% and 90%, respectively [34].

The authors' algorithm for obtaining CT-guided fine needle aspiration samples in pancreatic necrosis is shown in Fig. 4. There is no need for guided

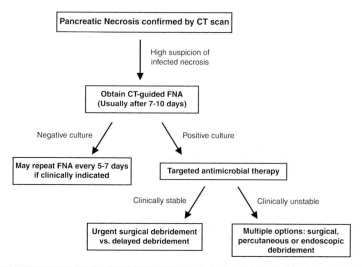

Fig. 4. Decision algorithm for infected pancreatic necrosis. FNA, fine needle aspiration.

percutaneous aspiration if there is sustained clinical improvement in the first 7 to 10 days of illness, with decreases in white blood cell count and temperature and resolution of organ failure. Even if these signs or symptoms persist, the initial aspiration usually is not performed until after the first 7 to 10 days of illness. There are two reasons for this delay. First, there is reasonable evidence that pancreatic infection rarely occurs during the first 7 to 10 days of illness [3]. Approximately one half of pancreatic infections are documented during the second and third week of illness, with the remaining cases identified at varying intervals thereafter. A second reason for delaying fine needle aspiration is that during the initial 7 to 10 days of acute pancreatitis, the development of fever, leukocytosis, and organ failure are caused by a severe inflammatory response and cytokine release.

If the initial aspirate after 7 to 10 days does not yield a positive culture, patients who have persistent fever, leukocytosis, or organ failure usually undergo CT-guided percutaneous aspiration every 5 to 7 days thereafter until positive culture is obtained or the patient improves clinically (see Fig. 4). Information is limited regarding the optimal timing of repeat fine needle aspiration in such cases.

Some clinicians do not believe that it is necessary to perform aspiration to distinguish sterile from infected necrosis because, in their view, all patients who have pancreatic necrosis should receive broad-spectrum antibiotic prophylaxis [35]. The rationale for their approach is threefold. First, if a patient who has infected necrosis has a false negative culture, antibiotics could be withheld inappropriately. Second, early identification of infection by guided percutaneous aspiration does not guide management because, in their view, surgical debridement should be delayed for several weeks in infected necrosis. Third, in their opinion, patients who remain persistently ill despite prophylactic antibiotics should undergo surgery regardless of whether the necrosis is sterile or infected.

An alternative point of view, which the authors support, is that microbiologic diagnosis by image-guided fine needle aspiration significantly aids the management of pancreatic necrosis [36] for the following reasons. First, in the authors' experience the false-negative rate for image-guided fine needle aspiration has been exceedingly low [3]. Generally, negative culture results are best interpreted as reflecting sterile necrosis, which warrants the prompt discontinuation of unnecessary antibiotics. If clinical suspicion for infection remains high after an initial negative culture, fine needle aspiration can be repeated in 5 to 7 days. Second, microbiologic results from fine needle aspiration guide appropriate selection of antibiotics. Selective use of antibiotics also may limit the development of resistant bacterial infections and fungal infections [20]. Third, a recent randomized prospective double-blind controlled trial did not support the use of prophylactic antibiotics for pancreatic necrosis [32]. Finally, the authors agree with the view of many surgeons that the clinical benefit of necrosectomy, in general, is limited to patients who have infected necrosis [37].

There are no prospective trials that compare the approach of universal antibiotics without fine needle aspiration with targeted antibiotics that are guided by results of aspiration. At the authors' institution, CT-guided fine needle aspiration remains integral to the management of necrotizing pancreatitis when pancreatic infection is suspected. The one exception, in the authors' view, is when symptoms, such as intractable abdominal pain or persistent malaise that is attributed to organized necrosis, necessitate debridement, whether the process is sterile or infected. In this case, there is no need to determine the presence of infection by aspiration.

ANTIMICROBIAL TREATMENT STRATEGIES FOR PANCREATIC NECROSIS
Prophylactic Antibiotic Therapy: Routine Use
Some investigators have suggested that all patients who have pancreatic necrosis should be treated with prophylactic antibiotics in an attempt to prevent pancreatic infection and associated mortality. Five randomized prospective, but not double-blind, studies evaluated whether prophylactic antibiotic administration (versus no antibiotic treatment) reduced the incidence of infected necrosis and decreased mortality. Four used intravenous antibiotics [38–41], and one examined selective decontamination of the digestive tract [42]. The choice of antibiotics differed in each trial, but included imipenem, ceftazidime, cefuroxime, amikacin, norfloxacin, Flagyl, and colistin. Some studies reported a statistically significant decrease in infected necrosis [40,42] whereas others did not [38,41]. In these studies, antibiotics were not shown to provide a statistically significant reduction in mortality in necrotizing pancreatitis. Two meta-analyses, including a Cochrane Review, evaluated different but overlapping groups of prophylactic antibiotic trials and came to different conclusions [43,44]. One meta-analysis concluded that antibiotic prophylaxis significantly reduced mortality [44], whereas the other concluded that it reduced the prevalence of pancreatic infection [43].

One year after the Cochrane Review, a prospective, double-blind, placebo-controlled trial was published in which 114 patients who had necrotizing pancreatitis were randomized to ciprofloxacin and metronidazole or no antibiotic therapy [32]. There was no reduction in the incidence of infected necrosis and no improvement in mortality in the group that received antibiotic treatment. The prevalence of pancreatic infection in both groups was low (<20%).

A recent editorial concluded that further clarification of the role of antibiotic therapy in necrotizing pancreatitis will require larger trials and improvement in study design [45]. Better standardization of criteria to assess the severity of acute pancreatitis will be needed to ensure that patients with equal severity are included in the antibiotic and placebo arms of studies. The editorial also acknowledged an increasing prevalence of superimposed fungal infections in necrotizing pancreatitis, and noted that this risk seems to correlate with the prolonged use of potent antibiotics [20]. Although there is some evidence that mortality may be increased significantly when there is superimposed fungal infection, additional information is needed to clarify this concern [20,46]. The role of prophylactic antifungal agents also remains unclear.

In the authors' view, until there is further evidence pertaining to the safety and efficacy of prophylactic antibiotic therapy, routine administration of prophylactic antibiotics is not recommended in necrotizing pancreatitis. It is worth noting, however, that other infections may arise in the setting of severe acute pancreatitis, such as pulmonary, urinary tract, and blood stream infections secondary to total parenteral nutrition. In all such cases, patients must be treated with appropriate antibiotic therapy.

Prophylactic Antibiotics: Selective Use

Routine use of prophylactic antibiotic therapy in the first 7 to 10 days of illness implies that all patients who have necrotizing pancreatitis, whether symptomatic or not, should be treated with antibiotics to prevent the development of pancreatic infection. The authors do not believe that there is sufficient evidence to adopt this protocol. It is difficult, however, to withhold antibiotic therapy in patients who have pancreatic necrosis who appear clinically septic with leukocytosis, fever, and in some cases, organ failure. Antibiotic therapy may be appropriate for these patients while a thorough investigation for sources of infection is ongoing. Workup should include cultures from the blood, urine, and sputum, as well as image-guided fine needle aspiration of the pancreas (usually after 7–10 days).

Once appropriate cultures are negative and no source of infection is identified, and particularly after image-guided fine needle aspiration provides assurance that there is no pancreatic infection, antibiotic therapy should be discontinued.

Targeted Antibiotic Therapy

Treatment of microbiologically confirmed pancreatic infection is guided by results of culture and sensitivity. Fluoroquinolones and carbapenems provide excellent gram-negative coverage and achieve adequate tissue concentration in the pancreas, whereas ampicillin and gentamicin do not attain effective therapeutic levels in the pancreatic tissue [47,48]. Metronidazole achieves excellent penetration as well, but is appropriate only as an adjunct agent for additional anaerobic coverage. Because the prevalence of gram-positive organisms seems to be increasing, with S enterococcus and S aureus accounting for 30% of isolates in one recent review of infected necrosis [6], appropriate coverage of these organisms, including resistant strains, is of increasing importance. Duration of antibiotic therapy after surgical debridement usually is determined in accordance with clinical judgment.

Although infected necrosis has long been considered to have a high mortality without operative intervention, several reports now support the concept that some patients may be treated successfully with antibiotics alone [39,49,50]. This approach has not been validated in prospective trials.

DEBRIDEMENT OF INFECTED NECROSIS

Surgical Debridement

Historically, standard of care for infected pancreatic necrosis has been prompt surgical debridement after guided percutaneous aspiration has confirmed the presence of infection [37,51]. The mortality that is associated with prompt surgical necrosectomy is minimal among patients who have infected necrosis who do not have organ failure or serious comorbid disease [5]. A delay of no more than 1 to 2 days before surgery is appropriate occasionally for patients who are in need of further medical stabilization and fluid resuscitation before debridement. Surgical debridement involves extensive finger dissection of pockets of semisolid pancreatic and peripancreatic necrosis, evacuation of discolored pancreatic and peripancreatic fluid, and copious lavage. The choice of surgical technique has varied among surgical centers. Approaches include necrosectomy with closed continuous irrigation by way of indwelling catheters, necrosectomy with open packing, and less frequently, necrosectomy with closed drainage without irrigation. No randomized prospective trial has compared these procedures. In general, all three procedures are considered to yield favorable results [37,52].

In recent years, the standard of care for infected pancreatic necrosis has evolved to include delaying surgical debridement for several weeks in clinically stable patients. This approach is based on several considerations [52]. First, a delay in surgical debridement may allow the acute inflammatory process in and around the pancreas to subside and then encapsulate as organized necrosis. Organized necrosis is removed more easily and safely in an operation that entails debridement of necrosis followed by anastomosis of the capsule to the stomach (cyst-gastrostomy) or the jejunum (Roux-en-y cyst-jejunostomy). Organized necrosis also can be debrided by laparoscopic and endoscopic approaches. Secondly, an additional benefit to delaying debridement is the possibility of avoiding surgery altogether should patients exhibit sustained clinical improvement with conversion of infected necrosis to sterile necrosis [39,49,50].

Until additional experience is published, and particularly until prospective trials are available that compare prompt surgery with delayed surgery, the authors believe that patients who are clinically stable and have infected pancreatic necrosis should undergo prompt surgical debridement.

The optimal treatment for patients who have infected necrosis and organ failure or significant comorbid disease remains a major concern. The mortality of infected necrosis that was complicated by multisystem organ failure was 48% in a recent study [5]. For unstable patients, it may not be possible to delay debridement for several weeks until organized necrosis forms. Because prompt open surgical debridement in these patients may pose unacceptable operative risks, several less invasive surgical procedures have been introduced.

One less invasive approach to debridement is laparoscopic necrosectomy with placement of large-caliber drains for irrigation [53,54]. Another technique is minimally invasive retroperitoneal necrosectomy, which uses percutaneous insertion of an operating nephroscope to access the area of pancreatic necrosis, followed by debridement, irrigation, and placement of catheters for continued retroperitoneal irrigation [55]. These techniques have not been compared with one another or with standard surgical debridement in prospective trials.

Percutaneous Debridement

Another option for patients who have infected necrosis and organ failure or significant comorbid disease are radiologically placed percutaneous catheters for drainage of infected necrosis [56,57]. This technique can be effective before or after the development of organized necrosis (see Fig. 2). Multiple catheters are required frequently as well as diligent, daily attention on the part of skilled radiologists. Continued care involves catheter irrigation several times a day, up-sizing of catheters if there is inadequate drainage of infected material, and placement of new catheters as needed.

The goal of percutaneous catheter placement for infected necrosis before the organized necrosis stage is to drain infected, necrotic material as a temporary measure. On occasion, the prolonged use of multiple catheters completely liquefied all infected necrotic tissue; surgical debridement was not required [57]. In the setting of organized necrosis, the goal of percutaneous catheter drainage is to provide definitive drainage so that surgery is not necessary. Percutaneous catheter drainage of infected organized necrosis may be ineffective—because of the inability to eliminate semisolid infected material completely—and necessitates eventual surgical debridement (see Fig. 2). Additional study is required to determine the value of this approach in larger groups of patients who have infected necrosis.

Endoscopic Debridement

Endoscopic necrosectomy is another emerging therapy for patients who have pancreatic necrosis. Unlike surgical and percutaneous approaches that can be used before or after the formation of organized necrosis, endoscopic therapy usually is reserved for the treatment of organized necrosis (see Fig. 3). The standard technique is to use endoscopic ultrasound to guide the site of puncture through the gastric or duodenal wall to avoid blood vessels and to enter the cystic structure accurately. The opening is enlarged by balloon dilatation and the endoscope is introduced into the cavity to facilitate evacuation of fluid and debridement of necrotic tissue. Multiple pigtail catheters are inserted to create a drainage pathway from the cyst to the stomach or duodenum. Repeated endoscopic debridement may be required at frequent (even daily) intervals until all fluid or necrotic debris is eliminated [58].

Endoscopic therapy has the advantage of being less invasive than surgical approaches, but it requires considerable expertise. A limitation of endoscopic treatment is difficulty in eliminating all necrotic tissue, with persistence of infection within the cavity. A second limitation is premature closure of the drainage pathway to the stomach. Under these circumstances, additional endoscopic therapy or percutaneous or surgical drainage may be required. Endoscopic debridement has not been compared with surgical approaches in prospective trials.

DIAGNOSIS AND MANAGEMENT OF OTHER PANCREATIC INFECTIONS

Infected extrapancreatic fluid collections also are diagnosed by image-guided fine needle aspiration. Microbiologically confirmed infected fluid collections should be treated with intravenous antibiotics and percutaneous catheter drainage. Persistent or loculated infected collections may require multiple radiologic drains. Less commonly, failure of drainage that is due to the presence of semisolid peripancreatic fat necrosis may necessitate surgical debridement of fat necrosis and infected peripancreatic fluid in patients who have continued pain or fever.

Diagnosis of infected pseudocysts also relies on image-guided fine needle aspiration. Microbiologic results should guide targeted antimicrobial therapy. For infected pseudocysts, image-guided percutaneous catheter placement is an effective intervention [59]. Endoscopic drainage also may be considered if the pseudocyst is compressing the stomach [60]. Surgery is reserved for patients who have symptoms, such as pain or fever, which are caused by inadequate drainage.

Pancreatic abscesses typically arise after 5 weeks as a late complication of pancreatic necrosis. Clinical manifestations may include fever, leukocytosis, and abdominal pain several weeks after a period of initial clinical improvement [61]. Pancreatic abscesses are diagnosed and managed similarly to infected pseudocysts with percutaneous catheter drainage and, if required, surgical debridement.

SUMMARY

The management of infected pancreatic necrosis is centered on image-guided fine needle aspiration followed by antibiotic therapy that is based on microbiologic culture results. The authors favor targeted antibiotic therapy rather than routine prophylactic antibiotic coverage. Prompt surgical debridement is recommended for patients who have infected necrosis who are suitable operative candidates. Newer surgical, percutaneous, and endoscopic techniques, as well as prolonged antibiotic therapy without intervention, are being evaluated as alternatives to operative debridement. Well-designed prospective trials will help to determine optimal treatment for patients who have infected pancreatic necrosis.

References

[1] Bradley EL III. A clinically based classification system for acute pancreatitis. Summary of the International Symposium on Acute Pancreatitis, Atlanta, Ga, September 11 through 13, 1992. Arch Surg 1993;128(5):586–90.
[2] Banks PA, Freeman ML. Practice guidelines in acute pancreatitis. Am J Gastroenterol, in press.
[3] Gerzof SG, Banks PA, Robbins AH, et al. Early diagnosis of pancreatic infection by computed tomography-guided aspiration. Gastroenterology 1987;93(6):1315–20.
[4] Rattner DW, Legermate DA, Lee MJ, et al. Early surgical debridement of symptomatic pancreatic necrosis is beneficial irrespective of infection. Am J Surg 1992;163(1):105–9. [discussion 109–10].
[5] Perez A, Whang EE, Brooks DC, et al. Is severity of necrotizing pancreatitis increased in extended necrosis and infected necrosis? Pancreas 2002;25(3):229–33.

[6] Beger HG, Rau B, Isenmann R, et al. Antibiotic prophylaxis in severe acute pancreatitis. Pancreatol 2005;5(1):10–9.
[7] Buchler MW, Gloor B, Muller CA, et al. Acute necrotizing pancreatitis: treatment strategy according to the status of infection. Ann Surg 2000;232(5):619–26.
[8] Beger HG, Bittner R, Block S, et al. Bacterial contamination of pancreatic necrosis. A prospective clinical study. Gastroenterology 1986;91(2):433–8.
[9] Isenmann R, Rau B, Beger HG. Bacterial infection and extent of necrosis are determinants of organ failure in patients with acute necrotizing pancreatitis. Br J Surg 1999;86(8): 1020–4.
[10] Foitzik T, Fernandez-del Castillo C, Ferraro MJ, et al. Pathogenesis and prevention of early pancreatic infection in experimental acute necrotizing pancreatitis. Ann Surg 1995;222(2):179–85.
[11] Byrne JJ, Joison J. Bacterial regurgitation in experimental pancreatitis. Am J Surg 1964;107: 317–20.
[12] Schmid SW, Uhl W, Friess H, et al. The role of infection in acute pancreatitis. Gut 1999;45(2):311–6.
[13] Widdison AL, Karanjia ND, Reber HA. Routes of spread of pathogens into the pancreas in a feline model of acute pancreatitis. Gut 1994;35(9):1306–10.
[14] Luiten EJ, Hop WC, Endtz HP, et al. Prognostic importance of gram-negative intestinal colonization preceding pancreatic infection in severe acute pancreatitis. Results of a controlled clinical trial of selective decontamination. Intensive Care Med 1998;24(5): 438–45.
[15] Sedman PC, Macfie J, Sagar P, et al. The prevalence of gut translocation in humans. Gastroenterology 1994;107(3):643–9.
[16] Jones CE, Polk HC Jr, Fulton RL. Pancreatic abscess. Am J Surg 1975;129(1):44–7.
[17] Medich DS, Lee TK, Melhem MF, et al. Pathogenesis of pancreatic sepsis. Am J Surg 1993;165(1):46–50 [discussion 51–2].
[18] Banks PA, Gerzof SG, Langevin RE, et al. CT-guided aspiration of suspected pancreatic infection: bacteriology and clinical outcome. Int J Pancreatol 1995;18(3):265–70.
[19] Gloor B, Muller CA, Worni M, et al. Pancreatic infection in severe pancreatitis: the role of fungus and multiresistant organisms. Arch Surg 2001;136(5):592–6.
[20] Isenmann R, Schwarz M, Rau B, et al. Characteristics of infection with Candida species in patients with necrotizing pancreatitis. World J Surg 2002;26(3):372–6.
[21] Muller CA, Uhl W, Printzen G, et al. Role of procalcitonin and granulocyte colony stimulating factor in the early prediction of infected necrosis in severe acute pancreatitis. Gut 2000;46(2):233–8.
[22] Riche FC, Cholley BP, Laisne MJ, et al. Inflammatory cytokines, C reactive protein, and procalcitonin as early predictors of necrosis infection in acute necrotizing pancreatitis. Surgery 2003;133(3):257–62.
[23] Christ-Crain M, Jaccard-Stolz D, Bingisser R, et al. Effect of procalcitonin-guided treatment on antibiotic use and outcome in lower respiratory tract infections: cluster-randomised, single-blinded intervention trial. Lancet 2004;363(9409):600–7.
[24] Simon L, Gauvin F, Amre DK, et al. Serum procalcitonin and C-reactive protein levels as markers of bacterial infection: a systematic review and meta-analysis. Clin Infect Dis 2004;39(2):206–17.
[25] Olah A, Belagyi T, Issekutz A, et al. Value of procalcitonin quick test in the differentiation between sterile and infected forms of acute pancreatitis. Hepatogastroenterology 2005; 52(61):243–5.
[26] Rau B, Steinbach G, Gansauge F, et al. The potential role of procalcitonin and interleukin 8 in the prediction of infected necrosis in acute pancreatitis. Gut 1997;41(6): 832–40.
[27] Le Mee J, Paye F, Sauvanet A, et al. Incidence and reversibility of organ failure in the course of sterile or infected necrotizing pancreatitis. Arch Surg 2001;136(12):1386–90.

[28] Balthazar EJ. Acute pancreatitis: assessment of severity with clinical and CT evaluation. Radiology 2002;223(3):603–13.

[29] Garg PK, Madan K, Pande GK, et al. Association of extent and infection of pancreatic necrosis with organ failure and death in acute necrotizing pancreatitis. Clin Gastroenterol Hepatol 2005;3(2):159–66.

[30] Gotzinger P, Sautner T, Kriwanek S, et al. Surgical treatment for severe acute pancreatitis: extent and surgical control of necrosis determine outcome. World J Surg 2002;26(4): 474–8.

[31] Lankisch PG, Pflichthofer D, Lehnick D. No strict correlation between necrosis and organ failure in acute pancreatitis. Pancreas 2000;20(3):319–22.

[32] Isenmann R, Runzi M, Kron M, et al. Prophylactic antibiotic treatment in patients with predicted severe acute pancreatitis: a placebo-controlled, double-blind trial. Gastroenterology 2004;126(4):997–1004.

[33] Casas JD, Diaz R, Valderas G, et al. Prognostic value of CT in the early assessment of patients with acute pancreatitis. AJR Am J Roentgenol 2004;182(3):569–74.

[34] Rau B, Pralle U, Mayer JM, et al. Role of ultrasonographically guided fine-needle aspiration cytology in the diagnosis of infected pancreatic necrosis. Br J Surg 1998;85(2):179–84.

[35] Pappas TN. Con: Computerized tomographic aspiration of infected pancreatic necrosis: the opinion against its routine use. Am J Gastroenterol 2005;100(11):2373–4.

[36] Banks PA. Pro: Computerized tomographic fine needle aspiration (CT-FNA) is valuable in the management of infected pancreatic necrosis. Am J Gastroenterol 2005;100(11): 2371–2.

[37] Uhl W, Warshaw A, Imrie C, et al. IAP Guidelines for the Surgical Management of Acute Pancreatitis. Pancreatol 2002;2(6):565–73.

[38] Delcenserie R, Yzet T, Ducroix JP. Prophylactic antibiotics in treatment of severe acute alcoholic pancreatitis. Pancreas 1996;13(2):198–201.

[39] Nordback I, Sand J, Saaristo R, et al. Early treatment with antibiotics reduces the need for surgery in acute necrotizing pancreatitis–a single-center randomized study. J Gastrointest Surg 2001;5(2):113–8 [discussion 118–20].

[40] Pederzoli P, Bassi C, Vesentini S, et al. A randomized multicenter clinical trial of antibiotic prophylaxis of septic complications in acute necrotizing pancreatitis with imipenem. Surg Gynecol Obstet 1993;176(5):480–3.

[41] Sainio V, Kemppainen E, Puolakkainen P, et al. Early antibiotic treatment in acute necrotising pancreatitis. Lancet 1995;346(8976):663–7.

[42] Luiten EJ, Hop WC, Lange JF, et al. Controlled clinical trial of selective decontamination for the treatment of severe acute pancreatitis. Ann Surg 1995;222(1):57–65.

[43] Bassi C, Larvin M, Villatoro E. Antibiotic therapy for prophylaxis against infection of pancreatic necrosis in acute pancreatitis. Cochrane Database Syst Rev 2003;(4):CD002941.

[44] Sharma VK, Howden CW. Prophylactic antibiotic administration reduces sepsis and mortality in acute necrotizing pancreatitis: a meta-analysis. Pancreas 2001;22(1):28–31.

[45] Brown A. Prophylactic antibiotic use in severe acute pancreatitis: hemlock, help, or hype? Gastroenterology 2004;126(4):1195–8.

[46] Connor S, Alexakis N, Neal T, et al. Fungal infection but not type of bacterial infection is associated with a high mortality in primary and secondary infected pancreatic necrosis. Dig Surg 2004;21(4):297–304.

[47] Buchler M, Malfertheiner P, Friess H, et al. Human pancreatic tissue concentration of bactericidal antibiotics. Gastroenterology 1992;103(6):1902–8.

[48] Bassi C, Pederzoli P, Vesentini S, et al. Behavior of antibiotics during human necrotizing pancreatitis. Antimicrob Agents Chemother 1994;38(4):830–6.

[49] Runzi M, Niebel W, Goebell H, et al. Severe acute pancreatitis: nonsurgical treatment of infected necroses. Pancreas 2005;30(3):195–9.

[50] Adler DG, Chari ST, Dahl TJ, et al. Conservative management of infected necrosis complicating severe acute pancreatitis. Am J Gastroenterol 2003;98(1):98–103.

[51] Werner J, Feuerbach S, Uhl W, et al. Management of acute pancreatitis: from surgery to interventional intensive care. Gut 2005;54(3):426–36.

[52] Heinrich S, Schafer M, Rousson V, et al. evidence-based treatment of acute pancreatitis: a look at established paradigms. Ann Surg 2006;243(2):154–68.

[53] Horvath KD, Kao LS, Wherry KL, et al. A technique for laparoscopic-assisted percutaneous drainage of infected pancreatic necrosis and pancreatic abscess. Surg Endosc 2001; 15(10):1221–5.

[54] Zhou ZG, Zheng YC, Shu Y, et al. Laparoscopic management of severe acute pancreatitis. Pancreas 2003;27(3):e46–50.

[55] Connor S, Ghaneh P, Raraty M, et al. Minimally invasive retroperitoneal pancreatic necrosectomy. Dig Surg 2003;20(4):270–7.

[56] Ashley SW, Perez A, Pierce EA, et al. Necrotizing pancreatitis: contemporary analysis of 99 consecutive cases. Ann Surg 2001;234(4):572–9 [discussion 579–80].

[57] Freeny PC, Hauptmann E, Althaus SJ, et al. Percutaneous CT-guided catheter drainage of infected acute necrotizing pancreatitis: techniques and results. AJR Am J Roentgenol 1998;170(4):969–75.

[58] Seewald S, Groth S, Omar S, et al. Aggressive endoscopic therapy for pancreatic necrosis and pancreatic abscess: a new safe and effective treatment algorithm (videos). Gastrointest Endosc 2005;62(1):92–100.

[59] Baril NB, Ralls PW, Wren SM, et al. Does an infected peripancreatic fluid collection or abscess mandate operation? Ann Surg 2000;231(3):361–7.

[60] Weckman L, Kylanpaa ML, Puolakkainen P, et al. Endoscopic treatment of pancreatic pseudocysts. Surg Endosc 2006;20:603–7.

[61] Bittner R, Block S, Buchler M, et al. Pancreatic abscess and infected pancreatic necrosis. Different local septic complications in acute pancreatitis. Dig Dis Sci 1987;32(10):1082–7.

Gastroenterol Clin N Am 35 (2006) 409–423

GASTROENTEROLOGY CLINICS
OF NORTH AMERICA

Approach to the Patient Who Has Suspected Acute Bacterial Cholangitis

Waqar A. Qureshi, MD

Department of Medicine, Baylor College of Medicine, 1709 Dryden, Suite 800,
Mail stop: BCM 620, Houston, TX 77030, USA

SUSPECTED ACUTE BACTERIAL CHOLANGITIS
Obstruction

Acute cholangitis refers to inflammation of the biliary ductal system from bacterial infection, usually in the setting of biliary obstruction. Other terms used are ascending cholangitis, suppurative cholangitis, and toxic cholangitis. The two important features are obstruction and bacterial infection. Important causes of biliary obstruction are listed in Table 1. The most common cause of biliary obstruction in the United States is gallstones. About one quarter of patients who have symptomatic gallstones present with a stone in the common bile duct (CBD) [1–3]. Fig. 1 illustrates a dilated biliary system with stones in the CBD leading to cholangitis. Fig. 2 shows the endoscopic retrograde cholangiopancreatography (ERCP) appearance of an impacted stone at the ampulla, and Fig. 3 shows pus drainage following stenting of the CBD. Malignant obstruction of the CBD is the second most common reason for cholangitis. The most common malignancies are pancreatic cancer, cholangiocarcinoma, cancer of the ampulla Vater, and metastatic cancer. Acute bacterial cholangitis is uncommon in malignant obstruction unless there has been some attempt at intervention. Instrumentation of the biliary tract with ERCP or percutaneous transhepatic cholangiography (PTC) may result in cholangitis if an attempt to decompress an obstructed biliary system is unsuccessful or only partially successful [4]. Nonmalignant fibrotic or inflammatory strictures are the cause of biliary obstruction due to a variety of causes (see Table 1) [5,6]. Primary biliary duct stones are unusual in the United States but are common in areas where biliary ductal parasitic infections are epidemic, such as southeast Asia and Hong Kong [7–10]. Parasites that infect the biliary tract include *Clonorchis sinensis*, *Opisthorchis felineus*, *Opisthorchis viverrini*, and *Fasciola hepatica* [11]. *Ascaris*

E-mail address: wqureshi@bcm.tcm.edu

0889-8553/06/$ – see front matter
doi:10.1016/j.gtc.2006.05.005

Table 1
Causes of biliary obstruction in acute cholangitis

Cause	Examples	Risk groups	Comments
Stones	Gallbladder stones migrated to common bile duct Primary bile duct stones	Same risk factors as for gallbladder stones Associated with bile duct stasis, strictures, parasites, or hemolysis	Most common cause of biliary obstruction with cholangitis
Neoplasms	Papillary tumors Pancreatic malignancy Cholangiocarcinoma Extrinsic compression by tumors in the hepatic hilum	Older age Hepatitis C (cholangiocarcinoma)	Biliary instrumentation increases risk for infection
Fibrotic stricture	Stone related Postsurgical Trauma Chronic pancreatitis Sclerosing cholangitis	Complicated stone disease History of surgery or trauma Alcohol, hereditary, autoimmune Ulcerative colitis	Acute infection is treated without surgery Chronic management often requires surgery
Parasitic	Ascaris lumbricoides Clonorchis sinensis Opisthorchis felineus Opisthorchis viverrini Fasciola hepatica	Immigrants from known endemic areas	Ascaris may have to be removed. May show only fibrosis and strictures; evidence of current parasitic infection may not be found

lumbricoides occasionally obstructs the biliary tree and leads to cholangitis [12]. Mass effect from echinococcal disease can cause biliary obstruction. Infections that complicate HIV disease (ie, cryptosporidium or microsporidium) result in AIDS cholangiopathy and may predispose to cholangitis [13].

Infection

The sphincter of Oddi regulates the direction of bile flow, and, along with the inherent bacteriostatic properties of bile salts normally maintains the sterility of bile [6,14]. A biliary system that is colonized by bacteria but not obstructed does not progress to cholangitis [15]. Infection is unusual when the obstruction is due to a malignant process in a patient who presents with jaundice [16]; however, intervention and instrumentation (eg, unsuccessful ERCP or PTC) can lead to bacterial contamination, proliferation, and cholangitis rapidly [17]. In most settings of acute cholangitis it is unclear exactly how bacteria enter an obstructed biliary. Some studies showed that the incidence of bacteremia or appearance of endotoxemia was related directly to the pressure within the biliary system [18–22]. Recent research has demonstrated that biliary obstruction is associated with increased intestinal permeability and disruption of intestinal integrity, which leads to an increased likelihood that bacteria enter the

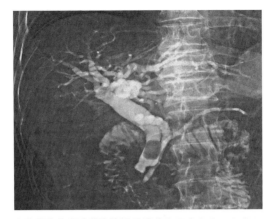

Fig. 1. Cholangiogram showing stone in the distal common bile duct. (Courtesy of John Baillie, BSc (Hons), MB, ChB, Winston-Salem, NC.)

blood or lymphatic system [23–25]. An obstructed biliary system promotes bacterial translocation to normally sterile sites [26–28].

Review of current literature reveals little new in the microbiology of cholangitis. Although a wider spectrum of antibiotics is now available, there is little evidence-based data to suggest a significantly superior efficacy over previous regimens. Gram-negative coverage is extremely important because most infections are due to *Escherichia coli* and to a lesser extent, *Klebsiella* spp. Gram-positive *Enterococcus* also is common. Other bacteria that are isolated from bile

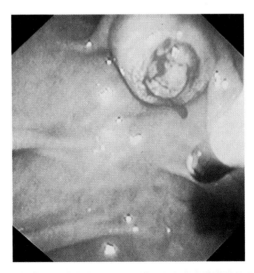

Fig. 2. An impacted stone is visible at the ampullary os at endoscopy.

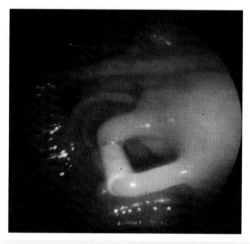

Fig. 3. Pus drainage following stent placement in the common bile duct in acute bacterial cholangitis.

in cholangitis include *Enterobacter* spp, *Proteus* spp, *Pseudomonas* spp, and anaerobes, such as *Clostridium* spp and *Bacteroides* spp [29–33]. Anaerobes are more likely in patients who have had previous biliary-intestinal anastomosis and in the elderly [27,34]. Anaerobes tend to be associated with a more severe infection than do aerobes [32]. Multiple organisms are identified frequently in infected bile, which highlights the importance of initial broad-spectrum coverage. Cholangitis that is caused by a combination of aerobic and anaerobic bacteria often is associated with a more serious clinical condition. Although *E coli* and *Klebsiella* spp are isolated frequently from blood cultures, it is unusual for enterococci or anaerobes to show up in blood cultures when the cholangitis is due to these bacteria [35].

Clinical Suspicion

Clinical findings in patients who have cholangitis can range from a mild illness in the early stages to a fulminant, overwhelming sepsis. Fever and jaundice are seen in more than 90% and more than 60% of patients who have cholangitis, respectively, which makes them the most common findings. The classic "Charcot's triad" of fever, right upper quadrant pain, and jaundice that was described by Charcot in 1877 is not necessarily seen in most cases of cholangitis. In fact, various studies put the presence of the triad of symptoms at between 15% and 70% [36–40]. In the elderly, acute cholangitis may not present with the usual symptoms, which leads to a delay in diagnosis with abnormal liver enzymes being a clue to the diagnosis [40]. The addition of septic shock and mental status change results in a much sicker patient with the so-called "Reynolds pentad" [41]. Chills resulting from intermittent bacteremia are prominent in about two thirds of patients, and this can be a clue in an atypical presentation [42,43].

The bilirubin and alkaline phosphatase levels are elevated in more than 90% of patients who have acute cholangitis. The total bilirubin levels are proportional to the severity of obstruction and length of illness, with higher levels being seen in malignant obstruction. The liver transaminases often are one to two times normal levels. Serum amylase may be increased in up to 40% of patients, but does not necessarily indicate pancreatitis. A leukocytosis is common although a leukopenia in a severely septic patient is a poor prognostic indicator.

APPROACH TO THE PATIENT WHO HAS SUSPECTED ACUTE CHOLANGITIS

Once there is suspicion of biliary obstruction with bacterial infection, a set of progressive diagnostic and treatment modalities is implemented. The exact sequence of events depends on the degree of diagnostic uncertainty, severity of illness, and existing comorbidities. Nevertheless, every case involves decisions about four crucial interventions: antibiotic therapy, diagnostic imaging, biliary drainage, and the role of surgery.

Antibiotic Therapy

Patients who have cholangitis require resuscitation with fluids, correction of electrolytes and coagulopathy, and prompt treatment with broad-spectrum empiric antibiotics after blood cultures have been obtained. Antibiotic treatment is given to control sepsis and local inflammation. Despite the significant morbidity and mortality form cholangitis, few randomized prospective trials have compared the various antimicrobials. The choice of antibiotic is based on the clinical picture (ie, severity of infection, age of patient, history of instrumentation or surgery, and some knowledge of local drug resistance patterns). Generally, antibiotic therapy is given for 7 to 10 days [44]. There is some evidence that once good drainage is established, 3 days of antibiotic treatment may be sufficient [45]. Although much is made of using antibiotics that are excreted into bile, little excretion can occur into an obstructed biliary system [46–49]. Antibiotics do not reach the biliary system until about 24 hours after drainage has been accomplished.

Broad-spectrum coverage is preferred and although the combination of ampicillin and gentamicin is popular, there are disadvantages: limited anaerobic coverage, frequent microbial resistance, and nephrotoxicity [50]. In extremely ill or elderly patients, anaerobic coverage is added because a mixed infection is likely. The ureidopenicillins have broad coverage that includes many anaerobes, enterococci, and pseudomonas. In a randomized trial by Gerecht and colleagues [51], mezlocillin alone was more effective than was the ampicillin-gentamicin combination in acute cholangitis. In a similar trial, piperacillin alone had equal efficacy to ampicillin plus tobramycin [52]. These single agents probably should be used with caution in areas of high β-lactam resistance. The piperacillin/tazobactam combination is a good alternative to the ampicillin/gentamicin combination. Cefepime has good gram-negative coverage, including *Pseudomonas* spp, as well as covering most of the important gram-positive bowel flora except *Enterococcus* spp. The need to cover *Enterococcus* spp is still debated. The role of quinolones in biliary sepsis is being studied. At least one randomized controlled trial showed ciprofloxacin to be as effective as ceftazidime-ampicillin-metronidazole triple combination [53]. Finally, the carbapenems, imipenem/cilastatin, ertapenem, or meropenem, although more expensive, are reasonable choices.

The response to antibiotic therapy (and other supportive interventions, such as intravenous fluids and cardiorespiratory support) usually determines the timing and method of other diagnostic and treatment modalities. Patients who develop normal vital signs rapidly after antibiotic therapy usually can be drained within 48 to 72 hours.

Diagnostic Imaging

Noninvasive imaging modalities to diagnose biliary ductal obstruction include routine transcutaneous abdominal ultrasound (US), CT, and MR cholangiography. The advantages and disadvantages of each modality in the setting of suspected biliary obstruction with infection is summarized in Table 2. US is a quick, inexpensive, and accurate way to look for dilated bile ducts with 96% accuracy for ductal dilation [54]. CT scan and magnetic resonance cholangiopancreatography (MRCP) may give more diagnostic information about the location and etiology of obstruction in comparison with US, but often are not crucial for the management of cholangitis. CT may be preferred if a tumor of the pancreas is suspected from the clinical presentation. MRCP is superior to transabdominal ultrasonography in the detection of ductal stones and in diagnosing the cause of the biliary obstruction [55]. Invasive imaging modalities that are useful in the setting of suspected biliary sepsis include ERCP, endoscopic US (EUS), and PTC. None of these is the initial diagnostic imaging modality. EUS enables accurate diagnosis of ductal dilation and choledocholithiasis [56–58]. Scheiman and colleagues [56] showed EUS to be more sensitive than MRCP (80% versus 40%) for the detection of choledocholithiasis. In this study, EUS was superior in diagnosing biliary stricture (specificity and positive predictive value [100%/100%]) compared with MRCP (76%/25%). The overall accuracy for detecting any abnormality was 61% (95% CI, 0.41–0.78) for MRCP and 89% (95% CI, 0.72–0.98) for EUS; however, EUS probably is not the procedure of choice in acute biliary sepsis because it does not allow for concomitant biliary drainage. If a patient responds to antibiotic therapy, EUS may offer superior diagnostic information as to the cause of obstruction in a stable patient (small CBD stone, benign or malignant stricture). EUS is gaining a role as a diagnostic test to use ERCP more selectively [57]. An example would be in suspected CBD stones in the setting of acute pancreatitis; however, its role in acute biliary sepsis is minimal.

A recent meta-analysis of 67 studies compared MRCP with ERCP, the gold standard, in suspected biliary disease. MRCP had an overall sensitivity of 95% (95% CI, 75%–99%) and specificity of 94% in all biliary disease. When

Table 2
Diagnostic imaging for suspected acute cholangitis

Tests	Advantages	Disadvantages	Comments
Abdominal ultrasound	Noninvasive Inexpensive Sensitive for detecting dilated ducts and gallbladder stones	Poor sensitivity for CBD stones and for diagnosing cause and location of obstruction	Common initial test for suspected biliary obstruction
CT	Noninvasive Usually good detail of location and cause of obstruction Useful when a neoplasm is suspected	Radiations risk in pregnant patients Nephrotoxic contrast required for best detail Cannot be used to establish drainage Cannot differentiate benign from malignant obstruction reliably	Superior detail of biliary tree compared with ultrasound but less sensitive for gallstones than ultrasound
MRI	Noninvasive Usually good detail of location and cause of obstruction Useful when a neoplasm is suspected Safe in pregnancy	Cannot be used in patients with implanted metallic devices Cannot be used to establish drainage	MRCP better than CT for stones in CBD
Endoscopic ultrasound	Very sensitive for choledocolithiasis	Invasive. Cannot be used to establish drainage	Role in acute cholangitis not established
PTC	High success for diagnosing location of obstruction while establishing drainage Biopsy or brushings of strictures or mass	Invasive Limited use in pregnant patients and those who have coagulopathy or ascites	Higher complication rate than ERCP More patient discomfort because of percutaneous catheter
ERCP	High success for diagnosing location of obstruction while establishing drainage Biopsy or brushings of strictures of mass Internal stent is comfortable	Invasive. Pancreatitis, bleeding, perforation	Most widely used procedure for diagnosis and urgent treatment

analyzed by disease process, MRCP was less sensitive for the diagnosis of stones when compared with ERCP (92% [95% CI, 80%–97%]). Its sensitivity for the differentiation of benign from malignant biliary obstruction was 88% (95% CI, 70%–96%). MRCP was better at diagnosing the presence of biliary obstruction and its level with sensitivities of 97% and 98%, respectively, than in diagnosing ductal stones [59].

ERCP has a major role in suspected biliary sepsis. It provides reliable diagnosis as to the location and etiology of the obstruction and can be used to establish drainage in most cases. PTC is an alternative when ERCP expertise is not available or technically is not possible.

Biliary Drainage

Many patients respond well to antibiotics and resuscitation, which makes biliary drainage a semielective procedure performed within the subsequent 72 hours. Some patients, however, will not respond to antibiotics or deteriorate over the next 12 to 24 hours and require urgent biliary decompression. Adequate biliary drainage remains the cornerstone of treatment of cholangitis because antibiotics alone often do not resolve the cholangitis in the presence of biliary obstruction. The timing of biliary drainage has not been studied in randomized trials but clearly, patients who are hypotensive on presentation have a high probability of needing urgent biliary decompression. The three modalities that are available for biliary drainage are ERCP, PTC, and open surgical drainage. Advantages and disadvantages of each technique are summarized in Table 3.

ERCP has become the procedure of choice for drainage of the biliary system in acute cholangitis. Lai and colleagues [60] showed that emergent endoscopic drainage was superior to endoscopic sphincterotomy (ES) in terms of morbidity (34% versus 66%) and mortality (10% versus 32%). This finding is supported by other studies [61–63]. It also is superior to PTC in terms of morbidity, length of hospitalization, and overall success rate [64,65]. ERCP is tolerated well and is safe at both extremes of age [66–68]. After access to the CBD has been achieved, several options exist to establish and maintain biliary drainage: sphincterotomy, nasobiliary tube drainage, stent drainage, stone removal, or a combination of these. Hui and colleagues [69] randomized 74 patients who had acute cholangitis into one group that was treated with ES and stenting and one group that was treated with stenting alone. There was no significant difference in the two groups with respect to success rates for stent insertion, complications, length of hospital stay, or resolution of jaundice. This study found that ES is not essential in this setting in which coagulopathy is common. In unstable patients, it is not crucial to clear the CBD of stones as long as a stent is placed to establish drainage. A more definitive procedure can be performed after the condition of the patient has improved. In one study by Chopra and colleagues [70], high-risk patients–elderly or with debilitating disease–were randomized to duct clearance or stent insertion only. At 72 hours, the group that had stent insertion had a complication rate of 7% and the group that underwent ductal clearance

Table 3
Biliary drainage procedures for acute cholangitis

Method	Advantage	Disadvantage	Comments
Endoscopic	Safer than surgery. Drainage usually established through combination of sphincterotomy, stent, or nasobiliary tube. Potential for stone removal and biopsy or brushings of strictures	Invasive. Pancreatitis, bleeding, perforation	ERCP most often is the procedure of choice
Transhepatic (radiologic)	Allows biliary drainage when ERCP is not possible	Invasive Higher complication rate than ERCP. Patient discomfort from percutaneous catheter	More likely needed in proximal malignant lesions involving the biliary system
Surgery	Cholecystectomy in stone disease. Allows biopsy diagnosis in magnancy. Definitive bypass procedure often possible	High morbidity and mortality	Surgery rarely is the procedure of choice in the setting of acute cholangitis

had a complication rate of 16% ($P = .18$); however, at a median of 20 months, the complication rate in the stented group was significantly higher than in the patients whose ducts were cleared. This study suggested that stent insertion alone was safe and effective and definitive treatment. Stone clearance may be performed electively when the patient is more stable [70]. In very sick or unstable patients, a nasobiliary catheter is preferred sometimes. It allows for a short procedure time, obviates a sphincterotomy in patients who are often coagulopathic, and allows for frequent lavage of the biliary system until the patient is more stable and a more definitive procedure can be performed. Nasobiliary drainage seems to be as effective as endoscopic sphincterotomy with CBD stenting in the management of acute cholangitis [71,72]. In one study 150 patients who had cholangitis were randomized to a 7F CBD stent or a 7F nasobiliary drain [72]. There was no difference in the outcome. Endoscopists who are comfortable with this procedure may prefer this option in selected patients.

PTC is achieved using local anesthesia. A small-gauge Chiba needle obtains access to the intrahepatic biliary system under fluoroscopic guidance. A wire can then be passed followed by a drainage catheter [73,74]. Although success rates are high (up to 90%), the morbidity and mortality are higher than with endoscopic drainage [64,70,75–77]. Complications include hemobilia, intraabdominal hemorrhage, septicemia, pneumothorax, hydrothorax, and bile leak. It is an option when ERCP expertise is lacking or the ampulla Vater is inaccessible because of previous bowel surgery or tumor. PTC-placed drains can be internalized by way of the so-called "combined or rendezvous" procedure with an interventional radiologist in patients who require palliative drainage. During this procedure, the radiologist provides a guide wire through the percutaneous drain that can be snared and pulled up by the duodenoscope, thus establishing access for CBD stent placement.

Open surgery rarely is the first-line therapy for biliary drainage because endoscopic and percutaneous drainage have lower morbidity and mortality [78–80]. In one retrospective view of 84 patients who had cholangitis and underwent CBD exploration, the overall complication and death rates were 50% and 20%, respectively. Multivariate analysis revealed that the complication and death rates increased to 91% and 55%, respectively, if three or more of the following risk factors were present at the time of surgery: concomitant medical problems, pH less than 7.4, total bilirubin greater than 90 μmol/L, platelet count less than 150 k/mm^3, and serum albumin less than 3 g/L. Surgical options include open choledochotomy, sphincteroplasty, T-tube placement, or biliary-enteric drainage procedures. Mortality from surgical drainage in acutely ill patients can be up to 50% [81]. This high mortality may reflect sicker patients who have failed endoscopic or percutaneous approaches; however, surgery is best done electively after initial nonoperative drainage and antibiotics, when the patient is more stable.

Biliary obstruction at the level of the hilum (Klatskin tumors) raise several issues. Should one keep injection of contrast to a minimum to avoid introducing infection into a sterile ductal system? Should the left and right hepatic ducts be stented and drained? Is a cholangiogram necessary? It has been shown that drainage of the left or the right hepatic duct is sufficient to drain and treat the obstruction, and it is not necessary to drain both sides [82,83]. De Palma and colleagues [82] found that a single metallic stent placed in whichever duct was easier to access achieved successful drainage in more than 96% of patients. Studies also suggest that selective MRCP or CT-targeted drainage without contrast injection may be more cost-effective than the traditional technique with bilateral stent drainage [84]. In practice, one should resist the urge to get a "good" cholangiogram in this setting. It is the author's practice to use a minimum amount of contrast, and then stent the side into which the guide wire goes. If the cholangitis does not resolve promptly following endoscopic stent placement, additional percutaneous drainage should be considered.

SUMMARY

Table 4 gives summary recommendations concerning the major decisions that are related to the diagnosis and management of suspected acute bacterial cholangitis. All of these decisions have to be made within the context of disease severity, degree of diagnostic uncertainty, and associated comorbidity. Although these recommendations are based on evidence, there are few

Table 4
Recommended approach to the patient who has suspected bacterial cholangitis

Intervention	Recommended	Alternative	Comments
Antibiotic therapy	Ampicillin + gentamicin ± metronidazole	Pipracillin + tobramycin ± metronidazole	
Diagnostic imaging	Abdominal ultrasound; CT scan or MRCP	CT scan or MRCP EUS	
Biliary drainage	ERCP	PTC	
Surgery	If definitive procedure (eg, Whipple's) is planned or palliative bypass in duodenal obstruction		

randomized controlled trials. Antibiotics that cover gram negatives and anaerobes, along with fluid and electrolyte correction, frequently stabilize the patient. Imaging studies frequently confirm the diagnosis and identify the location and etiology of the obstruction. With or without a definitive diagnosis, ERCP or PTC can be done emergently to establish drainage to control sepsis. Although endoscopic and percutaneous drainage techniques have lower morbidity and mortality than does emergent surgical decompression, optimal management of this potentially life-threatening condition requires close cooperation between the gastroenterologist, radiologist, and surgeon.

References

[1] Montariol T, Msika S, Charlier A, et al. Diagnosis of asymptomatic common bile duct stones: preoperative endoscopic ultrasonography versus intraoperative cholangiography—a multicenter, prospective controlled study. Surgery 1998;124(1):6–13.

[2] Gerber A, Apt MK. The case against routine operative cholangiography. Am J Surg 1982;143(6):734–6.

[3] Montariol T, Rey C, Charlier A, et al. Preoperative evaluation of the probability of common bile duct stones. J Am Coll Surg 1995;180(3):293–6.

[4] Deviere J, Motte S, Dumonceau JM, et al. Septicemia after endoscopic retrograde cholangiopancreatography. Endoscopy 1990;22:72–5.

[5] Born P, Rosch T, Bruhl K, et al. Long-term results of endoscopic and percutaneous transhepatic treatment of benign biliary strictures. Endoscopy 1999;31(9):725–31.

[6] Carpenter HA. Bacterial and parasitic cholangitis. Mayo Clin Proc 1998;73:473–8.

[7] Leung JW, Yu AS. Hepatolithiasis and biliary parasites. Bailleres Clin Gastroenterol 1997;11(4):681–706.

[8] Khuroo MS, Zargar SA, Mahajan R. Hepatobiliary and pancreatic ascariasis in India. Lancet 1990;335(8704):1503–6.

[9] Hurtado RM, Sahani DV, Kradin RL. Case records of the Massachusetts General Hospital. Case 9–2006. A 35-year-old woman with recurrent right-upper-quadrant pain. N Engl J Med 2006;354(12):1295–303.

[10] Horton J, Bilhartz L. Gallstone disease and its complications. In: Feldman M, Friedman L, Sleisenger M, editors. Sleisenger and Fordtran's gastrointestinal and liver disease: pathophysiology, diagnosis, management. Philadelphia: WB Saunders; 2002. p. 1065–90.

[11] Liu LX, Harinasuta KT. Liver and intestinal flukes. Gastroenterol Clin North Am 1996;25: 627–36.

[12] Sandouk F, Haffar S, Zada MM, et al. Pancreatic-biliary ascariasis: experience of 300 cases. Am J Gastroenterol 1997;92:2264–7.
[13] Ducreux M, Buffet C, Lamy P, et al. Diagnosis and prognosis of AIDS-related cholangitis. AIDS 1995;9:875–80.
[14] Csendes A, Fernandez M, Uribe P. Bacteriology of the gallbladder bile in normal subjects. Am J Surg 1975;129:629–31.
[15] Flemma RJ, Flint LM, Osterhout S, et al. Bacteriologic studies of biliary infection. Ann Surg 1967;166:563–72.
[16] Greig JD, Krukowski ZH, Matheson NA. Surgical morbidity and mortality in one hundred and twenty-nine patients with obstructive jaundice. Br J Surg 1988;75:216.
[17] Ozden I, Tekant Y, Bilge O, et al. Endoscopic and radiologic interventions as the leading causes of severe cholangitis in a tertiary referral center. Am J Surg 2005;189(6):702–6.
[18] Lygidakis NJ, Brummelkamp WH. The significance of intrabiliary pressure in acute cholangitis. Surg Gynecol Obstet 1985;161(5):465–9.
[19] Kodama T. [Experimental study on the development of endotoxemia in biliary tract infection with special reference to lymphatic pathway at controlled biliary duct pressure]. Nippon Geka Gakkai Zasshi 1988;89(12):1978–89 [in Japanese].
[20] Karsten TM, van Gulik TM, Spanjaard L, et al. Bacterial translocation from the biliary tract to blood and lymph in rats with obstructive jaundice. J Surg Res 1998;74(2):125–30.
[21] Hanau LH, Steigbigel NH. Acute (ascending) cholangitis. Infect Dis Clin North Am 2000;14:521–46.
[22] Csendes A, Sepulveda A, Burdiles P, et al. Common bile duct pressure in patients with common bile duct stones with or without acute suppurative cholangitis. Arch Surg 1988;123(4):697–9.
[23] Sileri P, Morini S, Sica GS, et al. Bacterial translocation and intestinal morphological findings in jaundiced rats. Dig Dis Sci 2002;47(4):929–34.
[24] Parks RW, Stuart Cameron CH, Gannon CD, et al. Changes in gastrointestinal morphology associated with obstructive jaundice. J Pathol 2000;192(4):526–32.
[25] Parks RW, Clements WD, Smye MG, et al. Intestinal barrier dysfunction in clinical and experimental obstructive jaundice and its reversal by internal biliary drainage. Br J Surg 1996;83(10):1345–9.
[26] Slocum MM, Sittig KM, Specian RD, et al. Absence of intestinal bile promotes bacterial translocation. Am Surg 1992;58(5):305–10.
[27] Kuzu MA, Kale IT, Col C, et al. Obstructive jaundice promotes bacterial translocation in humans. Hepatogastroenterology 1999;46(28):2159–64.
[28] White JS, Hoper M, Parks RW, et al. Patterns of bacterial translocation in experimental biliary obstruction. J Surg Res 2006;132(1):80–4.
[29] Pitt HA, Postier RG, Cameron JL. Biliary bacteria: significance and alterations after antibiotic therapy. Arch Surg 1982;117:445–9.
[30] Maluenda F, Csendes A, Burdiles P, et al. Bacteriological study of choledochal bile in patients with common bile duct stones, with or without suppurative cholangitis. Hepatogastroenterology 1989;36:132–5.
[31] Suzuki Y, Kobayashi A, Ohto M, et al. Bacteriological study of transhepatically aspirated bile: relation to cholangiographic findings in 295 patients. Dig Dis Sci 1984;29:109–15.
[32] Reiss R, Eliashiv A, Deutsch AA. Septic complications and bile cultures in 800 consecutive cholecystectomies. World J Surg 1982;6:195–9.
[33] Brook I. Aerobic and anaerobic microbiology of biliary tract disease. J Clin Microbiol 1989;27:2373–5.
[34] Bourgault A-M, England DM, Rosenblatt JE, et al. Clinical characteristics of anaerobic bactibilia. Arch Intern Med 1979;139:1346–9.
[35] Leung JW, Ling TK, Chan RC, et al. Antibiotics, biliary sepsis and CBD stones. Gastrointest Endosc 1994;40:716–21.

[36] Baker AR, Neoptolemos JP, Carr-Locke DL, et al. Sump syndrome following choledochoduo-denostomy and its endoscopic treatment. Br J Surg 1985;72:433–55.
[37] Leung JW, Chung SC, Sung JJ, et al. Urgent endoscopic drainage for acute suppurative chol-angitis. Lancet 1989;1:1307–9.
[38] Lois JF, Gomes AS, Grace PA, et al. Risks of percutaneous transhepatic drainage in patients with cholangitis. AJR Am J Roentgenol 1987;148:367–71.
[39] Lygidakis NJ. Incidence of bile infection in patients with choledocholithiasis. Am J Gastro-enterol 1982;77:12–7.
[40] Rahman SH, Larvin M, McMahon MJ, et al. Clinical presentation and delayed treatment of cholangitis in older people. Dig Dis Sci 2005;50(12):2207–10.
[41] Reynolds BM, Dargan EL. Acute obstructive cholangitis. A distinct clinical syndrome. Ann Surg 1959;150:299–303.
[42] Rector WG Jr. Fever, shock and chills in gram-negative bacillemia: clinical correlations in 100 cases. Johns Hopkins Med J 1981;149(5):175–8.
[43] Tokuda Y, Miyasato H, Stein GH, et al. The degree of chills for risk of bacteremia in acute febrile illness. Am J Med 2005;118(12):1417.
[44] Dooley JS, Hamilton-Miller JM, Brumfitt W, et al. Antibiotics in the treatment of biliary infec-tion. Gut 1984;25:988–98.
[45] van Lent AU, Bartelsman JF, Tytgat GN, et al. Duration of antibiotic therapy for cholangitis after successful endoscopic drainage of the biliary tract. Gastrointest Endosc 2002;55(4):518–22.
[46] Van Delden OM, van Leeuwen DJ. The relevance of biliary secretion and other features of antibiotics in biliary tract disease: some considerations. In: Tytagat GNJ, Huibregtse K, ed-itors. Bile and bile duct abnormalities: pathophysiology, diagnosis and management. New York: Thieme Medical Publishers; 1989. p. 15–20.
[47] Keighley MRB, Drysdale RB, Quoraishi AH, et al. Antibiotics in biliary disease: the relative importance of antibiotic concentrations in the bile and serum. Gut 1976;17:495–500.
[48] Leung JWC, Chan RCY, Cheung SW, et al. The effect of obstruction on the biliary excretion of cefoperazone and ceftazidime. J Antimicrob Chemother 1990;25:399–406.
[49] Mortimer PR, Mackie DB, Haynes S. Ampicillin levels in human bile in the presence of biliary tract disease. BMJ 1969;3:88–9.
[50] Desai TK, Tsan TK. Aminoglycoside nephrotoxicity in obstructive jaundice. Am J Med 1988;85:47–50.
[51] Gerecht WB, Henry NK, Hoffman WW, et al. Prospective randomized comparison of me-zlocillin therapy alone with combined ampicillin and gentamicin therapy for patients with cholangitis. Arch Intern Med 1989;149(6):1279–84.
[52] Thompson JE Jr, Pitt HA, Doty JE, et al. Broad spectrum penicillin as an adequate therapy for acute cholangitis. Surg Gynecol Obstet 1990;171(4):275–82.
[53] Sung JJ, Lyon DJ, Suen R, et al. Intravenous ciprofloxacin as treatment for patients with acute suppurative cholangitis: a randomized, controlled clinical trial. J Antimicrob Chemother 1995;35(6):855–64.
[54] Taylor KJW, Rosenfield AT, Spiro HM. Diagnostic accuracy of grey scale ultrasonography for the jaundiced patient. Arch Intern Med 1979;139:60–3.
[55] Hakansson K, Ekberg O, Hakansson HO, et al. MR and ultrasound in screening of patients with suspected biliary tract disease. Acta Radiol 2002;43:80–6.
[56] Scheiman JM, Carlos RC, Barnett JL, et al. Can endoscopic ultrasound or magnetic reso-nance cholangiopancreatography replace ERCP in patients with suspected biliary disease? A prospective trial and cost analysis. Am J Gastroenterol 2001;96(10):2900–4.
[57] Songur Y, Temucin G, Sahin B. Endoscopic ultrasonography in the evaluation of dilated common bile duct. J Clin Gastroenterol 2001;33(4):302–5.
[58] Kohut M, Nowakowska-Dulawa E, Marek T, et al. Accuracy of linear endoscopic ultraso-nography in the evaluation of patients with suspected common bile duct stones. Endoscopy 2002;34(4):299–303.

[59] Romagnuolo J, Bardou M, Rahme E, et al. Magnetic resonance cholangiopancreatography: a meta-analysis of test performance in suspected biliary disease. Ann Intern Med 2003;139:547–57.

[60] Lai EC, Mok FP, Tan ES, et al. Endoscopic biliary drainage for severe acute cholangitis. N Engl J Med 1992;326:1582–6.

[61] Leese T, Neoptolemos JP, Baker AR, et al. Management of acute cholangitis and the impact of endoscopic sphincterotomy. Br J Surg 1986;73:988–92.

[62] Chijiiwa K, Kozaki N, Naito T, et al. Treatment of choice for choledocholithiasis in patients with acute obstructive suppurative cholangitis and liver cirrhosis. Am J Surg 1995;170:356–60.

[63] Ditzel H, Schaffalitzky de Muckadell OB. Endoscopic sphincterotomy in acute cholangitis due to choledocholithiasis. Hepatogastroenterology 1990;37:204–7.

[64] Sugiyama M, Atomi Y. Treatment of acute cholangitis due to choledocholithiasis in elderly and younger patients. Arch Surg 1997;132:1129–33.

[65] Sugiyama M, Atomi Y. The benefits of endoscopic nasobiliary drainage without sphincterotomy for acute cholangitis. Am J Gastroenterol 1998;93:2065–8.

[66] Koklu S, Parlak E, Yuksel O, et al. Endoscopic retrograde cholangiopancreatography in the elderly: a prospective and comparative study. Age Ageing 2005;34(6):572–7.

[67] Huguet JM, Sempere J, Bort I, et al. Complications of endoscopic retrograde cholangiopancreatography in patient aged more than 90 years old. Gastroenterol Hepatol 2005;28(5):263–6.

[68] Cheng CL, Fogel EL, Sherman S, et al. Diagnostic and therapeutic endoscopic retrograde colangiopancreatography in children: a large series report. J Pediatr Gastroenterol Nutr 2005;41(4):445–53.

[69] Hui CK, Lai KC, Yuen MF, et al. Does the addition of endoscopic sphincterotomy to stent insertion improve drainage of the bile duct in acute suppurative cholangitis? Gastrointest Endosc 2003;58(4):500–4.

[70] Chopra KB, Peters RA, O'Toole PA, et al. Randomised study of endoscopic biliary endoprosthesis versus duct clearance fore bileduct stones in high-risk patients. Lancet 1996;348(9030):791–3.

[71] Lee DW, Chan AC, Lam YH, et al. Biliary decompression by nasobiliary catheter or biliary stent in acute suppurative cholangitis: a prospective randomized trial. Gastrointest Endosc 2002;56:361–5.

[72] Sharma BC, Kumar R, Agarwal N, et al. Endoscopic biliary drainage by nasobiliary drain or by stent placement in patients with acute cholangitis. Endoscopy 2005;37(5):439–43.

[73] Takada T, Yasuda H, Hanyu F. Technique and management of percutaneous transhepatic cholangial drainage for treating an obstructive jaundice. Hepatogastroenterology 1995;42:317–22.

[74] Laufer U, Kirchner J, Kickuth R, et al. A comparative study of CT fluoroscopy combined with fluoroscopy versus fluoroscopy alone for percutaneous transhepatic biliary drainage. Cardiovasc Intervent Radiol 2001;24(4):240–4.

[75] Joseph PK, Bizer LS, Sprayregen SS, et al. Percutaneous transhepatic biliary drainage: results and complications in 81 patients. JAMA 1986;255:2763–7.

[76] Kadakia SC. Biliary tract emergencies: acute cholecystitis, acute cholangitis, and acute pancreatitis. Med Clin North Am 1993;77:1015–36.

[77] Pessa ME, Hawkins IF, Vogel SB. The treatment of acute cholangitis: percutaneous transhepatic biliary drainage before definitive therapy. Ann Surg 1987;205:389–92.

[78] Boey JH, Way LW. Acute cholangitis. Ann Surg 1980;191:264–70.

[79] Lai EC, Tam PC, Paterson IA, et al. Emergency surgery for severe acute cholangitis: the high risk patients. Ann Surg 1990;211:55–9.

[80] Raraty MG, Finch M, Neoptolemos JP. Acute cholangitis and pancreatitis secondary to common duct stones: management update. World J Surg 1998;22:1155–61.

[81] O'Connor MH, Schwartz ML, McQuarrie DG, et al. Cholangitis due to malignant obstruction of biliary outflow. Ann Surg 1981;193:341.

[82] De Palma GD, Pezzullo A, Rega M, et al. Unilateral placement of metallic stents for malignant hilar obstruction: a prospective study. Gastrointest Endosc 2003;58(1):50–3.

[83] Freeman ML, Overby C. Selective MRCP and CT-targeted drainage of malignant hilar biliary obstruction with self-expanding metallic stents. Gastrointest Endosc 2003;58(1): 41–9.

[84] Harewood GC, Baron TH. Cost analysis of magnetic resonance cholangiography in the management of inoperable hilar biliary obstruction. Am J Gastroenterol 2002;97(5): 1152–8.

Gastroenterol Clin N Am 35 (2006) 425–461

GASTROENTEROLOGY CLINICS
OF NORTH AMERICA

ELSEVIER
SAUNDERS

Hepatitis B: The Pathway to Recovery Through Treatment

F. Blaine Hollinger, MD[a],*, Daryl T.-Y. Lau, MD, MSc, MPH[b,c]

[a]Departments of Medicine, Molecular Virology and Microbiology, Eugene B. Casey Hepatitis Research Center and Diagnostic Laboratory, Baylor College of Medicine, One Baylor Plaza, BCM-385, Houston, TX 77030–3498, USA
[b]Division of Gastroenterology and Hepatology, Department of Internal Medicine, The University of Texas Medical Branch at Galveston, 4.106 McCullough Building, 301 University Boulevard, Galveston, TX 77555–0764, USA
[c]Beth Israel Deaconess Medical Center, 330 Brooline Avenue, Boston, MA 02215, USA

Hepatitis B is a major public health problem in the world today. It is estimated that over 2 billion people have been infected with hepatitis B virus (HBV) resulting in 300 to 400 million carriers. During their lifetime, 25% of these persistently infected persons develop chronic hepatitis or hepatocellular carcinoma (HCC) resulting in 1.2 million deaths per year making hepatitis B the 10th leading cause of death worldwide. HCC is the third highest cause of death from cancer in the world, the fifth most common malignancy in males, and the eighth in females. Untreated, it yields a dismal 5-year survival between 2% and 6%.

In the United States, approximately 1.5 million people are infected with HBV. In 2003, the number of cases reported to the Centers for Disease Control and Prevention was 7526, a rate of 2.6 per 100,000 population [1]. This represents 46% of the cases of viral hepatitis reported, although it is estimated that the true incidence of hepatitis B is 15 to 30 times the reported rate. Since 1985, however, the number of reported cases has declined by over 75% (Fig. 1), presumably as a direct result of universal immunization of neonates, vaccination of at-risk populations, lifestyle or behavioral changes in high-risk groups, refinements in the screening of blood donors, and the use of virally inactivated or genetically engineered products in patients with bleeding disorders. In 2001, the authors screened over 450 Chinese-Americans in Houston, Texas, and noted an HBV carrier rate of 8.2% in that population.

This work was supported by the Eugene B. Casey Foundation and the William and Sonya Carpenter Fund, Baylor College of Medicine.

*Corresponding author. E-mail address: blaineh@bcm.tmc.edu (F.B. Hollinger).

0889-8553/06/$ – see front matter
doi:10.1016/j.gtc.2006.03.002

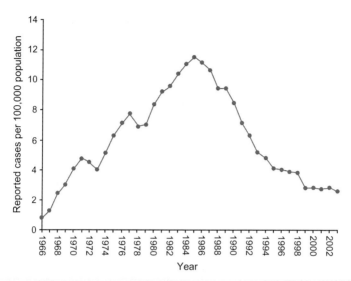

Fig. 1. Incidence of reported acute hepatitis B, United States, 1966–2003. (*Data from* Centers for Disease Control and Prevention. Hepatitis surveillance report No. 60. Atlanta (GA): US Department of Health and Human Services, Centers for Disease Control and Prevention; 2005.)

INFECTIOUS AGENT

HBV is an enveloped DNA virus that initiates an infection by binding to its receptor on the hepatocytes, penetrating the cellular membrane, followed by uncoating of the virion [2]. The nucleocapsid is translocated through nuclear pores into the nucleus of the cell where the genomic DNA is matured to the covalently closed, circular DNA [CCCDNA]. The CCCDNA is the power source for continuing replication of the virus and is amplified during the replicative cycle. The DNA is transcribed and the resulting RNAs translated in the cytoplasm to the various viral proteins. Pregenomic RNAs are encapsidated within subviral core particles in the cytoplasm along with a viral DNA polymerase enzyme for viral DNA synthesis. Unlike most DNA viruses, it replicates by reverse transcription of the genomic RNA template. This process includes polymerization of the minus-strand DNA, degradation of the RNA intermediate, and incomplete synthesis of the plus-strand. Progeny cores bud into the endoplasmic reticulum where they acquire their envelope before undergoing vesicular transport out of the cell.

During this process, HBV production may approach 10^{11} molecules per day, although during peak replication the production rate may increase 100 to 1000 times the basal rate, which suggests that there is considerable reserve replicative capacity. Ordinarily, DNA polymerases have excellent fidelity in reading DNA templates. Fidelity is defined as the frequency of correct nucleotide insertions per incorrect insertion. The reason for this enhanced fidelity is because when a mismatch is polymerized to the growing 3' end of a molecule, it retards the polymerase activity leaving the mismatched nucleotide at the 3' terminus. This delay allows spontaneous melting to occur and releases the 3' end to contact an exonuclease site, which then excises the incorrectly added nucleotides.

In contrast to that observed with other DNA viruses, the HBV DNA polymerase lacks either fidelity or proofreading function partly because exonuclease activity is either absent or deficient in HBV. As a result, the genome, and especially the envelope gene, is mutated with unusually high frequency during replication. The mutation rate of HBV lies somewhere between the RNA-containing retroviruses, such as HIV, and other DNA viruses that lack requirements for reverse transcriptase activity. The reasons for this are not entirely clear, but may be caused by the fact that mutations in HBV are not well tolerated because over 50% of the open reading frames in the HBV genome are overlapping. For example, the HBV viral polymerase gene overlaps the pre-S/S gene and covers approximately 80% of the genome. Therefore, any mutation that occurs during replication can affect more than one open reading frame.

Electron microscopy of sera from patients with hepatitis B infection reveals the presence of three distinct morphologic entities (Fig. 2). The more numerous forms (by a factor of 10^4 to 10^6) are small, hepatitis B surface antigen (HBsAg)–positive, pleomorphic spherical particles measuring 17 to 25 nm in diameter (mean of 20 nm). Tubular or filamentous forms of various lengths, but with a diameter similar to that of the smaller particles, also are observed. Neither of these forms contains viral-specific nucleic acid, which is found in a complex, double-shelled particle with a diameter of 42 nm that comprises the hepatitis B virion. It consists of a 27-nm core surrounded by a 7- to 8-nm viral protein coat called HBsAg. This protein is identical to that detected

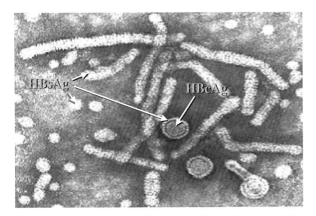

Fig. 2. Electron micrograph of hepatitis B virus. HBcAg, hepatitis B core antigen; HBsAg, hepatitis B surface antigen.

on the smaller particles and the filaments. It contains three related glycoproteins designated S or major, M or middle (pre-S1 + S), and L or large (pre-S1 + pre-S2 + S). These proteins are not distributed uniformly between the various HBV particles that circulate in the blood. For example, the more numerous 20-nm particles (by a factor of 10,000 to 1 million) are composed primarily of the S protein, with variable amounts of the M polypeptide and essentially none of the L chains. Conversely, the HBV virion contains relatively large amounts of the L chains to M or S chains. The L chains are believed to contain the recognition site for binding to hepatocytes and are important for viral assembly and infectivity. This arrangement may be evolutionary because it prevents the significantly more numerous, noninfectious 20-nm particles, which often lack L chains, from competing for receptor sites on the surface of hepatocytes thereby interfering with infection. Increased levels of L chains also seem to down-regulate the release of the 20-nm HBsAg particles. The nucleocapsid of the virion contains a single capsid protein called hepatitis B core antigen (HBcAg). The HBV DNA is encapsidated within the nucleocapsid as a relaxed circular, partially double-stranded DNA molecule.

The viral genome has four open reading frames that code for the viral polymerase; the structural protein of the nucleocapsid (HBcAg); the viral surface glycoproteins (HBsAg); and a complex regulatory protein (X protein) that is required for infectivity. Infected individuals develop antibodies to HBsAg (anti-HBs) and HBcAg (anti-HBc) and some also generate an antibody response to the X protein. The open reading frame that code for the core protein also codes for another protein known serologically as the hepatitis B e antigen (HBeAg). This product is not a part of the virion, and is secreted from the cell. Its accumulation in the serum is usually indicative of highly active replication of the virus. It often evokes its own antibody response (anti-HBe), which can signify a return to a less active state of viral replication. Mutant viruses with lesions in the pre-C or core promoter region of the HBV genome, however, can prevent the expression of HBeAg [3]. As a result, these patients are anti-HBe positive but may have viral replication rates that are higher than expected.

PATHOLOGY

HBV causes both acute and chronic liver disease. The pattern of liver injury is characterized by hepatocellular destruction, regeneration, and inflammatory infiltrates. Although these pathologic changes typically resolve completely after viral clearance, chronic infection is often accompanied by progressive fibrosis and architectural disarray that culminates in cirrhosis. The pattern of injury accompanying viral hepatitis has distinct features and may be distinguished from other forms of liver disease, such as cholestatic liver disease, autoimmune hepatitis, metabolic liver disease, drug-induced hepatitis, and steatohepatitis. The pattern of injury seen with acute hepatitis B, however, overlaps significantly with other causes of viral hepatitis.

Chronic Hepatitis

The histologic hallmark of chronic hepatitis B (CHB) is inflammatory destruction of hepatocytes accompanied by progressive fibrosis [4–6]. Because CHB takes decades to progress to end-stage liver disease, it is important to assess not only the pattern of injury but also the histologic severity and stage of hepatitis B. Most histologic classification systems have two scores: one based on inflammatory activities (grade) and the other on fibrosis (stage). The grade is indicative of ongoing disease activity, whereas the stage represents the cumulative effect of the disease. The inflammatory component is divided into three compartments: (1) the interface zone between the hepatocytes and the portal area (limiting plate); (2) the portal area; and (3) the hepatocellular parenchyma. Piecemeal necrosis or interface hepatitis describes the destruction of hepatocytes at the limiting plate, which forms a well-defined structure demarcating the hepatic parenchyma and the portal area. It may be focal, involving only one or two hepatocytes with little destruction of the limiting plate, or it may be extensive, involving the entire circumference of the portal area with penetration of the inflammatory cells to a depth of several hepatocytes. In more severe cases, the necroinflammatory process extends into the parenchyma, reaching to the terminal hepatic veins or to other portal areas (bridging necrosis). Lymphoid infiltrates can fill and expand the portal areas, and occasionally form aggregates of variable density.

Parenchymal inflammation in CHB generally consists of small foci of lymphocytes and macrophages surrounding apoptotic bodies or necrotic (dropout) hepatocytes. Plasma cells and eosinophils can sometimes be seen in these foci. The relative abundance of plasma cells serves to distinguish chronic hepatitis from acute hepatitis. When these foci of lobular necrosis are the dominant features of the inflammatory pattern, it often is difficult to distinguish chronic from acute hepatitis. Regardless, this pathologic feature can be seen in many patients with CHB, particularly those with HBeAg-negative mutant infection who experience periodic flares of symptoms and biochemical abnormalities [7]. Occasionally, more extensive lobular necroinflammation with confluent, bridging, or panlobular necrosis can be seen. Frequent and severe attacks can lead to more rapid progression to cirrhosis.

Although the pattern of inflammation characterizes the pathologic process of chronic hepatitis, it is the extent of fibrosis that determines the severity and prognosis of the disease. The earliest change is an expansion of the portal area by new collagen formation. Single hepatocytes or groups of hepatocytes are surrounded by newly formed connective tissue, forming active fibrous septa. These fibrous septations gradually extend from portal areas to other portal areas or to the terminal hepatic veins (bridging fibrosis). With continued inflammation, diffuse bridging fibrosis of varying width develops and, together with regenerative changes and acinar destruction, results in the distorted architectural pattern that is recognized as cirrhosis. Cirrhosis is defined as a diffuse change of the liver in which the normal architecture is replaced by regenerative nodules surrounded by bands of fibrosis. Once patients reach this stage, end-stage (decompensated) liver disease ensues with high morbidity and mortality.

DIAGNOSIS

Before reviewing the serologic changes that follow exposure to HBV, it is essential to have an understanding of the sensitivity of the current assays used to detect the various antigens, antibodies, and HBV DNA that circulate in the blood of infected individuals. Mass measurement units for HBsAg and HBV DNA proceed from micrograms, to nanograms, to picograms at 1000-fold intervals. Current licensed or newer enzyme immunoassays or chemiluminescent assays can detect <0.1 ng (0.1 IU or 100 pg) of HBsAg per milliliter of blood. Levels can approach 300 μg (300,000 ng) in many infected patients. However, the upper limit of detection for these assays is about 1 μg (1000 ng) per milliliter above which level saturation (a plateau) is reached. It has been estimated that you need at least 1000 20-nm HBsAg particles per milliliter of blood for current HBsAg tests to be reactive. Regardless, within the dynamic range of the test there is a direct correlation between the magnitude of the result and the concentration of antigen or antibody in the specimen, especially when paired samples are tested concurrently. If semiquantitation becomes necessary (eg, to predict resolution of the disease), the sample must be diluted until a value that falls within the dynamic range of the assay is obtained. Laboratories should report positive hepatitis serologic results in ratios in which levels ≥ 1 are considered reactive. A visit or call to the serology laboratory is often sufficient to obtain this information or to induce them to report the results as ratios. Confirmation of positive results is usually performed by showing that they are repeatable or, in the case of HBsAg, are specifically inhibited by unlabeled anti-HBs. Similar validation of HBsAg can be accomplished when anti-HBc (or HBV DNA, anti-HBe, or HBeAg) are detected. A common cause of nonspecific reactivity, especially with HBsAg, is usually manifested by a weakly positive response (ratios < 3) and occurs most often when testing blood that contains heparin or is from a patient with clotting abnormalities.

Nucleic acid hybridization procedures and other nucleic acid tests, such as the polymerase chain reaction (PCR) assay for the detection of HBV DNA in serum and tissue, have been important in unraveling some of the intricate immunopathogenetic mechanisms of HBV disease and for evaluating the response to antiviral therapy. Methodology for the detection of HBV DNA has gone through several innovative changes, and appreciation of their relative sensitivities is important when interpreting the published data. To place this information into perspective, it should be observed that 1 pg of HBV DNA is equivalent to about 283,000 copies or genomic-equivalents of HBV. The most sensitive assays are rapidly approaching the level of a single HBV DNA genome at least 50% of the time. For comparisons of sensitivities, it is important to convert everything to copies per milliliter or International Unit (IU) per milliliter rather than copies per reaction (or IU per reaction), because the amount of sample used to obtain a result is often different.

The dynamic range and lower limit of detection of nucleic acid assays, set at a level that detects at least 95% of the samples containing a designated amount of virus, are quite variable and, within similar products, widely divergent results can occur (Fig. 3). Results are reported in a confusing array of units including copies per milliliter, genome equivalents (gEq) per milliliter, megaequivalents (MEq) per milliliter, and IU per milliliter. The genome equivalents per milliliter or copies per milliliter differ for each assay. To resolve this, a World Health Organization International Standard was established and arbitrarily assigned a potency of 10^6 IU/mL [8]. Assays are now being normalized to this standard, such that 1 IU/mL equals approximately 4.2 to 6.8 gEq or copies per milliliter of HBV DNA or lower.

Nucleic acid tests are prone to false-positive and false-negative results, which clinicians must appreciate when monitoring their patients. In addition, clinicians must realize that a real-time test result performed on a single sample when compared with a previous real-time test result may differ by threefold to fivefold (0.5–0.7 $\log_{10}$) even when the results are, in reality, the same. This becomes an even greater problem if the test methodology is not the same. Batch testing, in which one test is performed on multiple stored samples from the same patient, can provide results that are considered disparate if they differ by more than threefold (0.5 $\log_{10}$).

Serology

With this background, an understanding of the various clinical and serologic patterns associated with acute hepatitis B and CHB is essential for interpreting the results of the various serologic tests as summarized in Table 1 [9]. In a typical case of acute transfusion-associated HBV infection, HBV DNA is detected 2 to 5 weeks after infection and up to 40 days before the appearance of HBsAg (average 6–15 days), although newer, more sensitive HBsAg assays are closing

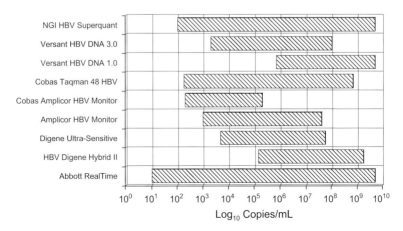

Fig. 3. Dynamic range of current and previous HBV DNA assays.

Table 1
Interpretation of hepatitis B virus serologic markers

HBV DNA	HBsAg	Anti-HBc	Anti-HBs	Interpretation
Pos	Neg	Neg	Neg	Preseroconversion window period; occult infection
Pos	**Pos**	Neg	Neg	Early acute infection
Pos	**Pos**	**Pos**	Neg	HBV infection, either acute or chronic
Neg	Neg	**Pos**	**Pos**	Previous infection with immunity (normal ALT)
Neg/**Pos**	Neg	**Pos**	Neg	Low-level carrier; early convalescent period; remote HBV infection; false-positive reaction; passive antibody
Neg	Neg	Neg	**Pos**	Vaccine-type response
Neg	Neg	Neg	Neg	Excludes HBV infection

Abbreviations: HBsAg, hepatitis B surface antigen; HBV, hepatitis B virus.
Data from Hollinger FB, Liang JT. Hepatitis B virus. In: Fields BN, Knipe DM, Howley PM, et al, editors. Fields Virology, 4th edition. Philadelphia: Lippincott Williams & Wilkins; 2001. p. 2971–3036.

this gap [10,11]. The HBV DNA rises slowly and circulates at relatively low levels during the early HBsAg seronegative window period (10^2–10^4 copies/mL). In contrast, viral concentrations exceeding 10^{10} HBV DNA copies per milliliter are often present during the prodromal, acute, or chronic phase of the infection. As anticipated, communicability is highest when concentrations of infectious virus attain their highest levels in the blood. This is especially true for nonparenteral (sexual) transmission. HBsAg is first detected 6 to 9 weeks after transfusion, which is 1 to 3 weeks before the alanine aminotransference (ALT) level becomes abnormal and 3 to 5 weeks before the onset of symptoms or jaundice. It reaches a peak concentration during the acute stage of the illness, and then slowly declines to undetectable levels within 4 to 6 months, although more sensitive assays can extend this time interval.

HBeAg and IgM-specific anti-HBc are usually detected subsequent to the appearance of HBsAg and concurrent with the onset of ALT abnormalities. Their appearance in the serum is indicative of ongoing viral replication. The IgM anti-HBc declines to undetectable levels regardless of whether the disease resolves or becomes chronic, but the antibody may reappear at relatively low levels as a 7S IgM fraction during reactivation of HBV as opposed to the 19S component that is present in acute disease [12,13]. IgG-specific anti-HBc generally remains detectable for a lifetime. There is no specific commercial IgG anti-HBc assay. Total anti-HBc assays measure both IgM and IgG anti-HBc.

Termination of acute HBV infection occurs with the disappearance of HBsAg and HBV DNA and the appearance of anti-HBs. Those patients who maintain high levels of HBsAg concentration throughout the infection, or those whose serum HBeAg persists 8 to 10 weeks after symptoms begin to resolve, are most likely to become chronic HBV carriers. In 21% to 32% of chronic carriers, anti-HBs also can be detected usually in relatively low concentrations [14–16]. Many of these patients have more serious liver disease, and either the antigenic specificity of the antibody is dissimilar to the HBsAg circulating in the blood or HBV may be mutated. Using highly sensitive PCR assays, HBV DNA usually remains detectable as long as HBsAg is present in the serum.

CLINICAL FEATURES

The clinical and serologic changes that occur following infection represent a complex interaction between the virus and the host associated with an immune response to the viral infection [9]. In addition to the inapparent or subclinical cases, patients may develop anicteric or icteric hepatitis (Table 2). The terms "inapparent hepatitis" and "anicteric hepatitis" often are used interchangeably. The term "anicteric hepatitis," however, should be reserved for those patients who develop clinical symptoms but who are not jaundiced. Patients with inapparent (subclinical) hepatitis have neither symptoms nor jaundice. Symptoms ranging from mild and transient to severe and prolonged may accompany clinical hepatitis. Patients may recover completely, progress to chronic hepatitis, or develop fulminant hepatitis and die. It is important to recognize that the frequency of clinical disease increases with age, whereas the percentage of carriers decreases [17]. In endemic regions, asymptomatic perinatal acquisition of disease from HBeAg-positive mothers results in a high carrier rate of 85% to 90% [18]. In contrast, symptomatic acute infection occurs in approximately 40% of the adult-acquired infection, but the carrier rate is only approximately 2% to 5% in the absence of immunodeficiency (see Table 2) [9].

The incubation period for hepatitis B virus ranges from 45 to 120 days. Incubation periods of less than 35 days or more than 150 days are unusual. A short prodromal or preicteric phase, varying from several days to more than a week, precedes the onset of jaundice in over 85% of the HBV cases.

Table 2	
Predicted outcome after an infection with hepatitis B virus	
Predicted parameter	**Outcome (%)**
Inapparent (subclinical) or anicteric disease	65–80
Icteric disease	20–35
Complete recovery	90–98
Chronic disease (% of total number infected)	2–5[a]
Mortality rate	
Based on infection	0.2–0.5
Based on icteric cases	0.5–1.5

[a]Data compiled for adults. Infection in the perinatal period leads to chronic disease in 80%–90% of infants born to HBeAg-positive carrier mothers.
Data from Holinger FB, Liang JT. Hepatitis B virus. In: Fields BN, Knipe DM, Howley PM, et al, editors. Fields Virology, 4th edition. Philadelphia: Lippincott Williams & Wilkins; 2001. p. 2971–3036.

Fever, if present, usually subsides after the first few days of jaundice. Occasionally, more extensive necrosis of the liver occurs. This entity, designated fulminant hepatitis B if it occurs during the first 8 weeks of illness, is characterized by the sudden onset of high fever, marked abdominal pain, vomiting, and jaundice, followed by the development of hepatic encephalopathy associated with deep coma and seizures and accompanied by severe impairment of hepatic synthetic processes, excretory functions, and detoxifying mechanisms. Although fulminant hepatitis is uncommon when compared with overall infection rates, it is observed in up to 4% of the hospitalized cases and leads to death in 70% to 90% of the patients in the absence of transplantation [19]. Recovery, when it occurs, is generally complex and without the development of chronicity.

At least one prospective study [17] indicates that higher proportions of individuals with subclinical hepatitis B are more likely to progress to chronic hepatitis (14.8% of 162) than are those who develop clinical hepatitis B (3.8% of 26). In general, chronic disease occurs in 2% to 5% of immunocompetent adults who are infected, whereas a higher rate is observed in immunocompromised patients. Previous reported higher rates of chronicity following acute hepatitis were probably inaccurate because of the fact that many of these cases were resulting from reactivation or exacerbation of unrecognized asymptomatic CHB.

Clinical Phases of Chronic Hepatitis B Virus Infection

Chronic HBV infection is defined by the persistence of HBsAg for 6 months or longer [20]. It can be classified into three major forms: (1) HBsAg carriers with inactive disease, (2) HBeAg-positive CHB, and (3) HBeAg-negative CHB. Most patients with chronic infection remain asymptomatic for many years. Some of these patients may have no clinical or biochemical evidence of liver disease. To distinguish this group from patients with chronic hepatitis, they are often categorized as asymptomatic hepatitis B carriers or simply HBsAg carriers. De Franchis and coworkers [21] recently studied the natural history of chronic HBV infection in a cohort of these patients. At baseline, 96% of 92 patients were anti-HBe positive and histologic abnormalities were normal or minimal in all but five who had only mild chronic hepatitis. During a mean follow-up of 130 months, liver enzymes remained normal in 85% of 68 patients who were extensively followed, and 13% of these patients cleared their HBsAg. Among 21 HBsAg carriers who showed no biochemical changes during 10 years of follow-up, there were no histologic changes; spontaneous reactivation was a rare event (4% of 68 patients); and no HCC was detected. Other investigators have reviewed the outcome of patients who have been histologically classified as having mild chronic hepatitis for up to 18 years [22,23]. Less than 1% of these patients progressed to cirrhosis.

CHB is the term used to describe HBeAg-positive or HBeAg-negative patients with significant chronic necroinflammatory disease of the liver associated with moderate to advanced fibrosis or cirrhosis caused by persistent HBV infection as found on liver biopsy. This is to distinguish them from the inactive (healthy) HBsAg carrier state described previously in which chronic HBV infection is present without significant ongoing necroinflammatory disease and no or minimal fibrosis on a biopsy. Patients with moderate to severe chronic hepatitis may have no symptoms, or they may be significantly incapacitated. At the time of the initial diagnosis, jaundice is uncommon, ascites and pedal edema are seen in approximately 20%, whereas fewer than 5% present with endogenous encephalopathy or variceal bleeding. Aminotransferases, bilirubin, and gamma globulin levels are mild to markedly elevated. During follow-up, there may be a series of remissions and relapses. Remissions may last a few months to several years. During a relapse, aminotransferases may be markedly elevated and jaundice may be present. Predictors of progression to cirrhosis include hepatic decompensation; repeated episodes of severe acute exacerbation with bridging hepatic necrosis or high alpha fetoprotein levels (greater than 100 ng/mL); acute exacerbations without HBeAg clearance; and HBV reactivation with the reappearance of HBeAg [24,25].

The frequency of HBV variants differs significantly in various regions of the world as a result of the geographic distribution of the HBV genotypes. HBeAg-negative CHB is common in Asia and the Middle East, accounting for about 70% to 80% of the chronic HBV cases in those regions [26]. In contrast, an overall low prevalence of HBeAg-negative chronic HBV infection (24%) was reported in the United States in 1996 [27]. The rate of these HBV variants may have preferentially increased in the different ethnic groups, however, especially among immigrant populations from the endemic areas. In a recent cross-sectional study conducted in 17 liver centers in the United States, Chu and coworkers [28] reported that 63% of the 530 study patients had HBeAg-negative CHB. Among them, 38% had precore variants, 51% had core promoter variants, and 19% had both HBV variants.

Patients with HBeAg-negative CHB display markedly different patterns of serum aminotransferase elevations: (1) continuous elevation of ALT level in approximately 24%, (2) fluctuating ALT levels in 48%, and (3) intermittent or relapsing activities in 28% [29]. Those patients with intermittent ALT elevations could be misdiagnosed as inactive HBV carriers in between flares of hepatitis. These observations underscore the importance of regular assessments of HBsAg-positive patients over time to confirm the diagnosis of HBeAg-negative CHB versus the inactive HBV carrier. In most cases, patients require a liver biopsy. Both HBeAg-positive and HBeAg-negative CHB with persistent or intermittent elevation of aminotransferases and HBV DNA levels, associated with histologic evidence of active hepatitis, should be considered for antiviral therapy.

In one series [25], the overall annual incidence for developing cirrhosis among a group of 684 HBsAg-positive patients with CHB was 2.4% among the HBeAg-positive group and 1.3% among the anti-HBe–positive subjects, but this was not statistically significant. Unfortunately, the outcome following grading and staging of the liver biopsy at baseline was not available. For patients who already have compensated cirrhosis, the 5-year probability of survival ranges from 80% to 86% [30–32] with the cause of death being liver failure in 53% and HCC in 35% (Fig. 4). The 5-year cumulative incidence of decompensation among compensated cirrhotics ranges from 16% to 20% [30,33] presenting as ascites in 49% or associated with jaundice in 30%. Once decompensation occurs, the prognosis is poor with 1- and 5-year survival rates ranging from 55% to 70% and 14% to 28%, respectively [30,31,34].

A proportion of hepatitis B patients, especially those who acquire the disease perinatally, are at risk of developing HCC, a tumor that is relatively slow growing with a median doubling time of 4 months (range of 1–14 months) [35,36]. Metastatic spread is uncommon, with the most frequent sites being the lung (36%); direct extension through the hepatic or portal venous systems (12%); adrenal glands (10%); skeletal tissue (10%); and brain (6%) [37]. Persons at high risk of developing HCC include adult male CHB patients with cirrhosis who contracted their disease in early childhood and who display serologic or histologic evidence of active HBV replication (HBV DNA, HBeAg, IgM anti-HBc, cytoplasmic HBcAg) [38,39]. Approximately 55% to 85% of hepatitis B patients with HCC have cirrhosis at the time of diagnosis [40,41]. Conversely, only about 5% of patients with cirrhosis develop HCC. The cumulative 5-year probability of developing HCC in HBV-infected patients with compensated cirrhosis is 9%; the incidence per 100 person-years is 2.2 [30,42]. Crockett and Keeffe [43] reviewed the relationship between various serologic patterns and the cumulative risk of HCC. The highest adjusted relative risk was found in HBsAg/HBeAg–positive patients with additional risk observed when these patients were found to be coinfected with HCV.

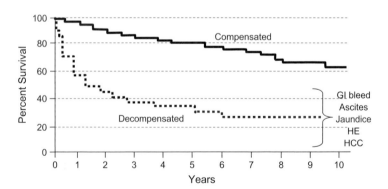

Fig. 4. Effect of decompensation on survival in patients with cirrhosis. GI, gastrointestinal; HCC, hepatocellular carcinoma; HE, hepatic encephalopathy. (*Data from* Realdi G, Fattovich G, Hadziyannis S, et al. Survival and prognostic factors in 366 patients with compensated cirrhosis type B: a multicenter study. The Investigators of the European Concerted Action on Viral Hepatitis (EUROHEP). J Hepatol 1994;21:656–66; and Fattovich G, Giustina G, Schalm SW, et al. Occurrence of hepatocellular carcinoma and decompensation in western European patients with cirrhosis type B. The EUROHEP Study Group on Hepatitis B Virus and Cirrhosis. Hepatology 1995;21:77–82.)

Recently, a great deal of interest has been generated concerning the relationship between a patient's HBV DNA level and the longer-term risk of liver cancer that is independent of HBeAg status, ALT level, and the presence of liver damage or cirrhosis [44,45]. Unfortunately, the patients in these studies usually did not have liver biopsies to document levels of fibrosis at baseline, so that the subset of patients who developed HCC within each of the HBV DNA categories could not be assessed as to risk based on histologic criteria. Chen and coworkers [44] conducted a long-term observational study on a large cohort of HBV carriers in Taiwan and found that the risk of HCC increased significantly proportional to the levels of serum HBV DNA $\geq 10^4$ copies per milliliter. It is not known, however, whether patients with low levels of HBV DNA, but relatively normal histology, are at risk, although previous studies do not support this hypothesis. It also is possible that the natural history of hepatitis B is different between endemic regions of the world where vertical and horizontal transmission is common at a young age and western countries where sexual transmission in adulthood predominates. In addition, the number of patients who acquired HCC was relatively small in this study even though the risk increased. For example, for those patients with HBV DNA levels $\leq 10,000$ copies per milliliter versus those with HBV DNA levels from 10,000 to 100,000 copies per milliliter, the difference in the cumulative incidence of HCC was only 2.2% (3.5%–1.37%) over 13 years. To capture this small subset of at-risk individuals requires the treatment of over 600 people to potentially salvage <7 additional cases of HCC, assuming that treatment of HBV lowers HBV DNA levels, normalizes ALT values, or achieves HBeAg seroconversion in these patients.

Another study implied that HBV replication, as manifested by the presence of HBeAg, is hazardous in terms of disease progression and HCC development (Fig. 5) [46]. This study, however, also did not examine histology at baseline or monitor ALT levels, clinical events, or HBeAg serology during follow-up. Critical subset analyses that take into account the other known risk factors for the development of HCC (age >40 years, male gender, HBeAg positivity, excessive alcohol consumption, elevated ALT level, increased fibrosis) are necessary to establish treatment decisions, especially in adult-acquired CHB patients who have persistently normal aminotransferases and mild histology.

THERAPY FOR CHRONIC HEPATITIS B

Currently, there are five antiviral agents that are approved for the treatment of CHB by the Food and Drug Administration (FDA) in the United States. They are pegylated (PEG) and standard interferon (IFN)-α, lamivudine, adefovir dipivoxil, and entecavir. This section focuses on the application of these compounds for both HBeAg-positive and HBeAg-negative CHB.

Goals of Therapy

Goals of antiviral therapy for CHB include sustained suppression of viral replication; delayed or arrested progression of liver injury; prevention of hepatic complications, such as liver failure and HCC; and increased survival.

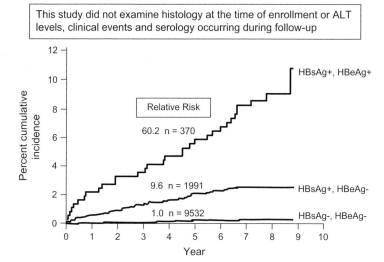

This study did not examine histology at the time of enrollment or ALT levels, clinical events and serology occurring during follow-up

Fig. 5. HBeAg and the risk of HCC. (*Data from* Yang HI, Lu SN, Liaw YF, et al. Hepatitis B e antigen and the risk of hepatocellular carcinoma. N Engl J Med 2002;347:168–74.)

Complete eradication of the HBV is difficult because it has a tendency to integrate into the host genome or remain latent as covalently closed, circular DNA. Patients who become HBsAg-negative and develop anti-HBs generally have resolution of liver disease. Thus, HBsAg seroconversion should be considered a complete therapeutic response, the most desired end point of therapy.

Basic Tenets of Therapy

The most important factors associated with the development of cirrhosis and HCC are disease activity (ALT and necroinflammation on biopsy) and viral load. Hepatitis B is unlikely to progress if the patient is anti-HBe–positive, has a persistently normal ALT level, and the HBV DNA is undetectable by PCR. Serum aminotransferases and HBV DNA levels can fluctuate, however, especially in those patients with HBeAg-negative CHB; thus, isolated ALT and HBV DNA levels cannot accurately determine active or inactive disease. Liver biopsy is valuable in assessing the severity of necroinflammatory activity and fibrosis, and to guide treatment decisions in HBeAg-negative CHB and in those with viral replication but near-normal aminotransferases.

The most important short and intermediate objectives of therapy are to select potent antiviral agents that maximize and maintain HBV DNA suppression. Sustained inhibition of HBV replication is associated with normalization of aminotransferases, histologic improvement, and reduced risk of drug resistance. The long-term and ultimate goal of therapy is HBsAg seroconversion that seems to be an immune-mediated process that likely requires an immunomodulatory agent in combination with an antiviral compound.

Interferons

Standard interferon-α

IFN-α was approved as therapy of CHB in the United States in 1992. The therapeutic effects of IFN-α are secondary to its direct antiviral function; antiproliferative effect (antiangiogenic and antitumor); immunomodulatory properties; and control of apoptosis. The immunomodulatory effects of IFN-α can be recognized clinically as flares of hepatitis defined as an increase in ALT level to at least twice the baseline level. The flare often precedes a virologic response [47]. The general recommended dosage regimen for IFN-α in adults is 5 million units (MU) daily or 10 MU thrice weekly (or every other day) for 16 to 24 weeks in HBeAg-positive patients and for 12 months in HBeAg-negative patients. Furthermore, there is evidence that continuing therapy for an additional 16 weeks for the HBeAg-positive patients may be beneficial if they achieved a significant fall in HBV DNA (<10 pg/mL) but remained HBeAg positive during the first 16 weeks of treatment [48].

Hepatitis B e antigen–positive patients

Traditionally, one of the most important treatment end points for patients with HBeAg-positive CHB is the loss of HBeAg. The efficacy of IFN-α for these patients was evaluated in a well-designed meta-analysis in 1993. Wong and coworkers [49] reviewed over 25 randomized controlled studies involving a total of 837 adult patients who received interferon in doses of 5 to 10 MU given daily to 3 times weekly for 4 to 6 months. Loss of HBeAg was significantly higher among treated patients (33%) compared with controls (12%) for a difference of 21%. Importantly, loss of HBsAg occurred in 6% more of the IFN-treated patients compared with controls.

A number of long-term follow-up studies of IFN-α therapy for HBeAg-positive hepatitis have been conducted in Asia, North America, and Europe. Most of these studies compared long-term clinical outcomes in treated patients versus historical controls or treatment responders with nonresponders. Because of the differences in study designs and definition of responses, direct comparisons of the study outcomes are not possible. Several trends emerge, however, in the follow-up studies from the different geographic regions [50–52]. Studies from North America and Europe reported that 95% to 100% of treatment responders (loss of HBeAg and HBV DNA, plus biochemical remission) continued to be HBeAg-negative after 5 to 10 years of follow-up and 30% to 86% of them eventually lost HBsAg. Liver-related complications and mortality were greater in nonresponders compared with responders, especially among those with pre-existing cirrhosis [50]. These studies demonstrated that the loss of HBeAg is a reliable treatment end point that is associated with long-term disease remission, and that interferon therapy is beneficial in preventing the progression to end-stage liver disease. In contrast, long-term follow-up of patients in Asian studies generally showed a lower rate of durable responses to IFN-α, and inconsistent rates of HBeAg and HBsAg clearance [53–55]. Despite the lower response, the study by Lin and coworkers [53] in Taiwan suggested that IFN therapy might prevent the development of HCC. These differences in long-term IFN-α treatment outcomes noted in the Eastern and Western countries could reflect differences in viral factors, such as genotypes, and in the natural history of the disease in high versus low endemic areas [17].

Several factors predict the likelihood of a favorable response to IFN-α treatment in patients with chronic HBV infection, the most important of these being a high baseline ALT and low serum HBV DNA levels [56]. A flare in liver aminotransferase during treatment with IFN-α also was found to be a predictor of good response. Lau and coworkers [57] observed that 39% of patients experienced hepatitis flare on treatment. In 52% of the cases, hepatitis flare resulted in a good virologic response. The flares with favorable treatment outcomes typically occurred within the first month of therapy and were associated with a significant decrease in HBV DNA to $<10^5$ copies per milliliter at the peak of ALT elevation. Another recent study demonstrated that the degree of aminotransferase elevation during treatment has a strong predictive value for response especially for those patients with high baseline serum HBV DNA levels [58]. Although a flare in aminotransferases predicts favorable response, the IFN-α–induced flare also could precipitate decompensation in patients with cirrhosis. For this reason, IFN-α is contraindicated for patients with significant reduced hepatic reserve.

Hepatitis B e antigen–negative patients

HBeAg-negative CHB is comprised of heterogeneous disease activities and patient populations that further complicate the analysis of clinical trials and the comparisons of study results. To date, there are approximately 20 published studies using IFN for HBeAg-negative CHB. The end point of most of these studies has been loss of HBV DNA detectable by molecular hybridization (HBV DNA $<10^{5.7}$ copies per milliliter) and normalization of serum ALT within 1 year after therapy. Similar to HBeAg-positive CHB, both end-of-treatment and sustained responses are superior in treated subjects [59]. Among the controlled trials, the sustained response rate was 10% to 47% in treated subjects compared with 0% in the controls. In view of the high relapse rate ($>50\%$), an important issue is to improve the durability of response. Of note, relapses can occur months to even years after therapy [59].

In a long-term follow-up study on HBeAg-negative CHB, Manesis and Hadziyannis [60] retrospectively analyzed the clinical outcomes of 216 patients treated with 3 MU IFN alfa-2b thrice weekly for 5 or 12 months. After a median follow-up of 7 years, 18% of the patients remained in biochemical and virologic remission after a single course of therapy. Longer treatment duration (12 months) and a biochemical response within the first 4 months of therapy were identified as predictors of long-term sustained response. Encouragingly, patients with sustained response also had significant improvement of liver histology, and 32% of them ultimately lost HBsAg. This study suggests that patients with HBeAg-negative CHB require a longer course of IFN therapy to achieve complete response.

Pegylated Interferon-α

The long-acting, once weekly PEG IFN α-2a was approved by the FDA for the treatment of CHB in 2005. Cooksley and coworkers [61] performed the first randomized controlled trial of PEG IFN α-2a on 143 patients with HBeAg-positive CHB. The treatment duration was 24 weeks with 24 weeks of follow-up. Treatment response, defined by the loss of HBeAg with serum HBV DNA level below 500,000 copies per milliliter and normal ALT at the end of follow-up, was 27%, 28%, and 19% among those who received 90, 180, or 270 μg/wk of the PEG IFN, respectively. The mean response rate for the three PEG IFN groups was twice as high (24%) as the 12% observed with standard IFN α-2a ($P = .036$). The safety profiles of PEG IFN and standard IFN were similar. This encouraging result led to the development of the subsequent clinical trials that further evaluated the efficacy of both PEG IFN α-2a (40-kd branched PEG molecule) and PEG IFN α-2b (12-kd linear PEG) either alone or in combination with lamivudine (see later). The advantages and disadvantages of PEG IFN versus other FDA-approved agents are compared in Table 3. The drug is contraindicated in decompensated cirrhotics and is ineffective in patients with normal aminotransferases and high HBV DNA level.

Nucleoside and Nucleotide Analogues

Nucleoside or nucleotide analogues compete with naturally occurring purines and pyrimidines for binding to HBV DNA polymerase. They require intracellular phosphorylation for their activity. Analogues lacking a 3'-OH group on the sugar moiety result in immediate chain termination. Many of these compounds are unnatural L-enantiomers. HBV has an unusual preference for these

Table 3
Advantages and disadvantages of Food and Drug Administration–approved agents

| | Nucleoside and nucleotide analogues | | |
Interferon	Lamivudine	Adefovir	Entecavir
Parenteral	Oral	Oral	Oral
Finite duration of therapy	Long duration	Long duration	Long duration
More durable response	Durability is limited by high rate of resistance	Suboptimal primary viral suppression in 25%	More potent than LAM
—	—	No resistance with LAM	Cross-resistance with LAM
No resistant mutants	Resistant mutants (Rx-naïve pts) 15%–30% y 1 70% y 5	Resistant mutants (Rx-naïve pts) 0% y 1, 25% y 5	Resistant mutants (Rx-naïve pts) 0% y 1 and 2
Frequent side effects	Hepatitis flares are common with resistance	Potential nephrotoxicity at high doses	Carcinogenic in rodents at very high doses only

Abbreviation: LAM, lamivudine.

products enhancing antiviral activity while diminishing cellular toxicity. The advantages and disadvantages of nucleoside and nucleotide analogues compared with IFN are listed in Table 3. Those drugs with a low resistance profile are preferable for treating patients with decompensated disease because IFN-based therapy is generally poorly tolerated.

Lamivudine

Lamivudine is a synthetic nucleoside analogue that was approved for the treatment of CHB in the United States in December 1998. Lamivudine is the (-) enantiomer of 2' -3' dideoxy-3'-thiacytidine. The phosphorylated form (3TC-TP) exerts its therapeutic action by competing with dCTP for incorporation into the growing viral DNA chains, causing chain termination. By inhibiting both the RNA- and DNA-dependent DNA polymerase activities, the synthesis of both the first strand and the second strand of HBV DNA are interrupted [62]. Lamivudine is an oral medication and its dose for CHB is 100 mg daily. This dose was chosen based on a preliminary trial published by Dienstag and coworkers [63] who randomly assigned 32 patients to receive 25, 100, or 300 mg of lamivudine daily for a total of 12 weeks. Lamivudine therapy was well tolerated, and a daily dose of 100 mg was more effective than 25 mg and was similar to 300 mg in reducing HBV DNA levels. The loss of HBV DNA was measured by molecular hybridization (HBV DNA $<10^6$ copies per milliliter) in the study, however, so it remains uncertain whether 300 mg causes a greater decline in HBV DNA levels compared with the 100-mg regimen.

Hepatitis B e antigen–positive chronic hepatitis B

There were two large placebo-controlled trials on treatment-naive, HBeAg-positive patients performed in North America and Asia, respectively [64,65]. In both studies, 1-year therapy with lamivudine was associated with a significantly better HBeAg seroconversion (defined as loss of HBeAg, with development of antibody to HBeAg) and undetectable HBV DNA in 16% and 17% of the patients compared with a 4% and 6% response, respectively, in the placebo groups. Fall in serum HBV DNA level of ~2 $\log_{10}$ occurred in virtually all patients who received lamivudine. Among the treated patients, sustained normalization of ALT levels occurred in 41% in the North American study and 72% in the Asian study. Of note, only 70% of the Asian patients had elevated ALT levels at baseline, whereas all the patients in the North American study had abnormal ALT levels. Furthermore, both studies demonstrated an improvement in the hepatic necroinflammatory activity defined as improvement of at least two points in the Knodell score. In contrast, worsening of inflammation occurred in 30% receiving placebo. No patient in the Asian study lost HBsAg during the study, and only 2% in the North American study had undetectable HBsAg at the end of 52 weeks of treatment.

In an Asian long-term lamivudine treatment study, an incremental HBeAg seroconversion from 17% at 1 year to 27% at 2 years was observed [66]. Continuous treatment with lamivudine for 3 and 4 years was associated with HBeAg seroconversion rates of 40% and 47%, respectively [67,68].

Importantly, HBeAg seroconversion increased linearly with increasing prether-apy ALT levels. For example, Liaw and coworkers [66] showed that patients with normal ALT levels did not have HBeAg seroconversion, whereas sero-conversion occurred in 23% and 80% of patients with ALT levels 2 to 5 times and >5 times the upper limit of normal, respectively. This finding was con-firmed in at least two other studies showing 1-year HBeAg seroconversion rates occurring in 4%, 15%, 26% to 28%, and 56% to 64% of patients with pretreat-ment ALT levels within normal, one to two times normal limits, two to five times normal, and more than five times normal, respectively [69,70]. Both Asians and whites have similar rates of HBeAg seroconversion at comparable ALT levels [71]. In addition to pretreatment ALT level, histologic activity in-dex score and body mass index have been identified as important predictors of HBeAg seroconversion during lamivudine therapy [69,70].

In another study by Liaw and coworkers [72], 436 HBV DNA–positive pa-tients with advanced fibrosis or cirrhosis were given continuous lamivudine treatment over a median of 32.4 months (0–42 months) (Fig. 6). Clinical pro-gression of disease was delayed by reducing the incidence of hepatic decompen-sation as seen by an increase in the Child-Pugh score (3.4% in the treated group versus 8.8% in those given a placebo; $P = .02$) and a decreased risk of HCC (3.9% for the lamivudine group versus 7.4% in the placebo group). YMDD mutations developed in 49% of the treated patients (versus 5% of the untreated group) and this was more likely to be associated with an increase in the Child-Pugh score. Indeed, 8 of 10 patients who died after reaching a clinical end point had evidence of YMDD mutations while receiving lamivudine.

Relapse rates after stopping lamivudine in patients who achieved HBeAg seroconversion are conflicting. Schiff and coworkers [71] observed a relapse of HBeAg in 19% of 42 patients with a response to lamivudine. In a recent study,

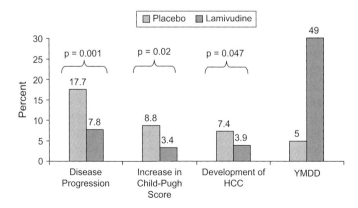

Fig. 6. Continuous treatment with lamivudine for a median of 32.4 months (0–42 months) de-lays the clinical progression of chronic hepatitis B. HCC, hepatocellular carcinoma. (*Data from* Liaw YF, Sung JJ, Chow WC, et al. Lamivudine for patients with chronic hepatitis B and ad-vanced liver disease. N Engl J Med 2004;351:1521–31.)

Dienstag and coworkers [73] followed 40 subjects with lamivudine-induced HBeAg seroconversion for a median duration of 36.6 (4.8–45.6) months. HBeAg relapse was observed at the last visit in 23% of 39 patients. Nine (22%) of 40 patients were found to be HBsAg-negative at the last assessment and 74% of 23 patients had sustained virologic and biochemical responses at the last visit. No safety issues of concern emerged. In contrast, in a retrospective Korean study in which a total of 98 patients were treated with 150 mg lamivudine daily for a mean duration of 9.3 ± 3 months, the cumulative relapse rates at 1 year and 2 years posttreatment were 38% and 49%, respectively [74]. Van Nunen and coworkers [75] combined data from 24 centers in 14 countries that yielded a total of 59 patients who responded to lamivudine therapy and showed a 3-year cumulative HBeAg relapse rate of 54% for the lamivudine-treated patients compared with 32% for IFN and 23% for those taking IFN-lamivudine combination therapy. Similarly, a Taiwanese study reported high cumulative relapse rates of 45% and 56% at 48 and 72 weeks posttreatment, respectively [76]. By multivariate analysis, pretreatment serum HBV DNA levels, pretreatment ALT levels, duration of additional lamivudine therapy after HBeAg seroconversion, and age (> 25 years) have been identified as important independent predictors of posttreatment relapse [74–76].

Hepatitis B e antigen–negative chronic hepatitis B

The efficacy and safety of lamivudine were evaluated in a number of studies in HBeAg-negative patients [77–80]. In a placebo-controlled, double-blind study, response rates in 60 patients receiving lamivudine for 52 weeks were compared with 65 patients receiving placebo. Among patients in the lamivudine group, 65% had both virologic and biochemical responses (HBV DNA <700,000 gEq/mL and normal ALT) that were significantly higher than the 6% observed in the placebo group ($P < .001$). At week 52, 60% of the lamivudine-treated patients also had histologic improvement ($\geq$2-point reduction in the Knodell necroinflammatory score) [77]. An Italian study had similar end-of-treatment biochemical and virologic responses in 87% of 15 patients at the end of 52 weeks of lamivudine therapy. All the patients relapsed within 1 to 12 months after stopping therapy, however, so sustained response was rare [78]. Hadziyannis and coworkers [79] assessed the long-term efficacy of 150 mg lamivudine daily for 24 months in 25 patients. Biochemical response was 96% at 12 months, but dropped to 60% by 24 months. Similarly, virologic response was 68% and 59% at 12 and 24 months, respectively. The decrease in rates of response over time was secondary to biochemical and virologic breakthrough [80]. Importantly, ALT increased to higher than the baseline levels in 70% of patients with a biochemical breakthrough reaching acute hepatitis levels in over 50%.

Lamivudine resistance

In general, lamivudine is well tolerated and safe even with long-term therapy in both HBeAg-positive and HBeAg-negative CHB. Unfortunately, the long-term effectiveness of lamivudine and durability of response have been compromised by the emergence of mutations in the HBV DNA polymerase, which confers to the variant virus a selective resistance to the drug [81]. Two main mutations have been associated with such resistance: a methionine-to-valine or isoleucine substitution in the YMDD motif of the catalytic "C" domain of HBV polymerase at position 204 (M204V/I, formerly M552V/I), and a leucine-to-methionine substitution at position 180 (L180M formerly L528M) upstream of the YMDD motif in the "B" domain (Fig. 7) [82–84]. Clinically, lamivudine resistance is defined as the presence of biochemical breakthrough (increase in ALT activity greater than 1.5 times the upper limit of normal after an initial biochemical response) and virologic breakthrough (reappearance or an increase of detectable serum HBV DNA by PCR after an initial virologic response). Typically, virologic breakthrough precedes biochemical breakthrough by a median of 4 to 6 months. Studies showed that the emergence of the YMDD variant can be detected as early as 49 days after taking lamivudine, but clinically important virologic and biochemical breakthrough does not occur before 6 months [85,86]. Withdrawal of lamivudine typically leads to reappearance of the wild-type species, and subsequent repeat treatment with lamivudine is associated with a more rapid reappearance of the HBV variant [85]. In a study by Liaw and coworkers [87], acute exacerbation of hepatitis B with significant elevation of the aminotransferases (defined as five times the upper limit of normal or to a level >300 IU/L) was observed in about 30% of patients 4 to 94 weeks (median, 24 weeks) after emergence of the YMDD mutation. There was no significant difference in baseline ALT or HBV DNA levels between those who did or did not experience exacerbations. Subsequent HBV DNA levels were, however, significantly higher in patients who developed an exacerbation ($P < .005$). Acute hepatitis B exacerbation with high HBV DNA and ALT levels also has been described with the withdrawal of lamivudine therapy, and a proportion of those patients developed hepatic decompensation [88].

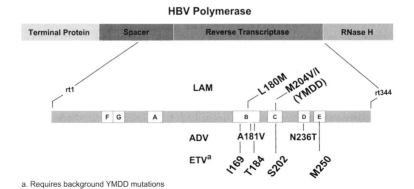

Fig. 7. Mutations in HBV polymerase related to lamivudine (LAM), adefovir (ADV), and entecavir (ETV) resistance.

In HBeAg-positive CHB, YMDD variants were reported to occur in approximately 14% of patients after 1 year of therapy [65]. With continuous treatment, the rates increased to 38% after 2 years, 53% after 3 years, and 67% after 4 years of therapy [67,68,89]. A long-term study by Leung and coworkers [67] assessed the clinical outcomes of continuous lamivudine therapy in the presence of YMDD variants in 33 patients. Fifteen of the patients who developed YMDD variants at year 2 and who continued to receive lamivudine experienced ALT flares of more than two times the upper limit of normal. Nine of the patients with lamivudine resistance had liver biopsies at baseline, 1 year, and 3 years. Worsening of the histologic activity index by 2 to 9 points was observed in six patients between the year 1 and year 3 biopsies. Approximately 25% of the patients, however, eventually achieved HBeAg seroconversion with continuous therapy despite the presence of the YMDD variants. Dienstag and coworkers [90] evaluated the histologic outcome during long-term lamivudine therapy. They found that after 3 years of continuous lamivudine treatment, 56% of 63 patients showed improvement, 33% no change, and 11% worsening. Those without YMDD variants, compared with those with, were more likely to improve (77% versus 44%) and less likely to deteriorate (5% versus 15%). Furthermore, patients with YMDD variants for more than 2 years were least likely to improve. Lau and coworkers [85] observed similar histologic responses in patients with lamivudine resistance on continuous therapy. The eight HBeAg-positive patients who developed lamivudine resistance before month 12 had no improvement in histologic activity index score. The pretreatment mean histologic activity index score was 12 compared with 11.3 at 1 year. These data suggest that continued therapy with lamivudine (up to 3 years) results in increased HBeAg seroconversion and improved histology. The studies also show, however, that continued treatment after the emergence of the YMDD variant could result in exacerbation of hepatitis, reversion of initial histologic benefits, and in some cases progression of liver disease.

In HBeAg-negative CHB, the reported rates of lamivudine resistance were variable. In a small United States study, Lau and coworkers [85] reported a low resistance rate of only 10% after 2 to 4 years of continuous therapy. In contrast, YMDD variants developed in approximately two thirds of patients within 3 years of therapy in the Mediterranean [80]. The differences could be related to the heterogeneity of the HBV. For example, most of the patients in the United States study had HBV genotypes B and C, whereas most of the study subjects in the Mediterranean had HBV genotype D. It is important to note that when the genotype D precore variant becomes YMDD-resistant, its replicative efficacy increases [91]. This observation may explain the frequent occurrence of severe virologic and biochemical breakthroughs in patients with HBeAg-negative CHB under lamivudine treatment that have been reported in studies from Greece, where there is a 95% predominance of HBV genotype D.

Papatheodoridis and coworkers [80] studied the course of virologic breakthroughs in 32 patients under long-term lamivudine monotherapy. After the onset of virologic breakthrough, the biochemical remission rate decreased from 44% at 6 months to 21% at 12 months, and 0% by 24 months. Follow-up histologic lesions in patients with biochemical breakthroughs did not differ from baseline findings. This study concludes that the emergence of viral resistance under long-term lamivudine monotherapy is usually a result of an increased HBV DNA level that culminates in the development of biochemical breakthroughs in most cases.

Predictive factors of the emergence of lamivudine resistance by multivariate analysis include high baseline HBV DNA, high baseline ALT, and high histologic activity index score [92]. Because lamivudine therapy can be associated with serious exacerbations of hepatitis, either during therapy caused by the development of drug resistance or after discontinuation of lamivudine therapy caused by relapse of wild-type HBV, patients should be closely monitored. They should have at least serum aminotransferases, and preferably also HBV DNA evaluations, every 3 months during treatment and for at least 1 year after discontinuation of therapy to allow early detection of hepatitis flares.

Adefovir Dipivoxil

Adefovir dipivoxil was approved by the FDA for treatment of CHB in September 2002. It is an oral diester prodrug of adefovir, a nucleotide adenosine analogue that, in its active form (adefovir diphosphate), inhibits HBV DNA polymerase. Because the acyclic nucleotide already contains a phosphate-mimetic group, it needs only two, instead of three, phosphorylation steps to reach the active metabolite stage. It does not depend on the virus-induced kinase to exert its antiviral action [93]. Adefovir dipivoxil has activity against wild-type, precore, and lamivudine-resistant HBV variants, and acts against a number of DNA viruses, in addition to HBV, and retroviruses (ie, HIV) [94].

Hepatitis B e antigen–positive chronic hepatitis B

In 2003, Marcellin and coworkers [95] reported results from a large phase III study involving 515 HBeAg-positive patients with CHB from 78 centers in North America, Europe, Australia, and Southeast Asia. Patients were randomized to receive either 10 or 30 mg of adefovir dipivoxil daily or a placebo for 48 weeks. Patients who received the 30 mg of adefovir had the most significant fall in serum HBV DNA levels: 4.76 log copies per milliliter compared with 3.52 log ($P < .001$) in the 10-mg dose group and 0.55 log in the placebo group. As a result, undetectable HBV DNA by PCR (less than 400 copies per milliliter) was achieved in 39% of those who received 30 mg of adefovir a day, in 21% of those who were given 10 mg a day, and in none of the placebo-treated patients. Similarly, normalization of alanine aminotransferase levels was higher in the treatment groups, 55% (30 mg) and 48% (10 mg), compared with 16% in the control group. HBeAg seroconversion occurred in 14% and 12% of the treated patients on 30 mg and 10 mg, respectively, and was infrequent (6%) in the placebo group. Most importantly, improvement in necroinflammatory and fibrosis scores was observed in 53% and 59% of the treated patients at the end of therapy compared with 25% with placebo. The safety profile of the 10-mg dose of adefovir was similar to that of placebo. In contrast, there was a slightly higher frequency of adverse events caused by renal laboratory abnormalities in the group given 30 mg of adefovir dipivoxil per day for 48 weeks. The major potential nephrotoxicity to adefovir dipivoxil is a Fanconi-like syndrome with phosphaturia and proteinuria. The cause of the renal toxicity is related to renal tubular damage, but the exact mechanisms are not well understood. Because the 10-mg dose has a favorable risk-benefit profile for long-term treatment, it is the FDA-recommended dose for CHB. Marcellin and coworkers [96] reported long-term efficacy data with 10 mg of adefovir daily for up to week 144. The antiviral effect was maintained and there was an encouraging trend of increased HBeAg seroconversion, HBV suppression, and ALT normalization with prolonged therapy. Furthermore, there were no significant adverse events; in particular, no increased risk of nephrotoxicity was observed with prolonged therapy.

Hepatitis B e antigen–negative chronic hepatitis B

A multicenter phase III clinical trial involving 185 patients with HBeAg-negative HBV was conducted in 32 international sites [97]. The patients were randomized to receive either 10 mg of adefovir dipivoxil or placebo once daily for 48 weeks in a 2:1 ratio and a double-blind manner. The primary end point was histologic improvement at the end of therapy. Similar to the HBeAg-positive patients, the treated patients had significant histologic improvement compared with the placebo-treated group (64% versus 33%, $P < .001$). The median decrease in log-transformed HBV DNA levels was greater with adefovir than with placebo (3.91 versus 1.35 log copies per milliliter, $P < .001$) comparable with the HBeAg-positive CHB trial. Serum HBV DNA levels were reduced to fewer than 400 copies per milliliter in 51% of the patients in the adefovir group but in none of the placebo group. Alanine aminotransferase levels had normalized at week 48 in 72% of treated patients as compared with 29% of those on placebo ($P < .001$). The safety profile of adefovir dipivoxil was similar to that of placebo. At 144 weeks of therapy, the antiviral effect and histologic alterations continued to show significant improvement and no significant side effects were observed, especially nephrotoxicity. A ranked histologic assessment in HBeAg-negative CHB patients treated for 4 or 5 years with adefovir showed that $< 5\%$ of the patients had worsening of their necroinflammation or fibrosis scores [98]. Among 12 patients with bridging fibrosis or cirrhosis, seven improved at least two or more fibrosis points (on a scale of 6) during year 4 or 5 of therapy. Switching patients from adefovir to a placebo after 48 weeks resulted in a reversal of the necroinflammatory improvement seen with adefovir, whereas changing from a placebo to adefovir resulted in an opposite effect.

Because CHB is a heterogeneous disease and genotypes may influence disease progression and antiviral response, a 48-week study was performed to analyze the antiviral efficacy of 10 mg adefovir dipivoxil with respect to HBV genotype, HBeAg serostatus, and race in patients from the two multinational phase III studies [99]. Regardless of geographic location, Asian patients were infected predominantly with genotypes B or C, whereas white patients were infected predominantly with A or D. In this study, adefovir resulted in reductions in serum HBV DNA levels independent of genotype, HBeAg status, or race. Similarly, there was no statistical difference in HBeAg seroconversion rates between genotypes.

Adefovir dipivoxil resistance

The primary site of adefovir-associated resistance mutation, N236T, is located in domain D of the HBV polymerase gene. There also is an upstream A181V substitution that is in proximity to the lamivudine L180V substitution (see Fig. 7). In vitro assays showed that HBV with the N236T substitution continues to be responsive to nucleoside analogues, such as lamivudine and entecavir [100]. In contrast, the A181V substitution had reduced responsiveness to nucleoside analogues in cell culture assays and was highly resistant to telbivudine, valtorcitabine and clevudine. It remained responsive, however, to tenofovir. These in vitro data suggest that resistance assays are necessary to identify the adefovir-induced substitutions and to guide the selection of the subsequent salvage therapy.

During the initial 48 weeks of therapy, there was no clinically important drug resistance noted in both the HBeAg-positive and HBeAg-negative CHB clinical trials [95,97,101]. In an ongoing program to monitor for the emergence of resistance in 124 patients who received continuous adefovir dipivoxil for 2 years, drug resistance developed in two (1.6%) patients [102]. With prolonged therapy, resistance was confirmed in 11%, 18%, and 28% of the study participants with HBeAg-negative CHB who continued treatment through years 3, 4, and 5, respectively [98,103]. Most of these patients exhibited viral rebound, but significant ALT flare was infrequent, and there was no worsening of liver function. Higher HBV DNA levels at year 1 are predictive of adefovir resistance development: 67% of those with HBV DNA > 6 logs at year 1 developed resistance at year 3 [104]. Conversely, resistance rates were less common with lower HBV DNA: 26% among those with 3 to 6 logs, and 4% in those with < 3 logs at year 1.

Entecavir

Entecavir, a cyclopentyl guanosine nucleoside analogue, is a selective inhibitor of HBV replication. It has no antiviral activity against HIV. Entecavir blocks all three polymerase steps involved in the replication process of the hepatitis B virus: (1) base priming, (2) reverse transcription of the negative strand from the pregenomic messenger RNA, and (3) synthesis of the positive strand of HBV DNA. It is more efficiently phosphorylated to its active triphosphate compound by cellular kinases compared with other nucleoside analogues. It is a potent inhibitor of wide-type HBV but is less effective against lamivudine-resistant HBV mutants [105].

In a 24-week, double-blind, randomized, phase II dose-finding clinical trial, 169 patients with CHB were evaluated [106]. The safety and efficacy of entecavir (0.01 mg/d, 0.1 mg/d, or 0.5 mg/d orally) were compared with lamivudine (100 mg/d orally). A dose-response relationship was observed with entecavir in HBV DNA suppression. At 22 weeks of therapy, 84% of patients treated with entecavir had an HBV DNA level below 0.7 MEq/mL by the branched DNA assay, compared with 58% treated with lamivudine ($P = .008$). Entecavir was well tolerated at all doses and the side effect profile was similar to lamivudine. Entecavir at 0.5 mg daily was subsequently chosen as an effective and safe dose for the treatment of naive patients and was further evaluated in phase III clinical trials.

Hepatitis B e antigen–positive chronic hepatitis B

A multinational phase III randomized, double-blind study was conducted in nucleoside therapy–naive patients with HBeAg-positive CHB [107]. Seven hundred and nine patients were randomized to entecavir, 0.5 mg once daily, or lamivudine, 100 mg once daily, for 48 weeks. The primary end point of the study was histologic improvement at week 48 of therapy. It was defined as ≥2-point decrease in the Knodell necroinflammatory score and no worsening of fibrosis from baseline. A significantly higher proportion of the patients in the entecavir treatment arm (72%) achieved this treatment end point when compared with the lamivudine arm (62%; $P = .0085$). Furthermore, 67% of the entecavir-treated patients had undetectable HBV DNA (< 300 copies per milliliter by PCR assay) at week 48 compared with 36% of those on lamivudine ($P < .0001$) (Fig. 8). Of note, the baseline HBV DNA levels were comparable in both groups: 9.62 and 9.69 log copies per milliliter in the entecavir and lamivudine arms, respectively. Entecavir also was superior to lamivudine for the

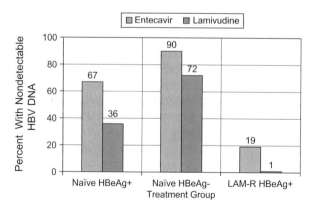

Fig. 8. Percent of chronic hepatitis B patients with nondetectable HBV DNA (<300 copies/mL) at week 48 of therapy with entecavir by HBeAg and lamivudine refractory status ($P \leq .001$). HBeAg, hepatitis B e antigen; LAM, lamivudine. *Data from* references 108, 110, and 112.

proportion of patients with ALT normalization ($\leq 1 \times$ upper limit of normal) at week 48 (68% versus 60%, respectively; $P = .02$). HBeAg seroconversion, however, was similar for both the entecavir (21%) and lamivudine (18%) treatment groups at week 48. With prolonged therapy at year 2, entecavir treatment was associated with an increased rate of HBeAg seroconversion to 31% compared to 26% with lamivudine. A higher proportion of the patients in the entecavir arm also achieved undetectable HBV DNA at year 2 compared with lamivudine, 31% versus 26% [108].

Hepatitis B e antigen–negative chronic hepatitis B
A multinational, randomized, double-blind study, investigated the safety and efficacy of entecavir versus lamivudine in 638 nucleoside-naive patients with chronic HBV infection who were HBeAg-negative [109]. The study design was similar to the HBeAg-positive trial. Patients were randomized to receive 0.5 mg entecavir once daily versus 100 mg lamivudine for 48 weeks. Histologic improvement at week 48 was observed in 70% of the entecavir-treated patients versus 61% of the lamivudine group ($P = .014$). The baseline HBV DNA levels were comparable in both groups: 7.6 and 7.55 log copies per milliliter, respectively. At week 48, entecavir treatment was associated with a significantly higher rate of HBV DNA suppression to < 300 copies per milliliter compared with lamivudine (90% versus 72% with $P < .0001$) (see Fig. 8). ALT normalization was 78% in the entecavir arm compared with 71% in the lamivudine arm ($P = .045$).

Entecavir resistance
The development of entecavir resistance requires pre-existing lamivudine resistance mutations and additional changes in the HBV polymerase: T184, I169 in domain B, S202 in domain C, or M250 in domain E (see Fig. 7) [110]. Among all the nucleoside treatment–naive patients in both the HBeAg-positive and HBeAg-negative CHB clinical trials who completed 2 years of entecavir therapy, there was no evidence of emerging entecavir substitutions. Among HBeAg-positive, lamivudine-refractory CHB patients who were switched to entecavir for 48 weeks (see Fig. 8), 19% had nondetectable HBV DNA (<300 copies per milliliter by PCR) versus only 1% in those continued on lamivudine [111]. For patients with lamivudine resistance who were subsequently switched to entecavir, virologic rebound (confirmed as $>1 \log_{10}$ increase from nadir by PCR) caused by resistance was observed in 1% of the patients in year 1 [112]. In all cases, entecavir mutants had pre-existing lamivudine resistance substitutions and emerging changes at T184 or S202. In contrast, although there was no evidence of entecavir resistance in nucleoside treatment–naive subjects, after 2 years of continuous therapy 10% of lamivudine-refractory patients experienced resistance to entecavir. Thus, phenotypic entecavir resistance seems to require the presence of pre-existing lamivudine resistance substitutions.

Combination Therapy
After evaluating the efficacy and limitations of each agent for the therapy of CHB, it is logical to examine a combination of the drugs with different

mechanisms of actions to optimize the suppression of HBV and to improve both the short- and long-term responses. Mathematical modeling of the HBV kinetics with nucleotide analogue therapy (adefovir) showed a biphasic decline of the HBV levels. The initial, faster phase of viral load decline reflects the clearance of HBV particles from plasma. The second, slower phase of viral load decline closely mirrors the rate-limiting process of infected cell loss [113]. Because the second phase of viral decline is likely to be induced by an immune-mediated process, the immune clearance of the virus should be up-regulated by immunomodulators, such as the IFNs. This suggests that there may be at least a theoretical advantage to the use of nucleoside and nucleotide analogues with IFN in combination.

Nucleoside analogues and pegylated interferon

There are a number of published multicenter clinical trials using a combination of lamivudine and PEG IFN-α. Two large randomized, controlled trials focused on HBeAg-positive patients and one on HBeAg-negative CHB [114–116]. In the study conducted by Janssen and coworkers [114], 307 HBeAg-positive patients were randomized to receive either a combination of PEG IFN α-2b, 100 μg/wk for 32 weeks then 50 μg/wk for 20 weeks, in combination with lamivudine, 100 mg/d, or PEG IFN α-2b with placebo. At 26 weeks follow-up, no difference in efficacy end points was found between the PEG IFN monotherapy and combination therapy, which used a relatively low dose of PEG IFN. Both groups achieved similar rates of HBV DNA suppression to <400 copies per milliliter (7% versus 9%); HBeAg loss (36% versus 35%); and ALT normalization (32% and 35%). Both regimens resulted in a relatively high rate of HBsAg loss at 7% in 1 year. Besides elevated baseline ALT levels, HBV genotype also was identified to be a predictor of response: 60% of the genotype A patients responded compared with 42% for genotype B, 32% for genotype C, and 28% for genotype D.

Lau and coworkers [115] reported results on another large randomized controlled trial comparing the efficacy and safety of PEG IFN α-2a (180 μg weekly), PEG IFN α-2a (180 μg weekly) with lamivudine (100 mg daily), and lamivudine (100 mg daily) alone for 48 weeks in 814 HBeAg-positive patients. At 24 weeks of follow-up, the two PEG IFN treatment arms (with or without lamivudine) showed the same efficacy, and were superior to that observed in the lamivudine arm alone (Fig. 9). Applying a similar study design, Marcellin and coworkers [116] evaluated the efficacy and the safety of PEG IFN alfa-2a alone or in combination with lamivudine versus lamivudine for 48 weeks in 537 patients with HBeAg-negative CHB. At the end of the 24-week posttreatment follow-up, the two PEG IFN treatment arms (with or without lamivudine) again showed similar efficacy and were superior to the lamivudine treatment (Fig. 10). Importantly, there was a higher rate of lamivudine resistance in the lamivudine monotherapy arm (18%) compared with the PEG IFN α-2a plus lamivudine combination arm (<1%) at week 48 ($P < .001$). These studies concluded that the combination of PEG IFN alfa-2a with

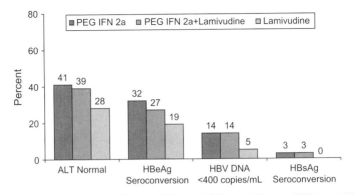

Fig. 9. Biochemical and virologic end points after 48 weeks of therapy and 24 weeks of follow-up in 814 HBeAg-positive chronic hepatitis B patients. HBeAg, hepatitis B e antigen, IFN, interferon; PEG, pegylated. (*Data from* Lau GK, Piratvisuth T, Luo KX, et al. Peginterferon alfa-2a, lamivudine, and the combination for HBeAg-positive chronic hepatitis B. N Engl J Med 2005;352:2682–95.)

lamivudine is not superior to PEG IFN alfa-2a alone. The PEG IFN combination, however, reduced the risk of lamivudine resistance.

Combined nucleoside and nucleotide analogues

To date, there have been limited data on the efficacy of combining nucleoside and nucleotide analogues. Lau and coworkers [117] evaluated combination therapy with lamivudine and famciclovir in 21 HBeAg-positive Chinese patients. They found that patients who received lamivudine, 150 mg daily, and famciclovir, 500 mg three times daily, had a more rapid fall in HBV DNA

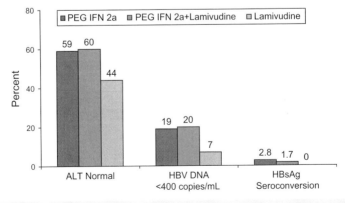

Fig. 10. Biochemical and virologic responses after 48 weeks of therapy and 24 weeks of follow-up in 537 HBeAg-negative chronic hepatitis B patients. HBsAg, hepatitis B surface antigen, IFN, interferon; PEG, pegylated. (*Data from* Marcellin P, Lau GK, Bonino F, et al. Peginterferon alfa-2a alone, lamivudine alone, and the two in combination in patients with HBeAg-negative chronic hepatitis B. N Engl J Med 2004;351:1206–17.)

levels and a higher rate of HBeAg loss compared with those on lamivudine monotherapy. A recent study compared the efficacy of adefovir with lamivudine versus lamivudine alone in 112 treatment-naive, predominantly HBeAg-positive patients [118]. The rates of undetectable HBV DNA by PCR (39% and 41%) and HBeAg loss (19% and 20%) were similar in the two arms. It is important to mention, however, that there was a significantly lower rate of lamivudine resistance in the combination group (2%) compared with lamivudine monotherapy (20%) ($P \leq .003$).

Although the combination regimens evaluated so far did not seem to improve efficacy, they did reduce the rates of resistance to nucleoside or nucleotide monotherapy (see previously). A number of promising nucleoside analogues, such as tenofovir, emtricitabine, clevudine, and valtorcitabine are being vigorously evaluated in national and international multicenter clinical trials to identify effective combination therapies. An optimal combination regimen should work synergistically in viral suppression, increase rates of HBeAg and HBsAg seroconversion, and prevent the occurrence of viral resistance. In view of an increased rate of viral mutation in immunocompromised hosts, a combination of tenofovir plus lamivudine or emtricitabine should be considered for HBV/HIV coinfected patients who require an antiretroviral regimen [94].

Current Treatment Recommendations

The goals of therapy for CHB are to achieve sustained viral suppression and improve clinical outcome, decreasing the risk of cirrhosis, HCC, and ultimately the complete resolution of liver disease. There are a number of published treatment guidelines for CHB [119,120]. It must be kept in mind, however, that treatment needs to be tailored to the individual patient because HBV is a heterogeneous disease with variable manifestations. The severity of liver disease, efficacy, potential complications, and cost of the therapeutic agents need to be considered carefully before initiating a course of therapy.

Table 4 presents the authors' perspective on the treatment of chronic hepatitis B based on the principles discussed in this article. It is important to point out that treatment decisions need to be governed by serial HBV DNA and ALT determinations rather than isolated laboratory values. The HBV DNA levels chosen are somewhat arbitrary and one must examine all the host and viral factors in decision making. Liver biopsy can be a valuable tool in the setting of fluctuating hepatitis, viral levels, or persistently normal or near-normal aminotransferases.

In the authors' opinion, lamivudine should no longer be used routinely as the first line of therapy because of its high rate of resistance. Lamivudine continues to have a role in the setting of shorter-term prophylaxis, such as the prevention of HBV reactivation during chemotherapy, or the vertical transmission of HBV in pregnant women with high levels of viremia in conjunction with hepatitis B immunoglobin and vaccine of their infants at birth to ensure optimal protection. Careful selection of a first-line agent is necessary to avoid not only resistance, but

Table 4
A perspective on the treatment of chronic hepatitis B

HBeAg	HBV DNA	ALT	Treatment strategy
+	+[a]	$\leq 2 \times$ ULN	Lower efficacy with current treatment Observe and consider treatment when ALT becomes elevated
+	+	$> 2 \times$ ULN	Peg-IFN-α, ADV or ETV; ADV or ETV for Peg-IFN-α NR/contraindications
−	+[b]	$> 2 \times$ ULN	Peg-IFN-α, ADV or ETV (oral agents may be preterred because of need for long-term treatment); ADV or ETV for Peg-IFN-α NR/contraindications
−	−	$\leq 2 \times$ ULN	No treatment needed; observe for hepatitis reactivation
+/−	Detectable	Cirrhosis	Compensated: ADV or ETV Decompensated:ADV or ETV; refer for liver transplant and coordinate treatment with transplant center
+/−	−	Cirrhosis	Compensated: observe and treat with oral agents if HBV DNA becomes positive Decompensated:refer for liver transplant

Abbreviations: ADV, adefovir; ETV, entecavir; HBeAg, hepatitis B e antigen; HBV, hepatitis B virus; IFN, interferon; NR, nonresponders; PEG, pegylated; ULN, upper limit of normal.
  [a]HBV DNA $> 10^4$ or $> 10^5$ copies/mL (arbitrary decision without unanimity).
  [b]HBV DNA $> 10^4$ copies/mL (arbitrarily chosen).

also the development of cross-resistance to other agents. When resistance to first-line therapy does develop, alternative therapy should be considered. In addition, surveillance of HCC in regular intervals should be considered even for those whose treatment is deferred, especially if they have risk factors.

Future hepatitis B consensus conferences will supplement these recommendations. Regardless, most experts would agree that the ideal end points to any therapy are to achieve permanently undetectable HBV DNA levels by PCR; a normal ALT level; HBeAg seroconversion (in HBeAg-positive patients); HBsAg seroconversion; and clearance of covalently closed, circular DNA from hepatocytes. With the increased number of new and potent antiviral agents being developed and evaluated, it provides hope and optimism for those who are chronically infected with HBV. One must not lose sight of the fact, however, that prevention remains the most effective strategy in the global management of HBV. Universal immunization programs will not only prevent HBV transmission and circumvent acute and chronic infection, but they will also interdict hepatitis delta infection and HCC.

References

[1] Centers for Disease Control and Prevention. Hepatitis surveillance report No. 60. Atlanta (GA): US Department of Health and Human Services, Centers for Disease Control and Prevention; 2005.

[2] Ganem D, Schneider RJ. Hepadnaviridae: the viruses and their replication. In: Fields BN, Knipe DM, Howley PM, et al, editors. Field Virology, 4th edition. Philadelphia: Lippincott Williams & Wilkins; 2001. p. 2923–69.

[3] Hadziyannis SJ, Vassilopoulos D. Hepatitis B e antigen-negative chronic hepatitis B. Hepatology 2001;34:617–24.

[4] Desmet VJ, Gerber M, Hoofnagle JH, et al. Classification of chronic hepatitis: diagnosis, grading and staging. Hepatology 1994;19:1513–20.

[5] Ishak K, Baptista A, Bianchi L, et al. Histological grading and staging of chronic hepatitis. J Hepatol 1995;22:696–9.

[6] Ludwig J. The nomenclature of chronic active hepatitis: an obituary. Gastroenterology 1993;105:274–8.

[7] Brunetto MR, Giarin MM, Oliveri F, et al. Wild-type and e antigen-minus hepatitis B viruses and course of chronic hepatitis. Proc Natl Acad Sci U S A 1991;88:4186–90.

[8] Saldanha J, Gerlich W, Lelie N, et al. An international collaborative study to establish a World Health Organization international standard for hepatitis B virus DNA nucleic acid amplification techniques. Vox Sang 2001;80:63–71.

[9] Hollinger FB, Liang JT. Hepatitis B virus. In: Fields BN, Knipe DM, Howley PM, et al, editors. Fields Virology, 4th edition. Philadelphia: Lippincott Williams & Wilkins; 2001. p. 2971–3036.

[10] Busch MP, Kleinman SH, Jackson B, et al. Committee report. Nucleic acid amplification testing of blood donors for transfusion-transmitted infectious diseases: report of the Interorganizational Task Force on Nucleic Acid Amplification Testing of Blood Donors. Transfusion 2000;40:143–59.

[11] Biswas R, Tabor E, Hsia CC, et al. Comparative sensitivity of HBV NATs and HBsAg assays for detection of acute HBV infection. Transfusion 2003;43:788–98.

[12] Sjogren MH, Lemon SM. Low-molecular-weight IgM antibody to hepatitis B core antigen in chronic infections with hepatitis B virus. J Infect Dis 1983;148:445–51.

[13] Tsuda F, Naito S, Takai E, et al. Low molecular weight (7s) immunoglobulin M antibody against hepatitis B core antigen in the serum for differentiating acute from persistent hepatitis B virus infection. Gastroenterology 1984;87:159–64.

[14] Shiels MT, Taswell HF, Czaja AJ, et al. Frequency and significance of concurrent hepatitis B surface antigen and antibody in acute and chronic hepatitis B. Gastroenterology 1987;93:675–80.

[15] Hayashi J, Noguchi A, Nakashima K, et al. Frequency of concurrence of hepatitis B surface antigen and antibody in a large number of carriers in Okinawa, Japan. Gastroenterol Jpn 1990;25:593–7.

[16] Wang YM, Ng WC, Lo SK. Detection of pre-S/S gene mutants in chronic hepatitis B carriers with concurrent hepatitis B surface antibody and hepatitis B surface antigen. J Gastroenterol 1999;34:600–6.

[17] McMahon BJ, Alward WL, Hall DB, et al. Acute hepatitis B virus infection: relation of age to the clinical expression of disease and subsequent development of the carrier state. J Infect Dis 1985;151:599–603.

[18] Beasley RP, Trepo C, Stevens CE, et al. The e antigen and vertical transmission of hepatitis B surface antigen. Am J Epidemiol 1977;105:94–8.

[19] Papaevangelou G, Tassopoulos N, Roumeliotou-Karayannis A, et al. Etiology of fulminant viral hepatitis in Greece. Hepatology 1984;4:369–72.

[20] Mast EE, Mahoney FJ, Alter MJ, et al. Progress toward elimination of hepatitis B virus transmission in the United States. Vaccine 1998;16:S48–51.

[21] de Franchis R, Meucci G, Vecchi M, et al. The natural history of asymptomatic hepatitis B surface antigen carriers. Ann Intern Med 1993;118:191–4.

[22] Redeker AG. Chronic viral hepatitis. In: Vyas GN, Perkins HA, Schmid R, editors. Hepatitis and blood transfusion. New York: Grune & Stratton; 1972. p. 55–60.

[23] Seeff LB, Zimmerman HJ, Wright EC, et al. Hepatic disease in asymptomatic parenteral narcotic drug abusers: a Veterans Administration collaborative study. Am J Med Sci 1975;270:41–7.

[24] Cooksley WG, Bradbear RA, Robinson W, et al. The prognosis of chronic active hepatitis without cirrhosis in relation to bridging necrosis. Hepatology 1986;6:345–8.

[25] Liaw YF, Tai DI, Chu CM, et al. The development of cirrhosis in patients with chronic type B hepatitis: a prospective study. Hepatology 1988;8:493–6.

[26] Schalm SW, Thomas HC, Hadziyannis SJ. Chronic hepatitis B. In: Popper H, Schaffner F, editors. Progress in liver disease. New York: WB Saunders; 1990. p. 443–62.

[27] Margolis HS, Alter MJ, Hadler SC. Hepatitis B: evolving epidemiology and implications for control. Semin Liver Dis 1991;11:84–92.

[28] Chu CJ, Keeffe EB, Han SH, et al. Prevalence of HBV precore/core promoter variants in the United States. Hepatology 2003;38:619–28.

[29] Brunetto MR, Oliveri F, Coco B, et al. Outcome of anti-HBe positive chronic hepatitis B in alpha-interferon treated and untreated patients: a long term cohort study. J Hepatol 2002;36:263–70.

[30] Fattovich G, Pantalena M, Zagni I, et al. Effect of hepatitis B and C virus infections on the natural history of compensated cirrhosis: a cohort study of 297 patients. Am J Gastroenterol 2002;97:2886–95.

[31] de Jongh FE, Janssen HL, de Man RA, et al. Survival and prognostic indicators in hepatitis B surface antigen-positive cirrhosis of the liver. Gastroenterology 1992;103:1630–5.

[32] Realdi G, Fattovich G, Hadziyannis S, et al. Survival and prognostic factors in 366 patients with compensated cirrhosis type B: a multicenter study. The Investigators of the European Concerted Action on Viral Hepatitis (EUROHEP). J Hepatol 1994;21:656–66.

[33] Liaw YF, Lin DY, Chen TJ, et al. Natural course after the development of cirrhosis in patients with chronic type B hepatitis: a prospective study. Liver 1989;9:235–41.

[34] Hui AY, Chan HL, Leung NW, et al. Survival and prognostic indicators in patients with hepatitis B virus-related cirrhosis after onset of hepatic decompensation. J Clin Gastroenterol 2002;34:569–72.

[35] Sheu JC, Sung JL, Chen DS, et al. Early detection of hepatocellular carcinoma by real-time ultrasonography: a prospective study. Cancer 1985;56:660–6.

[36] Sheu JC, Sung JL, Chen DS, et al. Growth rate of asymptomatic hepatocellular carcinoma and its clinical implications. Gastroenterology 1985;89:259–66.

[37] Ihde DC, Sherlock P, Winawer SJ, et al. Clinical manifestations of hepatoma: a review of 6 years' experience at a cancer hospital. Am J Med 1974;56:83–91.

[38] Di Bisceglie AM, Rustgi VK, Hoofnagle JH, et al. NIH conference: hepatocellular carcinoma. Ann Intern Med 1988;108:390–401.

[39] Sjogren MH, Lemon SM, Chung WK, et al. IgM antibody to hepatitis B core antigen in Korean patients with hepatocellular carcinoma. Hepatology 1984;4:615–8.

[40] Kew MC, Popper H. Relationship between hepatocellular carcinoma and cirrhosis. Semin Liver Dis 1984;4:136–46.

[41] Okuda K, Ohtsuki T, Obata H, et al. Natural history of hepatocellular carcinoma and prognosis in relation to treatment: study of 850 patients. Cancer 1985;56:918–28.

[42] Fattovich G. Natural history and prognosis of hepatitis B. Semin Liver Dis 2003;23:47–58.

[43] Crockett SD, Keeffe EB. Natural history and treatment of hepatitis B virus and hepatitis C virus coinfection. Ann Clin Microbiol Antimicrob 2005;4:13.

[44] Chen CJ, Yang HI, Su J, et al. Risk of hepatocellular carcinoma across a biological gradient of serum hepatitis B virus DNA level. JAMA 2006;295:65–73.

[45] Lai CL. State-of-the-Art Lecture, 2005. Available at: http://209.63.37.57/home/.

[46] Yang HI, Lu SN, Liaw YF, et al. Hepatitis B e antigen and the risk of hepatocellular carcinoma. N Engl J Med 2002;347:168–74.

[47] Perrillo RP. Acute flares in chronic hepatitis B: the natural and unnatural history of an immunologically mediated liver disease. Gastroenterology 2001;120: 1009–22.

[48] Janssen HL, Gerken G, Carreno V, et al. Interferon alfa for chronic hepatitis B infection: increased efficacy of prolonged treatment. The European Concerted Action on Viral Hepatitis (EUROHEP). Hepatology 1999;30:238–43.

[49] Wong DK, Cheung AM, O'Rourke K, et al. Effect of alpha-interferon treatment in patients with hepatitis B e antigen-positive chronic hepatitis B: a meta-analysis. Ann Intern Med 1993;119:312–23.

[50] Lau DT, Everhart J, Kleiner DE, et al. Long-term follow-up of patients with chronic hepatitis B treated with interferon alfa. Gastroenterology 1997;113:1660–7.

[51] Fattovich G, Giustina G, Realdi G, et al. Long-term outcome of hepatitis B e antigen-positive patients with compensated cirrhosis treated with interferon alfa. European Concerted Action on Viral Hepatitis (EUROHEP). Hepatology 1997;26: 1338–42.

[52] Niederau C, Heintges T, Lange S, et al. Long-term follow-up of HBeAg-positive patients treated with interferon alfa for chronic hepatitis B. N Engl J Med 1996;334: 1422–7.

[53] Lin SM, Sheen IS, Chien RN, et al. Long-term beneficial effect of interferon therapy in patients with chronic hepatitis B virus infection. Hepatology 1999;29:971–5.

[54] Yuen MF, Hui CK, Cheng CC, et al. Long-term follow-up of interferon alfa treatment in Chinese patients with chronic hepatitis B infection: the effect on hepatitis B e antigen seroconversion and the development of cirrhosis-related complications. Hepatology 2001;34: 139–45.

[55] Lok AS, Chung HT, Liu VW, et al. Long-term follow-up of chronic hepatitis B patients treated with interferon alfa. Gastroenterology 1993;105:1833–8.

[56] Brook MG, Karayiannis P, Thomas HC. Which patients with chronic hepatitis B virus infection will respond to alpha-interferon therapy? A statistical analysis of predictive factors. Hepatology 1989;10:761–3.

[57] Lau D, Kleiner DE, Park Y, et al. Flare of hepatitis B during alpha interferon therapy. Gastroenterology 1996;110:A1246.

[58] Nair S, Perrillo RP. Serum alanine aminotransferase flares during interferon treatment of chronic hepatitis B: is sustained clearance of HBV DNA dependent on levels of pretreatment viremia? Hepatology 2001;34:1021–6.

[59] Hadziyannis SJ, Papatheodoridis GV, Vassilopoulos D. Treatment of HBeAg-negative chronic hepatitis B. Semin Liver Dis 2003;23:81–8.

[60] Manesis EK, Hadziyannis SJ. Interferon alpha treatment and retreatment of hepatitis B e antigen-negative chronic hepatitis B. Gastroenterology 2001;121:101–9.

[61] Cooksley WG, Piratvisuth T, Lee SD, et al. Peginterferon alpha-2a (40 kDa): an advance in the treatment of hepatitis B e antigen-positive chronic hepatitis B. J Viral Hepatol 2003;10: 298–305.

[62] Lagget M, Rizzetto M. Current pharmacotherapy for the treatment of chronic hepatitis B. Expert Opin Pharmacother 2003;4:1821–7.

[63] Dienstag JL, Perrillo RP, Schiff ER, et al. A preliminary trial of lamivudine for chronic hepatitis B infection. N Engl J Med 1995;333:1657–61.

[64] Dienstag JL, Schiff ER, Wright TL, et al. Lamivudine as initial treatment for chronic hepatitis B in the United States. N Engl J Med 1999;341:1256–63.

[65] Lai CL, Chien RN, Leung NW, et al. A one-year trial of lamivudine for chronic hepatitis B. Asia Hepatitis Lamivudine Study Group. N Engl J Med 1998;339:61–8.

[66] Liaw YF, Leung NW, Chang TT, et al. Effects of extended lamivudine therapy in Asian patients with chronic hepatitis B. Asia Hepatitis Lamivudine Study Group. Gastroenterology 2000;119:172–80.

[67] Leung NW, Lai CL, Chang TT, et al. Extended lamivudine treatment in patients with chronic hepatitis B enhances hepatitis B e antigen seroconversion rates: results after 3 years of therapy. Hepatology 2001;33:1527–32.

[68] Chang TT, Lai CL, Liaw YF, et al. Incremental increases in HBeAg seroconversion and continued ALT normalization in Asian chronic HBV (CHB) patients treated with lamivudine for four years [abstract]. Antivir Ther 2000;5(Suppl 1):44.

[69] Perrillo RP, Lai CL, Liaw YF, et al. Predictors of HBeAg loss after lamivudine treatment for chronic hepatitis B. Hepatology 2002;36:186–94.

[70] Chien RN, Liaw YF, Atkins M. Pretherapy alanine transaminase level as a determinant for hepatitis B e antigen seroconversion during lamivudine therapy in patients with chronic hepatitis B. Asian Hepatitis Lamivudine Trial Group. Hepatology 1999;30:770–4.

[71] Schiff E, Cianciara J, Karayalcin S, et al. Durable HBeAg and HBsAg seroconversion after lamivudine for chronic hepatitis B (CHB). J Hepatol 2000;32(Suppl 2):99.

[72] Liaw YF, Sung JJ, Chow WC, et al. Lamivudine for patients with chronic hepatitis B and advanced liver disease. N Engl J Med 2004;351:1521–31.

[73] Dienstag JL, Cianciara J, Karayalcin S, et al. Durability of serologic response after lamivudine treatment of chronic hepatitis B. Hepatology 2003;37:748–55.

[74] Song BC, Suh DJ, Lee HC, et al. Hepatitis B e antigen seroconversion after lamivudine therapy is not durable in patients with chronic hepatitis B in Korea. Hepatology 2000;32:803–6.

[75] van Nunen AB, Hansen BE, Suh DJ, et al. Durability of HBeAg seroconversion following antiviral therapy for chronic hepatitis B: relation to type of therapy and pretreatment serum hepatitis B virus DNA and alanine aminotransferase. Gut 2003;52:420–4.

[76] Lee CM, Ong GY, Lu SN, et al. Durability of lamivudine-induced HBeAg seroconversion for chronic hepatitis B patients with acute exacerbation. J Hepatol 2002;37:669–74.

[77] Tassopoulos NC, Volpes R, Pastore G, et al. Efficacy of lamivudine in patients with hepatitis B e antigen-negative/hepatitis B virus DNA-positive (precore mutant) chronic hepatitis B. Lamivudine Precore Mutant Study Group. Hepatology 1999;29:889–96.

[78] Santantonio T, Mazzola M, Iacovazzi T, et al. Long-term follow-up of patients with anti-HBe/HBV DNA-positive chronic hepatitis B treated for 12 months with lamivudine. J Hepatol 2000;32:300–6.

[79] Hadziyannis SJ, Papatheodoridis GV, Dimou E, et al. Efficacy of long-term lamivudine monotherapy in patients with hepatitis B e antigen-negative chronic hepatitis B. Hepatology 2000;32:847–51.

[80] Papatheodoridis GV, Dimou E, Laras A, et al. Course of virologic breakthroughs under long-term lamivudine in HBeAg-negative precore mutant HBV liver disease. Hepatology 2002;36:219–26.

[81] Ono-Nita SK, Kato N, Shiratori Y, et al. YMDD motif in hepatitis B virus DNA polymerase influences on replication and lamivudine resistance: a study by in vitro full-length viral DNA transfection. Hepatology 1999;29:939–45.

[82] Wai CT, Lok AS. Treatment of hepatitis B. J Gastroenterol 2002;37:771–8.

[83] Lok AS, McMahon BJ. Chronic hepatitis B. Hepatology 2001;34:1225–41.

[84] Allen MI, Deslauriers M, Andrews CW, et al. Identification and characterization of mutations in hepatitis B virus resistant to lamivudine. Lamivudine Clinical Investigation Group. Hepatology 1998;27:1670–7.

[85] Lau DT, Khokhar MF, Doo E, et al. Long-term therapy of chronic hepatitis B with lamivudine. Hepatology 2000;32:828–34.

[86] Lewin SR, Ribeiro RM, Walters T, et al. Analysis of hepatitis B viral load decline under potent therapy: complex decay profiles observed. Hepatology 2001;34:1012–20.

[87] Liaw YF, Chien RN, Yeh CT, et al. Acute exacerbation and hepatitis B virus clearance after emergence of YMDD motif mutation during lamivudine therapy. Hepatology 1999;30:567–72.

[88] Honkoop P, de Man RA, Niesters HG, et al. Acute exacerbation of chronic hepatitis B virus infection after withdrawal of lamivudine therapy. Hepatology 2000;32:635–9.

[89] Guan R, Lai CL, Liaw YF. Efficacy and safety of 5 years lamivudine treatment in Chinese patients with chronic hepatitis B. J Gastroenterol Hepatol 2001;16:60.

[90] Dienstag JL, Goldin RD, Heathcote EJ, et al. Histological outcome during long-term lamivudine therapy. Gastroenterology 2003;124:105–17.

[91] Yuen MF, Sablon E, Hui CK, et al. Factors associated with hepatitis B virus DNA breakthrough in patients receiving prolonged lamivudine therapy. Hepatology 2001;34: 785–91.

[92] Chen RY, Edwards R, Shaw T, et al. Effect of the G1896A precore mutation on drug sensitivity and replication yield of lamivudine-resistant HBV in vitro. Hepatology 2003;37: 27–35.

[93] De Clercq E. Clinical potential of the acyclic nucleoside phosphonates cidofovir, adefovir, and tenofovir in treatment of DNA virus and retrovirus infections. Clin Microbiol Rev 2003;16:569–96.

[94] Benhamou Y: Treatment algorithm for chronic hepatitis B in HIV-infected patients. J Hepatol 2006;44S1:S90–4.

[95] Marcellin P, Chang TT, Lim SG, et al. Adefovir dipivoxil for the treatment of hepatitis B e antigen-positive chronic hepatitis B. N Engl J Med 2003;348:808–16.

[96] Marcellin P, Chang TT, Lim S, et al. Long term efficacy and safety of adefovir dipivoxil (ADV) 10 mg in HBeAg + chronic hepatitis B (CHB) patients: increasing serologic, virologic and biochemical response over time [abstract]. Hepatology 2004;40(Suppl 1):655A.

[97] Hadziyannis SJ, Tassopoulos NC, Heathcote EJ, et al. Adefovir dipivoxil for the treatment of hepatitis B e antigen-negative chronic hepatitis B. N Engl J Med 2003;348: 800–7.

[98] Hadziyannis SJ, Tassopoulos NC, Heathcote EJ, et al. Long-term therapy with adefovir dipivoxil for HBeAg-negative chronic hepatitis B. N Engl J Med 2005;352:2673–81.

[99] Westland C, Delaney W, Yang H, et al. Hepatitis B virus genotypes and virologic response in 694 patients in phase III studies of adefovir dipivoxil1. Gastroenterology 2003;125: 107–16.

[100] Qi X, Zhu Y, Curtis M, et al. In vitro cross-resistance analysis of the HBV polymerase mutation A181V. J Hepatol 2005;42(Suppl 2):194.

[101] Westland CE, Yang H, Delaney WE, et al. Week 48 resistance surveillance in two phase 3 clinical studies of adefovir dipivoxil for chronic hepatitis B. Hepatology 2003;38: 96–103.

[102] Gibbs CS, Xiong S, Yang H, et al. Resistance surveillance in HBeAg-negative chronic hepatitis B patients treated with adefovir dipivoxil for two years [abstract]. Antiviral Research 2003;57:A43.

[103] Hadziyannis S, Tassopoulos N, Chang TT, et al. Long-term adefovir dipivoxil treatment induces regression of liver fibrosis in patients with HBeAg-negative chronic hepatitis B: results after 5 years of therapy. Hepatology 2005;42:754A.

[104] Hadziyannis SJ, Tassopoulos N, Chang TT, et al. Adefovir dipivoxil (ADV) demonstrates sustained efficacy in HBeAg- chronic hepatitis B (CHB) patients. Gastroenterology 2005;128(Suppl 2):A693.

[105] Chang TT, Gish RG, Hadziyannis SJ, et al. A dose-ranging study of the efficacy and tolerability of entecavir in lamivudine-refractory chronic hepatitis B patients. Gastroenterology 2005;129:1198–209.

[106] Lai CL, Rosmawati M, Lao J, et al. Entecavir is superior to lamivudine in reducing hepatitis B virus DNA in patients with chronic hepatitis B infection. Gastroenterology 2002;123: 1831–8.

[107] Chang TT, Gish R, de Man R, et al. Entecavir is superior to lamivudine for the treatment of HBeAg(+) chronic hepatitis B: results of phase III study ETV-022 in nucleoside-naive patients. Hepatology 2004;40(Suppl 1):193A.

[108] Gish RG, Chang TT, de Man RA, et al. Entecavir results in substantial virologic and bio-chemical improvement and HBeAg seroconversion through 96 weeks of treatment in HBeAg(+) chronic hepatitis B patients (Study ETV-022) [abstract 181]. Hepatology 2005;42(Suppl 1):267A.

[109] Shouval D, Lai CL, Cheinquer H, et al. Entecavir demonstrates superior; histologic and vi-rologic efficacy over lamivudine in nucleoside-naive HBeAg(-) chronic hepatitis B: results of phase III trial ETV-027 [abstract LB 07]. Hepatology 2004;40(Suppl 1):728A.

[110] Tenney DJ, Levine SM, Rose RE, et al. Clinical emergence of entecavir-resistant hepatitis B virus requires additional substitutions in virus already resistant to Lamivudine. Antimicrob Agents Chemother 2004;48:3498–507.

[111] Sherman M, Yurdaydin C, Sollano J, et al. Entecavir is superior to continued lamivudine for the treatment of lamivudine-refractory, HBeAg(+) chronic hepatitis B: results of phase III study ETV-026 [abstract 1152]. Hepatology 2004;40(Suppl 1):664A.

[112] Colonno R, Rose R, Levine S, et al. Entecavir two year resistance update: no resistance ob-served in nucleoside naive patients and low frequency resistance emergence in lamivudine refractory patients [abstract 962]. Hepatology 2005;42(Suppl 1):573A.

[113] Tsiang M, Rooney JF, Toole JJ, et al. Biphasic clearance kinetics of hepatitis B virus from pa-tients during adefovir dipivoxil therapy. Hepatology 1999;29:1863–9.

[114] Janssen HL, van Zonneveld M, Senturk H, et al. Pegylated interferon alfa-2b alone or in combination with lamivudine for HBeAg-positive chronic hepatitis B: a randomised trial. Lancet 2005;365:123–9.

[115] Lau GK, Piratvisuth T, Luo KX, et al. Peginterferon alfa-2a, lamivudine, and the combination for HBeAg-positive chronic hepatitis B. N Engl J Med 2005;352:2682–95.

[116] Marcellin P, Lau GK, Bonino F, et al. Peginterferon alfa-2a alone, lamivudine alone, and the two in combination in patients with HBeAg-negative chronic hepatitis B. N Engl J Med 2004;351:1206–17.

[117] Lau GK, Tsiang M, Hou J, et al. Combination therapy with lamivudine and famciclovir for chronic hepatitis B-infected Chinese patients: a viral dynamics study. Hepatology 2000;32:394–9.

[118] Sung JJY, Lai JY, Zeuzem S, et al. A randomised double-blind phase II study of lamivudine (LAM) compared to lamivudine plus adefovir (ADV) for treatment naive patients with chronic hepatitis B (CHB): Week 52 analysis. J Hepatol 2003;38:A4313.

[119] Lok AS, McMahon BJ. Chronic hepatitis B: update of recommendations. Hepatology 2004;39:857–61.

[120] Keeffe EB, Dieterich DT, Han SH, et al. A treatment algorithm for the management of chronic hepatitis B virus infection in the United States. Clin Gastroenterol Hepatol 2004;2:87–106.

Gastroenterol Clin N Am 35 (2006) 463–486

GASTROENTEROLOGY CLINICS
OF NORTH AMERICA

Treatment of Hepatitis C Infection

Rise Stribling, MD[a], Norman Sussman, MD[a],
John M. Vierling, MD[b],*

[a]Departments of Medicine and Surgery, Baylor College of Medicine, 1709 Dryden,
Suite 1500, Houston, TX 77030, USA
[b]Baylor Liver Health, Baylor College of Medicine, 1709 Dryden, Suite 1500, Houston,
TX 77030, USA

nfection with the hepatitis C virus (HCV) is a global health problem that causes chronic hepatitis, cirrhosis, liver failure, and hepatocellular carcinoma (HCC). Approximately 125 million persons are infected chronically worldwide, including 3 million Americans [1]. Despite the fact that risk factors for HCV infection have been identified, only a minority of HCV-infected persons has been diagnosed, and even a smaller percentage has ever been treated. In the United States HCV infection accounts for nearly 40% of all chronic liver disease and is the leading indication for orthotopic liver transplantation (OLT). Among the estimated 3 million infected individuals in the United States, only approximately 500,000 have been treated. Computerized simulation of American population for 2010–2019 indicates dramatic increases in morbidity, mortality, and costs associated with chronic HCV infection in the absence of treatment. Estimates include 165,000 deaths due to associated liver disease, 27,200 deaths due to HCC, and direct medical costs of $10.7 billion [2–5]. This is of grave concern, because therapies for HCV are curative in responding patients. This article summarizes published information on the treatment of chronic HCV infection using combination therapy with pegylated interferons (PEG-IFNs) and ribavirin, reviews the efficacy and safety of therapy for subsets of patients, and notes the new antiviral agents that are being introduced into clinical trials.

DIAGNOSTIC SCREENING AND SELECTION OF TREATMENT CANDIDATES
Anti–Hepatitis C Virus Antibodies and Molecular Testing for Hepatitis C Virus RNA
Diagnostic testing with an anti-HCV antibody test is indicated for anyone with risk factors for acquisition of infection (Box 1). Any person testing positive for

*Corresponding author. E-mail address: vierling@bcm.tmc.edu (J.M. Vierling).

0889-8553/06/$ – see front matter
doi:10.1016/j.gtc.2006.05.003

Box 1: Risk factors for hepatitis C virus infection

Injection drug use

Intranasal cocaine use

Sex with multiple partners

Body piercing

Chronic hemodialysis

Occupational exposure (eg, needle stick, scalpel cut)

Vietnam era veteran

Maternal-newborn exposure

Recipient of clotting factors before 1987

Recipient of blood products or organ transplantation before 1992

anti-HCV antibodies should have a molecular test to detect HCV RNA, using a qualitative polymerase chain reaction (PCR).

Genotypes

Genotyping should be performed in all viremic patients because it is predictive of the likelihood of achieving a sustained virological response (SVR), which is defined as the absence of detectable HCV RNA using PCR at least 24 weeks after cessation of antiviral therapy, and it determines the duration of therapy. Among the six genotypes, most American patients have genotype 1 infections (70%–80%), whereas infections with genotype 2 or 3 account for 20% to 30% of cases [6–8]. Small numbers of patients in the United States have genotypes 4 (North Africa or Middle East), 5 (South Africa), or 6 (Hong Kong and Vietnam). The probability of achieving an SVR with combination therapy using PEG-IFNs and ribavirin exhibits a genotypic hierarchy: $2 > 3 > 5 > 6 > 4 > 1$.

Role of Liver Biopsy

The absence of optimal antiviral therapies that are free of adverse events and capable of curing all HCV infections has led to intense debate about the selection of appropriate candidates for therapy. Liver biopsy has been recommended to determine the need for antiviral therapy based on the degree of inflammation and amount of fibrosis [9]. Because current therapies are associated with the risk for multiple adverse events and require prolonged periods of treatment and monitoring, the emphasis is on treating patients who have progressive disease, which is characterized by stages 2 to 4 fibrosis scores on liver biopsy [10]. Biopsy also is useful in detecting nonalcoholic fatty liver disease, which can accelerate fibrogenesis and is a negative predictor of response to antiviral therapy in genotypes 1 and 3 infections [11,12]; however, the superior rates of SVRs in patients who are infected with HCV genotypes 2 and 3 warrant therapy for all eligible candidates, which makes liver biopsy optional [10,13,14].

Progress is being made in research to identify surrogate tests for hepatic fibrosis to identify patients who have progressive hepatitis C without a biopsy and to monitor the natural history [15,16]. As yet, none of these tests has supplanted liver biopsy. Therapy can be provided to any individual who desires it, but refuses a biopsy.

MONITORING THERAPEUTIC RESPONSES
Because the response of individual patients to antiviral therapy for HCV infection varies considerably and cannot be predicted, it is desirable to monitor the effect of therapy on HCV replication (Box 2) to determine the probability that continued therapy will produce a SVR. Thus, before initiation of therapy, a baseline HCV RNA concentration should be measured using a quantitative amplification assay with a broad dynamic range. It is particularly important that the upper range of the assay encompass values up to 10^7 IU/mL, because early virological response (EVR) within 12 weeks of initiation of therapy is defined as at least a 2 $\log_{10}$ reduction in HCV RNA [17,18]. Failure to quantify accurately the baseline viral load could lead to false negative conclusions regarding EVR.

GOALS OF THERAPY
The risk of cirrhosis among untreated persons who are infected chronically with HCV is approximately 5% to 25% over a period of 20 to 30 years [19–22]. Among cirrhotics, the risk for decompensation is 30% after 10 years and the annual incidence of HCC is 1% to 2% [23]. Thus, the primary goal of therapy is eradication of HCV infection. Secondary goals include prevention of histopathologic progression, regression of fibrosis, and prevention of hepatic decompensation and HCC. Because the host immune response to persistent HCV infection plays a dominant role in the progression to cirrhosis and decompensation, the eradication of HCV should be accompanied by termination of HCV-specific hepatic necroinflammation and fibrogenesis [24].

COMBINATION PEGYLATED INTERFERON AND RIBAVIRIN: CURRENT STANDARD OF CARE
Three pivotal, randomized, controlled trials (RCTs) have provided evidence of the safety and efficacy of treatment with PEG-IFNα2a (fixed dose of 180 μg)

Box 2: Quantitative hepatitis C virus RNA and monitoring response to therapy

Early virological response (EVR): at least a 2$\log_{10}$ decrease from pretreatment baseline HCV RNA or absence of detectable HCV RNA within 12 weeks after the initiation of therapy

End of treatment response (ETR): absence of detectable HCV RNA at the completion of therapy

Sustained virological response (SVR): absence of HCV RNA at least 24 weeks after cessation of therapy

[18,25] or PEG-IFNα2b (weight-based dosing of 1.5 µg/kg) [26] injected subcutaneously once weekly plus oral ribavirin twice daily. Rates of SVR overall were 54% to 56%. The genotype-specific SVR rates were 42% to 46% for genotype 1 and 76% to 82% for genotypes 2 and 3. The overall results were statistically significantly superior to those of control patients who were treated with non–PEG-IFNα2b, 3 million units subcutaneously three times per week, and oral ribavirin daily. Combination therapy with PEG-IFN and ribavirin also was superior for genotype 1 infections, but the SVR rates for genotype 2 and 3 infections were comparable among patients who were treated with pegylated or nonpegylated IFN; however, the ease of a weekly injection with PEG-IFN makes it preferable for the treatment of all genotypes. Although predictors of response to these therapies have been identified using multivariate logistic regression analyses (Table 1), clinicians should keep in mind that no predictor precludes an individual from achieving an SVR. Thus, predictors of response should not be regarded as absolutes when making decisions about specific patients. Dose reductions because of adverse events (see later discussion) were required in 36% to 45% of patients in these three registration trials, whereas discontinuation of therapy was necessary in 5% to 16%.

Questions about the comparative safety and effectiveness of the two PEG-IFNs abound; however, none can be answered definitively because of the significant differences among the studies [18,25,26]. First, the proportion of patients with genotype 1 infections and viral loads of more than 2 million copies/mL varied between the registration trials: 40% for PEG-IFNα2a/ribavirin and 50% PEG-IFNα2b/ribavirin. Second, the PEG-IFNα2a/ribavirin registration trial included a smaller proportion of patients (12%) who had

Table 1
Predictors of sustained virological response to treatment of previously untreated, immunocompetent patients who have compensated chronic hepatitis C with pegylated interferon and ribavirin combination therapy

Predictor	PEGα2a[a]	PEGα2b[b]	PEGα2a[c]
Non-1 genotype	P < .001	p < .0001	p < .001
Absence of bridging fibrosis or cirrhosis	NS	p < .01	NS
HCV RNA ≤2 × 10⁶ copies/mL	NS	p < .0001	p < .034
Age ≤40 y	P < .001	p < .01	NS
Weight ≤75 kg	P < .002	NS	NS

Abbreviation: NS, not significant.

[a] Data from Fried MW, Shiffman ML, Reddy KR, et al. Peginterferon alfa-2a plus ribavirin for chronic hepatitis C infection. N Engl J Med 2002;347(13):957–82.

[b] Data from Manns MP, McHutchinson JG, Gordon SC, et al. Peginterferon alfa-2b plus ribavirin compared with interferon alfa-2b plus ribavirin for initial treatment of chronic hepatitis C: a randomized trial. Lancet 2001;358(928b):958–65.

[c] Data from Hadziyannis SJ, Sette H Jr, Morgan TR, et al. Peginterferon-alpha2a and ribavirin combination therapy in chronic hepatitis C: a randomized study of treatment duration and ribavirin dose. Ann Intern Med 2004;140(5):346–55.

bridging fibrosis (stage 3) or cirrhosis (stage 4) than did the PEG-IFNα2b/ribavirin registration trial (29%). Third, American patients accounted for 41% of the population in the PEG-IFNα2a/ribavirin study and 68% of the population in the PEG-IFNα2b/ribavirin trial. Fourth, the mean weight of patients also differed between the trials: 79.8 kg for the PEG-IFNα2a/ribavirin trial and 82 kg for the PEG-IFNα2b/ribavirin trial. Theoretically, this difference would have favored outcomes with PEG-IFNα2a/ribavirin, because rates of SVR are lower for patients who weigh more than 75 kg. An RCT is being conducted to compare the effectiveness of PEG-IFNα2a (fixed dosage of 180 µg/wk) or PEG-IFNα2b (weight-based dosages of 1.0 µg/kg/wk or 1.5 µg/kg/wk) combined with ribavirin.

Duration of Therapy and Ribavirin Dosing

In the two original registration trials, all patients were treated for 48 weeks, regardless of genotype [18,26]. In the subsequent registration trial of PEG-IFNα2a (180 µg/wk) plus ribavirin, patients were randomized to 24 or 48 weeks of therapy with ribavirin at a fixed dose of 800 mg or weight-based dosing (1000 mg/d for up to 74 kg/d or 1200 mg for at least 75 kg/d) [25]. The results (Table 2) showed that the highest rate of SVR for genotype 1 infections occurred with 48 weeks of therapy and weight-based dosing of ribavirin. A post-hoc analysis of the PEG-IFNα2ab/ribavirin registration trial that used ribavirin at a fixed dosage of 800 mg/d showed an SVR of 61% in the subgroup of patients whose dosage of ribavirin was greater than 10.6 mg/kg/d [26].

In contrast, the rates of SVR in genotype 2 or 3 infections were comparable among groups (see Table 2), which proved that treatment for 24 weeks was effective, regardless of the dosage of ribavirin. The responses of the 36 patients with genotype 4 to treatment with PEG-IFNα2a/ribavirin indicated that an SVR in genotype 4 infections is more likely than with genotype 1 infections, but full-dose, full-duration therapy is required [25]. A subsequent RCT of 24 weeks versus 48 weeks of therapy with PEG-IFNα2b/ribavirin for genotypes 2 or 3 confirmed that treatment for 24 weeks is sufficient [27].

EARLY VIROLOGICAL RESPONSE AS A PREDICTOR OF SUSTAINED VIROLOGICAL RESPONSES

Reduction of serum HCV RNA that is induced by interferon therapy exhibits biphasic kinetics [28–31]. Modeling analysis has shown that the rapid decrease during the first 2 to 3 days of therapy is due to inhibition of HCV replication. The second, slower phase of reduction (lasting weeks to months) is believed to be due to the elimination of HCV-infected hepatocytes, which presumably is mediated by the host immune response. Evidence that more rapid reductions of serum levels of HCV RNA correlated with increases in SVR led to multiple studies of induction therapy using higher initial dosages of IFN or more frequent administration [32,33]. The results did not support the hypothesis that induction regimens would increase the rates of SVR, and led to the abandonment of such protocols. In contrast, assessment of EVR during standard IFN-based therapy has proven to be useful in predicting the likelihood of SVR and

Table 2
Effects of duration of therapy and dose of ribavirin on sustained virological response rates using combination therapy with pegylated interferon2a/ribavirin for genotypes 1 through 4

Ribavirin dosage (mg/d)	N	Duration of therapy (wk)	Genotype 1 SVR	Genotype 2 and 3 SVR	Genotype 4 SVR (n = 36)
800	207	24	29%	84%	0/5 (0%)
1000/1200	280	24	42%	81%	8/12 (67%)
800	361	48	41%	79%	5/8 (63%)
100/1200	436	48	52%	80%	9/11 (82%)

making decisions about continuation of therapy [17,18,34]. Retrospective analysis of pooled data from the registration trials of PEG-IFNα/ribavirin showed that SVR occurred in 70% of patients who met the definition of an EVR of at least a 2-$\log_{10}$ reduction of HCV RNA within 12 weeks of starting therapy. Among 380 patients with at least a 2-$\log_{10}$ reduction of HCV RNA by 12 weeks, SVR was achieved in 84% of those with undetectable HCV RNA, but in only 21% of those with detectable HCV RNA [17]. Thus, the most positive predictor of SVR is an undetectable HCV RNA by PCR after 12 weeks of therapy. Failure to achieve an EVR has excellent negative predictive value with a probability of SVR of 0% to 2%. Thus, discontinuation of antiviral therapy is appropriate for treated patients who fail to achieve an EVR.

ADHERENCE AS A PREDICTOR OF SUSTAINED VIROLOGICAL RESPONSE

Retrospective analysis of the registration trials of non–PEG-IFNα2b/ribavirin showed that SVR (especially for genotype 1 infections) was more likely in patients who had received at least 80% of planned IFN injections and at least 80% of planned ribavirin capsules for at least 80% of the anticipated duration of therapy [35]. To prevent reductions in dosages of IFN and ribavirin that could compromise an SVR, some clinicians use granulocyte colony-stimulating factor and erythropoietin to maintain adequate levels of neutrophils and hemoglobin.

EFFECT OF ANTIVIRAL THERAPY ON HISTOPATHOLOGY AND CLINICAL OUTCOMES

Analysis of data from combined trials of PEG-IFNα2b with or without ribavirin showed that treatment was associated with reversal of cirrhosis [36]. Similarly, a meta-analysis of three RCTs of PEG-IFNα2a versus standard IFNα2a showed that PEG-IFNα2a significantly reduced fibrosis in patients who achieved an SVR [37]. Improvements in the grade of necroinflammation or stage of fibrosis also have been reported in nonresponders [38,39], with or without reductions in HCV RNA levels during therapy [40]. The Cochrane Collaboration systematic review, which reported the histologic response of treatment-naive patients to combination therapy with IFNα/ribavirin versus

IFNα monotherapy, found that combination therapy reduced the necroinflammatory grade but was not superior to IFNα monotherapy in reducing the fibrosis stage [41]. In addition, differences in the reduction of fibrosis were not observed among relapsers and nonresponders. Unfortunately, posttreatment biopsies were not included in the two RCTs of PEG-IFNα2a/ribavirin; however, analyses of paired biopsies in patients who were treated with PEG-IFNα2b alone or in combination with ribavirin showed reductions in necroinflammation (hepatic activity index inflammation grade −1.5 to −3.4, respectively) but insignificant decreases in fibrosis (hepatic activity index fibrosis score +0.1 to −0.1, respectively).

Trials of therapy with durations of up to 48 weeks and 24 weeks of posttreatment observation are designed to assess the rates of SVR, but beg the question of the long-term impact of response on disease progression, morbidity, and mortality [10]. The Cochrane Collaboration systematic review identified no differences in liver-related morbidity or all-cause mortality for patients who were treated with a combination of non–PEG-IFNα/ribavirin or IFNα monotherapy [41]; however, successful therapy with IFNα has been associated with prolonged survival, a reduction in complications, and improvement in the quality of life [42,43]. Decision analyses that were based on the natural history of chronic HCV infection and the efficacy of antiviral therapy also showed that IFNα-based therapy is cost effective for patients who have even mild grades of HCV infection [44–48]. Specifically, therapy reduced the estimated direct medical costs, which are surrogate measures for a beneficial impact of therapy on morbidity and mortality.

Results of analyses to determine whether antiviral therapy affects the occurrence of HCC remain controversial [49–55]. This is primarily due to the fact that most of the studies were nonrandomized or retrospective with a significant risk for lead-time bias in favor of the treatment of patients who had early stages of disease. In the single, prospective RCT, the extraordinarily high rate (38%) of HCC in the untreated control group compromised the certainty of the conclusions, and suggested that IFNα may have reduced the incidence of HCC in responders and nonresponders [53]. Among cirrhotic patients, in whom the incidence of HCC is highest, retrospective and prospective studies have not demonstrated any reduction in HCC following IFNα2a therapy [23,56,57].

SIDE EFFECTS OF COMBINATION THERAPY

The side effects that are associated with IFNα and PEG-IFNα are identical and can be classified into five categories [18,26]. First, flulike symptoms of malaise, myalgia, headache, and fever occur in approximately 85% of individuals. Second, bone marrow suppression causes specific reductions in neutrophils and platelets of unpredictable magnitude. Third, neuropsychiatric side effects include depression in approximately 20% to 30% of patients, irritability, disturbed memory, difficulty concentrating, and insomnia. Fourth, IFN can stimulate preexisting autoimmune or immune-mediated inflammatory diseases, such as systemic lupus erythematosus, rheumatoid arthritis, psoriasis, sarcoidosis, colitis, or pancreatitis. Additionally, IFN treatment causes autoimmune thyroiditis that results in hypothyroidism in approximately 4% of patients [58]. Fifth, IFN therapy is associated with a variety of systemic adverse events, such as fatigue, asthenia, alopecia, dyspepsia, altered vision (including retinal hemorrhages observed more commonly in patients with diabetic or hypertensive retinopathy), impaired hearing, and interstitial pneumonitis.

The principal adverse event that is associated with ribavirin is hemolytic anemia because of the deleterious effect of intracellular ribavirin triphosphate on erythrocyte survival [59]; however, a systematic review of ribavirin in combination with IFN showed that ribavirin also increased the risk for several adverse events above those observed in patients who were treated with IFN monotherapy [41]. The increased relative risks of combining ribavirin with IFN included anemia (16.67; CI, 5.68–48.9); leukopenia (4.52; CI, 1.55–13.23); rash (2.3; CI, 1.58–3.56); pruritus (2.32; CI, 1.75–3.08); dyspnea (2.03; CI, 1.49–2.77); dyspepsia (1.72; CI, 1.17–2.54); cough (1.66; CI, 1.19–2.31); and pharyngitis (1.55; CI, 1.14–2.12). Ribavirin also is associated with sinusitis, and can precipitate attacks of gout.

As a result of the increased intensity and diversity of adverse events that are observed with combination therapy with IFN and ribavirin, it is not surprising that dose reductions and discontinuation of therapy for adverse events were more common in patients who were treated with combination therapy than in those who were treated with IFN monotherapy. In a systematic review, the relative risk for dose reduction for combination therapy was 2.44 (CI, 1.58–3.75) and of discontinuation was 1.28 (CI, 1.07–1.52) [41]. In the registration trials for PEG-IFNα/ribavirin, using strict guidelines for dose reductions due to neutropenia, thrombocytopenia, or anemia, 36% to 45% of patients had dosages reduced because of side effects or laboratory abnormalities and 5% to 16% required drug discontinuation [18,25,26]. Thresholds for dose reductions that were established in registration trials are summarized in Table 3.

Ribavirin is teratogenic in animals [60]. This mandates that strict contraception must be practiced by both partners during, and, for 6 months after, therapy. Before starting therapy, women of childbearing age must have a negative pregnancy test. Most clinicians repeat pregnancy testing and document the specific contraceptive practices of both partners during each clinical visit.

CONTRAINDICATIONS

Current contraindications to therapy with PEG-IFNα/ribavirin are summarized in Box 3. Treatment of some conditions that are relative contraindications for therapy may permit the safe use of PEG-IFNα/ribavirin in individuals who are monitored carefully.

Anemia

Combination therapy is contraindicated in patients who have preexisting, severe anemia. It is also contraindicated in persons who have coronary artery disease or cerebrovascular disease because of their inability to tolerate anemia.

Table 3
Recommendations for dose reductions for cytopenias induced by combination therapy with pegylated interferon/ribavirin therapy

Cytopenia	Recommended dose reduction
Absolute neutrophil counts	
500–750/mm^3	Reduce PEG-IFNα2a to 135 µg/wk
	Reduce PEG-IFNα2b by 50%
<500/mm^3	Stop PEG-IFNα2a/2b
Platelet counts	
80,000/mm^3	Reduce PEG-IFNα2b by 50%
25,000–50,000/mm^3	Reduce PEG-IFNα2a to 90 µg/wk; stop PEG-IFNα2b
<25,000/mm^3	Stop PEG-IFNα2a
Hemoglobin	
≤10 g/dL	For PEG-IFNα2b, reduce ribavirin dose by 200 mg
	For PEG-IFNα2a, reduce ribavirin to 600 mg
≤8.5 g/dL	Stop ribavirin

Several preliminary studies showed that injection of erythropoietin prevented the need for ribavirin dose reductions and improved symptomatic anemia, fatigue, and quality of life [61–63].

Neutropenia

The effect of combination therapy on the absolute neutrophil count is unpredictable. Because recommended dose reductions of PEG-IFNα (see Table 3) may compromise the ability to achieve an SVR, off-label, short-term use of granulocyte colony-stimulating factor to maintain adequate neutrophil counts has become popular [64,65].

Neuropsychiatric Conditions

Combination therapy may alter neuropsychiatric functions and result in depression, irritability, and insomnia. Because mental illnesses are associated with high-risk behaviors, such as injection drug use, chronic hepatitis C is associated with higher rates of depression, bipolar disorder, and other psychiatric illnesses. Precipitation or worsening of preexisting depression is of special concern, because a small minority has developed severe depression with suicidal ideation and suicide attempts. Depression was the most common cause for discontinuation of therapy in the three registration trials of IFN/ribavirin, PEG-IFNα monotherapy, and PEG-IFNα/ribavirin [18,25,26]. Two deaths that were due to suicide were reported during therapeutic trials [25,66]. Recognizing that 20% to 30% of patients may be at risk for depression on therapy, a detailed history of symptoms of depression or a previous diagnosis is mandatory. In one study, the magnitude of the self-rating depression score was a strong predictor of intolerance to therapy and failure to achieve SVR [67]. Because patients who are on stable doses of antidepressant medications are

Box 3: Contraindications to combination therapy with pegylated interferonα/ribavirin

Pregnancy

Breastfeeding

Inability to practice birth control

Uncontrolled depression or severe mental illness

Active substance abuse without participation in a concurrent rehabilitation program

Advanced cardiac disease

Advanced pulmonary disease

Severe anemia, leukopenia, or thrombocytopenia

Uncontrolled diabetes mellitus

Uncontrolled hypertension

Retinopathy

Seizure disorder

Treatment with immunosuppressive drugs

Autoimmune or immune-mediated inflammatory disorders

Decompensated cirrhosis

Other uncontrolled comorbid conditions

Hypersensitivity reactions to the antiviral drugs

less likely to experience worsening depression on therapy, most clinicians respond to a history of depression by prescribing antidepressants for 6 to 8 weeks before starting PEG-IFNα/ribavirin [68]. Psychiatric consultation is recommended for patients who have severe depression, bipolar disorder, or other psychiatric illness before deciding to treat. If therapy is recommended, the psychiatrist should remain involved actively.

Renal Insufficiency

Ribavirin is excreted in the urine, and decreased glomerular filtration rates result in ribavirin accumulation and an increased risk for severe hemolytic anemia; however, two studies showed that dose reductions based on calculated creatinine clearance (Cockcroft-Gault equation) achieved desired serum levels of ribavirin in patients with estimated creatinine clearances as low as 20 mL/min [69,70]. Treatment remains contraindicated for patients who require chronic hemodialysis because of the accumulation of ribavirin, which is not dialyzed.

Decompensated Cirrhosis

IFN-based therapy has been associated with life-threatening adverse events in patients who had decompensated cirrhosis, defined as total bilirubin of greater than 1.5 mg/dL, prothrombin time international normalized ratio of at least 1.7, albumin less than 3.4 g/dL, and history of ascites, variceal hemorrhage, or hepatic encephalopathy. Antiviral therapy is contraindicated in such patients who should be referred for evaluation as candidates for OLT [71,72]. Trials of low-dose, escalating therapy in patients who are listed for OLT are in progress to determine if absence of viremia at the time of OLT can prevent HCV infection of the allograft [73].

TREATMENT RECOMMENDATIONS

Chronic Hepatitis C, Genotype 1, Naive to Treatment

Genotype 1 accounts for 70% to 75% of chronic HCV infections in North America. PEG-IFNα/ribavirin is indicated for therapy in naive to treatment patients with circulating HCV RNA, consistently or intermittently elevated ALT levels, and biopsy evidence of chronic hepatitis [10,13,14,72]. The most important candidates for therapy are patients who have progressive disease whose biopsies show moderate to severe inflammation and significant fibrosis (eg, METAVIR stage at least F2, Ishak stage at least 3, septal or bridging fibrosis, or cirrhosis). In the absence of contraindications, PEG-IFNα/ribavirin treatment is recommended for all patients who have advanced fibrosis or compensated cirrhosis.

The dosages of PEG-IFN2a and PEG-IFNα2a are 180 μg/wk and 1.5 μg/kg/wk, respectively. Most clinicians use weight-based dosing of ribavirin (1000 mg for weight up to 75 kg and 1200 mg for more than 75 kg) with either pegylated IFN, although the registration trial that used 1.5 μg/kg/wk of PEG-IFNα2b used a fixed dosage of 800 mg of ribavirin [26].

A quantitative HCV RNA should be obtained at baseline and after 12 weeks of therapy to determine if the patient has achieved an EVR. Failure to achieve an EVR predicts the ultimate absence of an SVR with virtual certainty; however, some authorities recommend continued treatment for an additional 12 weeks because histopathologic improvement can occur in the absence of an SVR [38,39,74]. Therapy should be discontinued in any patient with detectable levels of HCV RNA at week 24, because an SVR cannot be achieved.

Chronic Hepatitis C, Genotypes 2 or 3, Naive to Treatment

Treatment should be recommended for all patients with HCV genotype 2 or 3 infections because of the high probability of SVR. Biopsy is optional, because the decision for therapy will not be influenced by the histopathologic grade and stage. RCTs support treatment with PEG-IFNα/ribavirin for 24 weeks, using 800 mg of ribavirin daily [25,27]. The preliminary evidence that indicated that patients with genotype 2 or 3 infections could achieve SVRs with only 12 weeks of therapy if they had undetectable HCV RNA at week 4 is being studied further in ongoing controlled trials [75].

Chronic Hepatitis C, Genotypes 4, 5, and 6, Naive to Treatment

These genotypes, which are rare in North America, are observed primarily in immigrants from Egypt and the Middle East (genotype 4), South Africa (genotype 5), and Southeast Asia (genotype 6). Optimal responses for genotype 4 infections require full-dose therapy with PEG-IFNα/ribavirin for 48 weeks (see Table 2) [25]. The rate of SVR for genotype 5 infections that were treated with combination therapy for 48 weeks is similar to that of genotypes 2 or 3 [25,76]. Thus, liver biopsy also is optional for patients with this genotype. Patients who had genotype 6 infections who were treated with standard IFN, 5 mouse units (MU) three times per week, and weight-based ribavirin for 12 months achieved an SVR of 63% [25,76,77]. It is reasonable to treat patients who have genotype 6 infections with combination PEG-IFNα/ribavirin therapy.

Chronic Hepatitis C with Persistently Normal Alanine Aminotransferase Levels

Serial liver biopsies that were performed over intervals of up to 5 years have documented low rates of progression to advanced fibrosis or cirrhosis in patients with persistently normal levels of ALT. During observation, however, ALT levels became abnormal in up to 25% of patients, which indicated that serial testing is required to define such patients. Initial trials of IFN monotherapy for patients with normal ALT levels resulted in low rates of response and unexpected elevations of ALT [78]. In contrast, subsequent trials of IFN/ribavirin or PEG-IFNα/ribavirin showed SVRs comparable to those achieved in patients with abnormal ALT levels and more advanced histopathology [78–82]. Elevations of ALT during therapy were not observed. Modeling also demonstrated that treatment of such patients is cost-effective [44,46]. Decisions about therapy should be based on genotype, the level of concern of the patient, symptoms, occupation, age, and weight. Some authorities advocate observation and a repeat biopsy every 3 to 5 years to assess for progression, but data on the optimal interval between biopsies are lacking.

Relapse After Interferon-Based Therapy

Relapse is defined as detectable HCV RNA within 24 weeks after an ETR with documented absence of HCV RNA. The outcomes of retreatment vary depending on the nature of the original therapy and the regimen for retreatment. For example, an SVR of 50% was achieved by treating patients with IFNα/ribavirin who had relapsed after IFN monotherapy [66]. Retreatment with PEG-IFNα2b/ribavirin achieved an SVR of 42% in patients who had relapsed after treatment with IFN monotherapy or combination IFN/ribavirin [83]. The probability of SVR also is greater following treatment with combination PEG-IFNα/ribavirin than with PEG-IFNα monotherapy. Thus, retreatment with PEG-IFNα/ribavirin should be considered for patients who relapsed after IFN monotherapy, combination IFN/ribavirin of PEG-IFNα monotherapy.

Nonresponse to Interferon-Based Therapy

Nonresponse, which is defined as a failure to eliminate circulating HCV RNA by the end of a course of therapy, encompasses three populations of patients. The first, which is characterized by insignificant reductions of HCV RNA during therapy, is truly nonresponsive to IFN. The second group is characterized by therapeutic decreases of HCV RNA, even to undetectable levels, which are followed by a breakthrough increase in HCV RNA during therapy. This is indicative of resistance. The characteristic of the third group is a declining HCV RNA that remains detectable after 24 weeks of therapy. This is indicative of a slow or incomplete response that might benefit from therapy of longer duration. It is important to distinguish among these groups when assessing data regarding the safety and efficacy of retreatment.

Retreatment trials have focused on the use of combination therapy with high-dose, non-PEG alfacon-1 IFN/ribavirin or PEG-IFNα/ribavirin. Preliminary studies of alfacon-1 IFN/ribavirin showed benefit for the retreatment of nonresponders to IFN/ribavirin and PEG-IFN/ribavirin [84]. The National Institutes of Health (NIH) Hepatitis C Antivirus Longterm Treatment Against Cirrhosis (HALT-C) study of the safety and efficacy of PEG-IFNα2a/ribavirin for the retreatment of nonresponders to IFN, with or without ribavirin, has provided the most comprehensive information [85,86]. In the lead-in phase, 604 nonresponder patients who had advanced fibrosis or cirrhosis were treated with PEG-IFNα2a/ribavirin. Although the ETR at the end of 48 weeks of therapy was 35%, subsequent relapse resulted in an SVR of only 18%. Of note, 98% of the relapses occurred in the first 12 weeks after cessation of therapy. Among patients who achieved an EVR, 33% achieved an SVR. In contrast, the SVR was only 1% in the absence of an EVR. The rate of SVR was associated with the ability to maintain ribavirin dosing during the first 20 weeks of therapy. The SVR was 21% for patients who were tolerant of at least 80% of their target dose, compared with 11% in those who required reductions to up to 69% of target doses. Multivariate regression analysis of independent factors that are associated with SVR identified factors that are useful in decision making about retreatment of nonresponders who have advanced, compensated disease (Table 4).

Acute Hepatitis C

Patients who have acute hepatitis C rarely seek medical care because of the paucity of symptoms and the rarity of jaundice. Thus, data regarding the efficacy of antiviral therapy in preventing the high rate of chronicity of acute HCV infection are limited. Meta-analyses of short-term, randomized, placebo-controlled trials of IFNα2b or IFNβ (reviewed in [10]) showed a significant reduction in chronicity among treated patients. The most compelling study of efficacy was the prospective, open-label trial of IFNα2b treatment of 44 consecutive German patients approximately 3 months after initial diagnosis [87]. The treatment regimen consisted of 5 MU daily for 4 weeks, followed by 5 MU three times per week for 20 weeks. Forty-three (98%) of the patients achieved an SVR 26 weeks after the completion of therapy, compared with a spontaneous resolution rate of 52% for symptomatic acute hepatitis C among noncontemporaneous German controls [88]. The role for PEG-IFNα, with or without ribavirin, remains unclear. In one report, PEG-IFNα monotherapy for 24 weeks was as successful as the high-dose IFNα2b regimen that was

Table 4
Factors determining sustained virological response in nonresponders who have advanced fibrosis or cirrhosis treated with pegylated interferonα2a/ribavirin

Factors	Rate of SVR
Previous treatment with IFN monotherapy versus IFNα/ribavirin	28% vs. 12%
Caucasian versus African American	20% vs. 6%
Age <60 y versus ≥60 y	19% vs. 6%
Genotype 1 versus non-genotype 1	14% vs. 65%
HCV RNA≤1.5 × 10^6 versus 1.5 × 10^6 IU/mL	27% vs. 15%
Cirrhosis versus advanced fibrosis	11% vs. 23%
Ratio of AST:ALT ≤1 versus >1	21% vs. 6%
EVR present versus absent	34% vs. 1%

Factors that are predictive of SVR included gender, weight, body mass index, and histologic activity index score.

Data from Hadziyannis SJ, Sette H Jr, Morgan TR, et al. Peginterferon-alpha2a and ribavirin combination therapy in chronic hepatitis C: a randomized study of treatment duration and ribavirin dose. Ann Intern Med 2004;140(5):346–55.

used in the German trial [89]. Among 40 patients who were randomized to receive PEG-IFNα monotherapy or PEG-IFNα/ribavirin for 24 weeks, the SVRs were 80% and 85%, respectively. Although it is clear that therapy for acute hepatitis C is effective, the optimal regimen, dose, time for initiation of therapy, and the benefit of ribavirin remain unclear. Most authorities favor initiation of a 24-week course of PEG-IFNα/ribavirin therapy within 3 months of the onset of acute infection to provide for activation of the host immune responses and the possibility of spontaneous clearance.

Children

Children are infected with HCV less frequently than are adults, and their rate of progression seems to be slower [90–92]. The SVRs that were reported in children who were treated with IFN monotherapy or IFN/ribavirin combination therapy have been comparable to those that were observed in adults [91,93–96]. Therapy is not recommended under 3 years of age. The approved pediatric regimen consists of IFNα2b, 3 MU/m², and ribavirin (available as an oral suspension or capsules). Controlled trials of the safety and efficacy of PEG-IFNα/ribavirin are in progress.

African Americans

Recent studies have confirmed that African Americans respond less well than do whites to treatment with PEG-IFNα2a/ribavirin combination therapy. Comparison of the responses of 100 African Americans and 100 non-Hispanic whites to combination therapy with PEG-IFNα2b/ribavirin showed an SVR of only 19% in African Americans versus 52% in whites [97]. Another study of 78 African Americans and 28 whites who were treated with a combination of PEG-IFNα2a/ribavirin showed an SVR of 26% in African Americans compared with 39% in whites [98]. The recent NIH ViraHepC trial of combination PEG-IFNα2a/ribavirin therapy for genotype 1 HCV infections in 196 African

Americans and 205 whites also showed a significantly lower SVR in African Americans of 28% compared with 52% in whites [99]. This was primarily due to a lower ETR, because relapse rates were comparable. Racial differences in virological responses were evident as early as week 4, and breakthrough viremia was more frequent among African Americans. Despite lower response rates, African Americans with histopathologic features of progressive hepatitis should be treated.

Hepatitis C Virus and HIV Coinfection

Patients who have HIV are coinfected frequently with HCV because of shared routes of parenteral transmission Nearly 40% of HIV-infected Americans and up to 90% of injection drug users who have HIV are coinfected with HCV [100,101]. The prolonged survival of HIV-infected patients who are treated with highly active antiretroviral therapy has been accompanied by an increased deleterious impact of HCV coinfection, including evidence of accelerated rates of fibrosis, development of decompensated cirrhosis, liver failure, and HCC [102–106]. Thus, HCV infection rapidly has become a major cause of morbidity and mortality in persons who have HIV. As a result, it is imperative that all persons who have HIV infection be tested for HCV infection.

Coinfected individuals should be considered as candidates for therapy with combination PEG-IFNα/ribavirin after the HIV infection is controlled. This recommendation is based on the results of large, RCTs that demonstrated the relative safety and efficacy of antiviral therapy in HCV-HIV coinfected persons (Table 5) [107–110]. The reason for lower SVR rates in coinfected patients is unknown, but a diminished immune response to IFN during HIV infection has been postulated.

End-Stage Renal Disease

Dialyzed patients who have end-stage renal disease have an increased prevalence of HCV infection, an increased risk for progressive liver disease, and reduced graft and patient survival after kidney transplantation [111–113]. When considering kidney transplantation in a patient who has chronic hepatitis C, a liver biopsy should be performed to define the stage of fibrosis, because

Table 5
Results of randomized, controlled trials of pegylated interferon/ribavirin standard interferon/ribavirin in patients coninfected with HIV and hepatitis C virus

	ACTG 5071 [108]	RIBAVIC [107]	APRICOT [110]	Barcelona [109]
Duration	48 wk	48 wk	48 wk	48/24[a] wk
PEG-IFNα	α2b	α2b	α2a	α2b
SVR (genotypes 1, 4)[b]	14%	17%	29%	38%
SVR (genotypes 2, 3)	73%	44%	62%	53%
Discontinuation[c]	12%	39%	25%	15%

[a] 48 wk for genotypes 1 and 4 and 24 wk for genotypes 2 and 3 with HCV RNA <8 × 105 IU/ML.
[b] Data only for significantly superior PEG-IFNα/ribavirin arm.
[c] Combined from both treatment arms, because discontinuation rates are comparable.

advanced fibrosis or cirrhosis is associated specifically with reduced graft and patient survival.

Safe and effective therapeutic regimens have not been established [114]. Combination therapy with usual doses of ribavirin is contraindicated because ribavirin is excreted by the kidney and is not cleared by dialysis. Treatment has been restricted largely to IFN monotherapy [115], but pilot trials of combination therapy using low-dose ribavirin also have been conducted [116]. The manufacturer of PEG-IFNα2a recommends a dose reduction to 135 µg/wk for patients who have renal failure. No dose reduction is recommended for PEG-IFNα2b. Trials of PEG-IFNα with low doses of ribavirin are being conducted.

Extrahepatic Diseases

Chronic hepatitis C is associated with the rare occurrence of extrahepatic disease manifestations that are due to immune complexes, porphyria cutanea tarda, or sicca syndrome [117]. Cutaneous vasculitis, glomerulonephritis, and arthritis that are associated with mixed essential cryoglobulinemia in HCV infection should be treated. Whenever possible, combination therapy with PEG-IFNα/ribavirin should be used to achieve an SVR. The goal of preventing the formation of immune complexes and reducing manifestations of porphyria cutanea tarda can be achieved with IFN or PEG-IFNα monotherapy to reduce HCV replication and the concentration of HCV antigens; however, indefinite maintenance therapy may be required.

Maintenance Therapy for Nonresponders

Patients who fail to achieve an SVR remain at risk for progression until new therapies become available. Previous studies indicated that the anti-inflammatory and antifibrotic effects of IFN improved histopathology at the end of therapy in 75% of cases, although only a small minority achieved an SVR [74]. These observations indicated that it might be possible to treat the histopathologic disease process effectively in the absence of a virological response. The results of two small, randomized studies supported this hypothesis by showing that continuation of IFN monotherapy significantly reduced the fibrosis stage or necroinflammation compared with controls who were observed after completion of therapy [39,118]. These findings provided the impetus for the initiation of three prospective RCTs. The lead-in phase of the NIH HALT-C study demonstrated that combination therapy with PEG-IFNα2a/ribavirin produced an SVR of 18% among patients who had advanced fibrosis or cirrhosis who were nonresponders to previous IFN therapy, with or without ribavirin [86]. Those without an SVR were randomized to observation or treatment with PEG-IFNα2a maintenance monotherapy. The study is in progress, and the Data and Safety Monitoring Board recommended continuation after review of the 2-year data. The Colchicine versus PEG-INTRON Long-Term trial is an RCT that is comparing the long-term effect of PEG-IFNα2b, 0.5 µg/kg/wk, with colchicine on disease progression and development of complications in patients who have bridging fibrosis or cirrhosis. Evaluation of PEG-INTRON in Control of Hepatitis C is a multinational, RCT.

Recurrent Hepatitis C After Liver Transplantation

Infection of the allograft after OLT is universal in viremic patients [119]. Initial graft and patient survival are good, with the exception of the infrequent recipient who develops rapidly progressive fibrosing cholestatic hepatitis. Progression to advanced fibrosis, cirrhosis, or decompensation ultimately occurs in up to 28% of patients after 5 to 7 years, and survival is reduced significantly compared with other indications for OLT [120,121]. Controlled and uncontrolled trials have shown reduced tolerance for full doses of IFN, IFN/ribavirin, PEG-IFNα, or PEG-IFNα/ribavirin [122]. Moreover, the probability of achieving an SVR is no more than 20% when calculated on an intention-to-treat basis [123].

FUTURE THERAPIES

Adjunctive Therapies

A variety of agents has been used in combination with IFN or IFN/ribavirin, including amantadine, rimantadine, ursodeoxycholic acid, nonsteroidal anti-inflammatory drugs, and thymosinα [124–127]; however, none has increased the probability of SVR conclusively. Sylimarin, the active ingredient in milk thistle, has no antiviral effect on HCV replication or sustained impact on aminotransferase levels [128].

Hepatitis C Virus Molecular Targets

As a result of a more precise understanding of the details of HCV replication in cell culture, multiple therapeutic targets for the treatment of chronic hepatitis C have been identified (Box 4). Recently, several new agents were introduced

---

Box 4: Molecular targets for future hepatitis C virus therapeutics

HCV RNA
RNA interference
Antisense oligonucleotides
RNA decoys
Ribozymes

HCV enzymes
NS2-3 protease
NS3-4A protease
NS3 helicase
NS5B RNA-dependent RNA polymerase

Other HCV Proteins
NS4B
NS5A

into clinical studies, including a prodrug of a nucleoside inhibitor of NSB5 RNA-dependent RNA polymerase (valopicitabine, NM283), and two NS3-4A protease inhibitors (VX-950 and SCH503034). Trials of BILN-2061, a potent NS3 protease inhibitor in phase 1 trials [129], were abandoned because of concerns about cardiotoxicity.

SUMMARY

HCV infection is one of the leading causes of chronic liver disease worldwide, and it results in cirrhosis, liver failure, and HCC. As a result, hepatitis C cirrhosis has become the principal indication for liver transplantation. Ironically, HCV infection can be cured with available antiviral therapies, but only a minority of infected persons has ever been treated. The current standard of therapy is a combination of PEG-IFNα and ribavirin, which produces high rates of SVRs (absence of detectable HCV RNA at least 24 weeks after cessation of therapy): 42% to 56% in genotype 1 and 75% to 84% in genotypes 2 and 3. Recent reports indicate that the less frequent genotypes 4, 5, and 6 also are responsive to combination therapy. Recommendations for treatment of conventional and special patient populations were reviewed in detail. Newer therapeutics that are entering clinical trials provide hope that SVRs may be possible in patients who are difficult to treat and in nonresponders to current therapy.

References

[1] Shepard CW, Finelli L, Alter MJ. Global epidemiology of hepatitis C virus infection. Lancet Infect Dis 2005;5(9):558–67.
[2] Davis GL, Albright JE, Cook SF, et al. Projecting future complications of chronic hepatitis C in the United States. Liver Transpl 2003;9(4):331–8.
[3] Kim WR, Gross JB Jr, Poterucha JJ, et al. Outcome of hospital care of liver disease associated with hepatitis C in the United States. Hepatology 2001;33(1):201–6.
[4] Kim WR. The burden of hepatitis C in the United States. Hepatology 2002;36 (5)(Suppl 1): S30–4.
[5] Wong JB, McQuillan GM, McHutchison JG, et al. Estimating future hepatitis C morbidity, mortality, and costs in the United States. Am J Public Health 2000;90(10):1562–9.
[6] Simmonds P, Holmes EC, Cha TA, et al. Classification of hepatitis C virus into six major genotypes and a series of subtypes by phylogenetic analysis of the NS-5 region. J Gen Virol 1993;74(Pt 11):2391–9.
[7] Simmonds P, Alberti A, Alter HJ, et al. A proposed system for the nomenclature of hepatitis C viral genotypes. Hepatology 1994;19(5):1321–4.
[8] Simmonds P. Variability of hepatitis C virus. Hepatology 1995;21(2):570–83.
[9] Dienstag JL. The role of liver biopsy in chronic hepatitis C. Hepatology 2002;36 (5)(Suppl 1): S152–60.
[10] Dienstag JL, McHutchison JG. American Gastroenterological Association technical review on the management of hepatitis C. Gastroenterology 2006;130(1):231–64.
[11] Patton HM, Patel K, Behling C, et al. The impact of steatosis on disease progression and early and sustained treatment response in chronic hepatitis C patients. J Hepatol 2004;40(3):484–90.
[12] Westin J, Nordlinder H, Lagging M, et al. Steatosis accelerates fibrosis development over time in hepatitis C virus genotype 3 infected patients. J Hepatol 2002;37(6):837–42.
[13] Heathcote J, Main J. Treatment of hepatitis C. J Viral Hepat 2005;12(3):223–35.
[14] Kim AI, Saab S. Treatment of hepatitis C. Am J Med 2005;118(8):808–15.

[15] Poynard T, Imbert-Bismut F, Munteanu M, et al. Overview of the diagnostic value of bio-chemical markers of liver fibrosis (FibroTest, HCV FibroSure) and necrosis (ActiTest) in patients with chronic hepatitis C. Comp Hepatol 2004;3(1):8.

[16] Zeremski M, Talal AH. Noninvasive markers of hepatic fibrosis: are they ready for prime time in the management of HIV/HCV co-infected patients? J Hepatol 2005;43(1): 2–5.

[17] Davis GL, Wong JB, McHutchison JG, et al. Early virologic response to treatment with peginterferon alfa-2b plus ribavirin in patients with chronic hepatitis C. Hepatology 2003;38(3):645–52.

[18] Fried MW, Shiffman ML, Reddy KR, et al. Peginterferon alfa-2a plus ribavirin for chronic hepatitis C virus infection. N Engl J Med 2002;347(13):975–82.

[19] Mathurin P, Moussalli J, Cadranel JF, et al. Slow progression rate of fibrosis in hepatitis C virus patients with persistently normal alanine transaminase activity. Hepatology 1998;27(3):868–72.

[20] Poynard T, Bedossa P, Opolon P. Natural history of liver fibrosis progression in patients with chronic hepatitis C. The OBSVIRC, METAVIR, CLINIVIR, and DOSVIRC groups. Lancet 1997;349(9055):825–32.

[21] Poynard T, Ratziu V, Benmanov Y, et al. Fibrosis in patients with chronic hepatitis C: detection and significance. Semin Liver Dis 2000;20(1):47–55.

[22] Strader DB, Seeff LB. The natural history of chronic hepatitis C infection. Eur J Gastroenterol Hepatol 1996;8(4):324–8.

[23] Fattovich G, Giustina G, Degos F, et al. Morbidity and mortality in compensated cirrhosis type C: a retrospective follow-up study of 384 patients. Gastroenterology 1997;112(2): 463–72.

[24] Chang KM. Immunopathogenesis of hepatitis C virus infection. Clin Liver Dis 2003;7(1): 89–105.

[25] Hadziyannis SJ, Sette H Jr, Morgan TR, et al. Peginterferon-alpha2a and ribavirin combination therapy in chronic hepatitis C: a randomized study of treatment duration and ribavirin dose. Ann Intern Med 2004;140(5):346–55.

[26] Manns MP, McHutchison JG, Gordon SC, et al. Peginterferon alfa-2b plus ribavirin compared with interferon alfa-2b plus ribavirin for initial treatment of chronic hepatitis C: a randomised trial. Lancet 2001;358(9286):958–65.

[27] Zeuzem S, Hultcrantz R, Bourliere M, et al. Peginterferon alfa-2b plus ribavirin for treatment of chronic hepatitis C in previously untreated patients infected with HCV genotypes 2 or 3. J Hepatol 2004;40(6):993–9.

[28] Buti M, Sanchez-Avila F, Lurie Y, et al. Viral kinetics in genotype 1 chronic hepatitis C patients during therapy with 2 different doses of peginterferon alfa-2b plus ribavirin. Hepatology 2002;35(4):930–6.

[29] Neumann AU, Lam NP, Dahari H, et al. Hepatitis C viral dynamics in vivo and the antiviral efficacy of interferon-alpha therapy. Science 1998;282(5386):103–7.

[30] Zeuzem S, Schmidt JM, Lee JH, et al. Hepatitis C virus dynamics in vivo: effect of ribavirin and interferon alfa on viral turnover. Hepatology 1998;28(1):245–52.

[31] Zeuzem S, Herrmann E, Lee JH, et al. Viral kinetics in patients with chronic hepatitis C treated with standard or peginterferon alpha2a. Gastroenterology 2001;120(6): 1438–47.

[32] Layden TJ, Layden JE, Reddy KR, et al. Induction therapy with consensus interferon (CIFN) does not improve sustained virologic response in chronic hepatitis C. J Viral Hepat 2002;9(5):334–9.

[33] Senturk H, Ersoz G, Ozaras R, et al. Interferon-alpha2b induction treatment with or without ribavirin in chronic hepatitis C: a multicenter, randomized, controlled trial. Dig Dis Sci 2003;48(6):1124–9.

[34] Davis GL. Monitoring of viral levels during therapy of hepatitis C. Hepatology 2002;36 (5)(Suppl 1):S145–51.

[35] McHutchison JG, Manns M, Patel K, et al. Adherence to combination therapy enhances sustained response in genotype-1-infected patients with chronic hepatitis C. Gastroenterology 2002;123(4):1061–9.

[36] Poynard T, McHutchison J, Manns M, et al. Impact of pegylated interferon alfa-2b and ribavirin on liver fibrosis in patients with chronic hepatitis C. Gastroenterology 2002;122(5):1303–13.

[37] Camma C, Di BD, Schepis F, et al. Effect of peginterferon alfa-2a on liver histology in chronic hepatitis C: a meta-analysis of individual patient data. Hepatology 2004;39(2): 333–42.

[38] Shiffman ML, Hofmann CM, Thompson EB, et al. Relationship between biochemical, virological, and histological response during interferon treatment of chronic hepatitis C. Hepatology 1997;26(3):780–5.

[39] Shiffman ML, Hofmann CM, Contos MJ, et al. A randomized, controlled trial of maintenance interferon therapy for patients with chronic hepatitis C virus and persistent viremia. Gastroenterology 1999;117(5):1164–72.

[40] Poynard T, McHutchison J, Davis GL, et al. Impact of interferon alfa-2b and ribavirin on progression of liver fibrosis in patients with chronic hepatitis C. Hepatology 2000;32(5): 1131–7.

[41] Kjaergard LL, Krogsgaard K, Gluud C. Interferon alfa with or without ribavirin for chronic hepatitis C: systematic review of randomised trials. BMJ 2001;323(7322):1151–5.

[42] Yoshida H, Arakawa Y, Sata M, et al. Interferon therapy prolonged life expectancy among chronic hepatitis C patients. Gastroenterology 2002;123(2):483–91.

[43] Kasahara A, Tanaka H, Okanoue T, et al. Interferon treatment improves survival in chronic hepatitis C patients showing biochemical as well as virological responses by preventing liver-related death. J Viral Hepat 2004;11(2):148–56.

[44] Bennett WG, Inoue Y, Beck JR, et al. Estimates of the cost-effectiveness of a single course of interferon-alpha 2b in patients with histologically mild chronic hepatitis C. Ann Intern Med 1997;127(10):855–65.

[45] Buti M, San MR, Brosa M, et al. Estimating the impact of hepatitis C virus therapy on future liver-related morbidity, mortality and costs related to chronic hepatitis C. J Hepatol 2005;42(5):639–45.

[46] Salomon JA, Weinstein MC, Hammitt JK, et al. Cost-effectiveness of treatment for chronic hepatitis C infection in an evolving patient population. JAMA 2003;290(2):228–37.

[47] Wong JB, Koff RS. Watchful waiting with periodic liver biopsy versus immediate empirical therapy for histologically mild chronic hepatitis C. A cost-effectiveness analysis. Ann Intern Med 2000;133(9):665–75.

[48] Younossi ZM, Singer ME, McHutchison JG, et al. Cost effectiveness of interferon alpha2b combined with ribavirin for the treatment of chronic hepatitis C. Hepatology 1999;30(5): 1318–24.

[49] El-Serag HB. Hepatocellular carcinoma and hepatitis C in the United States. Hepatology 2002;36 (5)(Suppl 1):S74–83.

[50] Ikeda K, Arase Y, Saitoh S, et al. Interferon beta prevents recurrence of hepatocellular carcinoma after complete resection or ablation of the primary tumor-A prospective randomized study of hepatitis C virus-related liver cancer. Hepatology 2000;32(2):228–32.

[51] Ikeda K, Saitoh S, Kobayashi M, et al. Long-term interferon therapy for 1 year or longer reduces the hepatocellular carcinogenesis rate in patients with liver cirrhosis caused by hepatitis C virus: a pilot study. J Gastroenterol Hepatol 2001;16(4):406–15.

[52] Mazzella G, Accogli E, Sottili S, et al. Alpha interferon treatment may prevent hepatocellular carcinoma in HCV-related liver cirrhosis. J Hepatol 1996;24(2):141–7.

[53] Nishiguchi S, Kuroki T, Nakatani S, et al. Randomised trial of effects of interferon-alpha on incidence of hepatocellular carcinoma in chronic active hepatitis C with cirrhosis. Lancet 1995;346(8982):1051–5.

[54] Serfaty L, Aumaitre H, Chazouilleres O, et al. Determinants of outcome of compensated hepatitis C virus-related cirrhosis. Hepatology 1998;27(5):1435–40.

[55] Yoshida H, Shiratori Y, Moriyama M, et al. Interferon therapy reduces the risk for hepatocellular carcinoma: national surveillance program of cirrhotic and noncirrhotic patients with chronic hepatitis C in Japan. IHIT Study Group. Inhibition of Hepatocarcinogenesis by Interferon Therapy. Ann Intern Med 1999;131(3):174–81.

[56] Bernardinello E, Cavalletto L, Chemello L, et al. Long-term clinical outcome after beta-interferon therapy in cirrhotic patients with chronic hepatitis C. TVVH Study Group. Hepatogastroenterology 1999;46(30):3216–22.

[57] Fattovich G, Giustina G, Degos F, et al. Effectiveness of interferon alfa on incidence of hepatocellular carcinoma and decompensation in cirrhosis type C. European Concerted Action on Viral Hepatitis (EUROHEP). J Hepatol 1997;27(1):201–5.

[58] Prummel MF, Laurberg P, Mazziotti G, et al. Interferon-alpha and autoimmune thyroid disease. Thyroid 2003;13(6):547–51.

[59] Bodenheimer HC Jr, Lindsay KL, Davis GL, et al. Tolerance and efficacy of oral ribavirin treatment of chronic hepatitis C: a multicenter trial. Hepatology 1997;26(2):473–7.

[60] Kochhar DM, Penner JD, Knudsen TB. Embryotoxic, teratogenic, and metabolic effects of ribavirin in mice. Toxicol Appl Pharmacol 1980;52(1):99–112.

[61] Afdhal NH, Dieterich DT, Pockros PJ, et al. Epoetin alfa maintains ribavirin dose in HCV-infected patients: a prospective, double-blind, randomized controlled study. Gastroenterology 2004;126(5):1302–11.

[62] Dieterich DT, Wasserman R, Brau N, et al. Once-weekly epoetin alfa improves anemia and facilitates maintenance of ribavirin dosing in hepatitis C virus-infected patients receiving ribavirin plus interferon alfa. Am J Gastroenterol 2003;98(11):2491–9.

[63] Dieterich DT, Spivak JL. Hematologic disorders associated with hepatitis C virus infection and their management. Clin Infect Dis 2003;37(4):533–41.

[64] Curry MP, Afdhal NH. Use of growth factors with antiviral therapy for chronic hepatitis C. Clin Liver Dis 2005;9(3):439–51.

[65] Lebray P, Nalpas B, Vallet-Pichard A, et al. The impact of haematopoietic growth factors on the management and efficacy of antiviral treatment in patients with hepatitis C virus. Antivir Ther 2005;10(6):769–76.

[66] Davis GL, Esteban-Mur R, Rustgi V, et al. Interferon alfa-2b alone or in combination with ribavirin for the treatment of relapse of chronic hepatitis C. International Hepatitis Interventional Therapy Group. N Engl J Med 1998;339(21):1493–9.

[67] Raison CL, Broadwell SD, Borisov AS, et al. Depressive symptoms and viral clearance in patients receiving interferon-alpha and ribavirin for hepatitis C. Brain Behav Immun 2005;19(1):23–7.

[68] Fried MW. Side effects of therapy of hepatitis C and their management. Hepatology 2002;36 (5)(Suppl 1):S237–44.

[69] Bruchfeld A, Lindahl K, Schvarcz R, et al. Dosage of ribavirin in patients with hepatitis C should be based on renal function: a population pharmacokinetic analysis. Ther Drug Monit 2002;24(6):701–8.

[70] Kamar N, Chatelut E, Manolis E, et al. Ribavirin pharmacokinetics in renal and liver transplant patients: evidence that it depends on renal function. Am J Kidney Dis 2004;43(1):140–6.

[71] Crippin JS, McCashland T, Terrault N, et al. A pilot study of the tolerability and efficacy of antiviral therapy in hepatitis C virus-infected patients awaiting liver transplantation. Liver Transpl 2002;8(4):350–5.

[72] Strader DB, Wright T, Thomas DL, et al. Diagnosis, management, and treatment of hepatitis C. Hepatology 2004;39(4):1147–71.

[73] Everson GT, Trotter J, Forman L, et al. Treatment of advanced hepatitis C with a low accelerating dosage regimen of antiviral therapy. Hepatology 2005;42(2):255–62.

[74] Carithers RL Jr, Emerson SS. Therapy of hepatitis C: meta-analysis of interferon alfa-2b tri-als. Hepatology 1997;26 (3)(Suppl 1):83S–8S.

[75] Mangia A, Santoro R, Minerva N, et al. Peginterferon alfa-2b and ribavirin for 12 vs. 24 weeks in HCV genotype 2 or 3. N Engl J Med 2005;352(25):2609–17.

[76] Nguyen MH, Keeffe EB. Prevalence and treatment of hepatitis C virus genotypes 4, 5, and 6. Clin Gastroenterol Hepatol 2005;3 (10)(Suppl 2):S97–101.

[77] Yuen MF, Lai CL. Response to combined interferon and ribavirin is better in patients infected with hepatitis C virus genotype 6 than genotype 1 in Hong Kong. Intervirology 2006;49(1–2):96–8.

[78] Ahmed A, Keeffe EB. Chronic hepatitis C with normal aminotransferase levels. Gastroen-terology 2004;126(5):1409–15.

[79] Bacon BR. Treatment of patients with hepatitis C and normal serum aminotransferase levels. Hepatology 2002;36 (5)(Suppl 1):S179–84.

[80] Gordon SC, Fang JW, Silverman AL, et al. The significance of baseline serum alanine ami-notransferase on pretreatment disease characteristics and response to antiviral therapy in chronic hepatitis C. Hepatology 2000;32(2):400–4.

[81] Lee SS, Sherman M. Pilot study of interferon-alpha and ribavirin treatment in patients with chronic hepatitis C and normal transaminase values. J Viral Hepat 2001;8(3):202–5.

[82] Zeuzem S, Diago M, Gane E, et al. Peginterferon alfa-2a (40 kilodaltons) and ribavirin in patients with chronic hepatitis C and normal aminotransferase levels. Gastroenterology 2004;127(6):1724–32.

[83] Jacobson IM, Gonzalez SA, Ahmed F, et al. A randomized trial of pegylated interferon al-pha-2b plus ribavirin in the retreatment of chronic hepatitis C. Am J Gastroenterol 2005;100(11):2453–62.

[84] Kaiser S, Hass H, Gregor M. Successful retreatment of peginterferon nonresponder pa-tients with chronic hepatitis C with high dose consensus interferon induction therapy [ab-stract]. Gastroenterology 2004;126:125.

[85] Shiffman ML. Retreatment of patients who do not respond to initial therapy for chronic hep-atitis C. Cleve Clin J Med 2004;71(Suppl 3):S13–6.

[86] Shiffman ML, Di Bisceglie AM, Lindsay KL, et al. Peginterferon alfa-2a and ribavirin in pa-tients with chronic hepatitis C who have failed prior treatment. Gastroenterology 2004;126(4):1015–23.

[87] Jaeckel E, Cornberg M, Wedemeyer H, et al. Treatment of acute hepatitis C with interferon alfa-2b. N Engl J Med 2001;345(20):1452–7.

[88] Gerlach JT, Diepolder HM, Zachoval R, et al. Acute hepatitis C: high rate of both sponta-neous and treatment-induced viral clearance. Gastroenterology 2003;125(1):80–8.

[89] Wedemeyer H, Jackel E, Wiegand J, et al. Whom? When? How? Another piece of evi-dence for early treatment of acute hepatitis C. Hepatology 2004;39(5):1201–3.

[90] Jonas MM. Children with hepatitis C. Hepatology 2002;36 (5)(suppl 1):S173–8.

[91] Schwimmer JB, Balistreri WF. Transmission, natural history, and treatment of hepatitis C virus infection in the pediatric population. Semin Liver Dis 2000;20(1):37–46.

[92] Vogt M, Lang T, Frosner G, et al. Prevalence and clinical outcome of hepatitis C infection in children who underwent cardiac surgery before the implementation of blood-donor screen-ing. N Engl J Med 1999;341(12):866–70.

[93] Alberti A, Benvegnu L. Management of hepatitis C. J Hepatol 2003;38(Suppl 1): S104–18.

[94] Jacobson KR, Murray K, Zellos A, et al. An analysis of published trials of interferon mono-therapy in children with chronic hepatitis C. J Pediatr Gastroenterol Nutr 2002;34(1): 52–8.

[95] Jonas MM. Treatment of chronic hepatitis C in pediatric patients. Clin Liver Dis 1999;3(4): 855–67.

[96] Jonas MM. Challenges in the treatment of hepatitis C in children. Clin Liver Dis 2001;5(4): 1063–71.

[97] Muir AJ, Bornstein JD, Killenberg PG. Peginterferon alfa-2b and ribavirin for the treatment of chronic hepatitis C in blacks and non-Hispanic whites. N Engl J Med 2004;350(22): 2265–71.

[98] Jeffers LJ, Cassidy W, Howell CD, et al. Peginterferon alfa-2a (40 kd) and ribavirin for black American patients with chronic HCV genotype 1. Hepatology 2004;39(6):1702–8.

[99] Conjeevaram HS, Fried MW, Jeffers LJ, et al. Peginterferon and ribavirin treatment in African American and Caucasian American patients with hepatitis C genotype 1. Gastroenterology, in press.

[100] Tien PC. Management and treatment of hepatitis C virus infection in HIV-infected adults: recommendations from the Veterans Affairs Hepatitis C Resource Center Program and National Hepatitis C Program Office. Am J Gastroenterol 2005;100(10):2338–54.

[101] Thomas DL. Hepatitis C and human immunodeficiency virus infection. Hepatology 2002;36 (5)(Suppl 1):S201–9.

[102] Lesens O, Deschenes M, Steben M, et al. Hepatitis C virus is related to progressive liver disease in human immunodeficiency virus-positive hemophiliacs and should be treated as an opportunistic infection. J Infect Dis 1999;179(5):1254–8.

[103] Monga HK, Rodriguez-Barradas MC, Breaux K, et al. Hepatitis C virus infection-related morbidity and mortality among patients with human immunodeficiency virus infection. Clin Infect Dis 2001;33(2):240–7.

[104] Rosenthal E, Poiree M, Pradier C, et al. Mortality due to hepatitis C-related liver disease in HIV-infected patients in France (Mortavic 2001 study). AIDS 2003;17(12):1803–9.

[105] Sulkowski MS. Hepatitis C virus infection in HIV-infected patients. Curr HIV/AIDS Rep 2004;1(3):128–35.

[106] Tedaldi EM, Baker RK, Moorman AC, et al. Influence of coinfection with hepatitis C virus on morbidity and mortality due to human immunodeficiency virus infection in the era of highly active antiretroviral therapy. Clin Infect Dis 2003;36(3):363–7.

[107] Carrat F, Bani-Sadr F, Pol S, et al. Pegylated interferon alfa-2b vs standard interferon alfa-2b, plus ribavirin, for chronic hepatitis C in HIV-infected patients: a randomized controlled trial. JAMA 2004;292(23):2839–48.

[108] Chung RT, Andersen J, Volberding P, et al. Peginterferon alfa-2a plus ribavirin versus interferon alfa-2a plus ribavirin for chronic hepatitis C in HIV-coinfected persons. N Engl J Med 2004;351(5):451–9.

[109] Laguno M, Murillas J, Blanco JL, et al. Peginterferon alfa-2b plus ribavirin compared with interferon alfa-2b plus ribavirin for treatment of HIV/HCV co-infected patients. AIDS 2004;18(13):F27–36.

[110] Torriani FJ, Rodriguez-Torres M, Rockstroh JK, et al. Peginterferon alfa-2a plus ribavirin for chronic hepatitis C virus infection in HIV-infected patients. N Engl J Med 2004;351(5): 438–50.

[111] Chan TM, Lok AS, Cheng IK, et al. Chronic hepatitis C after renal transplantation. Treatment with alpha-interferon. Transplantation 1993;56(5):1095–8.

[112] Gentil MA, Rocha JL, Rodriguez-Algarra G, et al. Impaired kidney transplant survival in patients with antibodies to hepatitis C virus. Nephrol Dial Transplant 1999;14(10): 2455–60.

[113] Rostaing L, Modesto A, Baron E, et al. Acute renal failure in kidney transplant patients treated with interferon alpha 2b for chronic hepatitis C. Nephron 1996;74(3):512–6.

[114] Martin P, Fabrizi F. Treatment of chronic hepatitis C infection in patients with renal failure. Clin Gastroenterol Hepatol 2005;3 (10)(Suppl 2):S113–7.

[115] Strader DB. Understudied populations with hepatitis C. Hepatology 2002;36 (5)(suppl 1)S226–36.

[116] Bruchfeld A, Stahle L, Andersson J, et al. Ribavirin treatment in dialysis patients with chronic hepatitis C virus infection–a pilot study. J Viral Hepat 2001;8(4):287–92.

[117] Sterling RK, Bralow S. Extrahepatic manifestations of hepatitis C virus. Curr Gastroenterol Rep 2006;8(1):53–9.

[118] Alri L, Duffaut M, Selves J, et al. Maintenance therapy with gradual reduction of the inter-
      feron dose over one year improves histological response in patients with chronic hepatitis
      C with biochemical response: results of a randomized trial. J Hepatol 2001;35(2):272–8.
[119] Gane E. The natural history and outcome of liver transplantation in hepatitis C virus-in-
      fected recipients. Liver Transpl 2003;9(11):S28–34.
[120] Gane EJ, Portmann BC, Naoumov NV, et al. Long-term outcome of hepatitis C infection af-
      ter liver transplantation. N Engl J Med 1996;334(13):815–20.
[121] Forman LM, Lewis JD, Berlin JA, et al. The association between hepatitis C infection and
      survival after orthotopic liver transplantation. Gastroenterology 2002;122(4):889–96.
[122] Roche B, Samuel D. Treatment of hepatitis B and C after liver transplantation. Part 2, hep-
      atitis C. Transpl Int 2005;17(12):759–66.
[123] Braun M, Vierling JM. The clinical and immunologic impact of using interferon and ribavi-
      rin in the immunosuppressed host. Liver Transpl 2003;9(11):S79–89.
[124] Khokhar N. Treatment of interferon non-responsive chronic hepatitis C with triple therapy
      with interferon, ribavirin, and amantidine can be encouraging. Gut 2004;53(3):468–9.
[125] Jubin R, Murray MG, Howe AY, et al. Amantadine and rimantadine have no direct inhib-
      itory effects against hepatitis C viral protease, helicase, ATPase, polymerase, and internal
      ribosomal entry site-mediated translation. J Infect Dis 2000;181(1):331–4.
[126] Younossi ZM, Perrillo RP. The roles of amantadine, rimantadine, ursodeoxycholic acid,
      and NSAIDs, alone or in combination with alpha interferons, in the treatment of chronic
      hepatitis C. Semin Liver Dis 1999;19(Suppl 1):95–102.
[127] Rustgi VK. Thymalfasin for the treatment of chronic hepatitis C infection. Expert Rev Anti
      Infect Ther 2005;3(6):885–92.
[128] Huber R, Futter I, Ludtke R. Oral silymarin for chronic hepatitis C—a retrospective analysis
      comparing three dose regimens. Eur J Med Res 2005;10(2):68–70.
[129] Hinrichsen H, Benhamou Y, Wedemeyer H, et al. Short-term antiviral efficacy of BILN
      2061, a hepatitis C virus serine protease inhibitor, in hepatitis C genotype 1 patients. Gas-
      troenterology 2004;127(5):1347–55.

Gastroenterol Clin N Am 35 (2006) 487–505

GASTROENTEROLOGY CLINICS
OF NORTH AMERICA

HIV-Related Liver Disease: Infections Versus Drugs

Homayon Sidiq, MD[a], Victor Ankoma-Sey, MD[b,c,*]

[a]St. Luke's Episcopal Hospital Center for Liver Disease, 6620 Main St. 15051, Houston, TX 77301, USA
[b]Department of Medicine, University of Texas Medical School, 6431 Fannin Street, Houston, TX 77030, USA
[c]Liver Associates of Texas, P.A., 6410 Fannin Street, Suite 225, Houston, TX 77030, USA

HEPATITIS C AND HIV

Introduction

Hepatitis C virus (HCV) infection has emerged as a significant health concern in HIV- infected subjects. It is well established that the introduction of highly active antiretroviral therapy (HAART) in the mid 1990s has resulted in a dramatic decline in mortality in the patient who has AIDS, and has extended the life expectancy by at least 10 years [1]. This improvement in patient survival has resulted in the emergence of HCV as an opportunistic infection in patients who have HIV. In addition to HIV and HCV infection being major health issues, there are many other important similarities between the two. Both viruses possess a single-strand RNA genome and result in a subclinical chronic infection. Both are evasive against the host's immune system because of high genetic variability and resistance to eradication through the use of current available therapies. Furthermore, the replication rate of each virus is on the order of billion virions per day.

Impact of Hepatitis C Virus in the HIV-Infected Population

Mortality and morbidity are increased in HIV-infected patients who have chronic HCV infection [2]. A 5-year study of an HIV-infected cohort in Canada during the HAART era found an increased mortality in HIV/HCV-coinfected patients compared with HIV-monoinfected patients, with a mortality of 6.7 versus 2.3 per 100 person-years (risk ratio, 11.7; $P = .05$). Patients who had HIV and HCV coinfection had more hospitalizations as compared with HCV-negative patients who had HIV (15.0 versus 6.8 per 100 person-years) [3]. Coinfection with HCV may limit life expectancy because it can lead to serious liver disease, including decompensated liver cirrhosis and hepatocellular

*Corresponding author. Liver Associates of Texas, P.A., 6410 Fannin Street, Suite 225, Houston, TX 77030. E-mail address: akobot@aol.com (V. Ankoma-Sey).

0889-8553/06/$ – see front matter
doi:10.1016/j.gtc.2006.05.001

carcinoma (HCC) [4]. A decline in mortality from all causes from 2.0% to 0.9% was seen in a large French cohort study of more than 17,000 HIV-infected outpatients that compared mortality in 1995 (pre-HAART) with 1997 (HAART era). Deaths that were related to cirrhosis or HCC increased from 6.5% to 10% of all deaths, however [5]. Liver disease now accounts for greater than 50% of the deaths among patients with a CD4 count of greater than 200 cells/mL or an undetectable HIV viral load in some studies [6,7].

Prevalence and Transmission

The prevalence of HCV infection in HIV-infected individuals shows a wide variation that depends largely on the mode of transmission of HIV itself. The risk for transmission is higher in patients who acquire HIV infection through the parenteral route as compared with the sexual mode of transmission. Of the one million HIV-infected individuals in the United States, up to 30% are coinfected with HCV [4,8]. Prevalence rates (HIV/HCV coinfection) of 70% to 90% were reported in persons with increased blood exposure, such as intravenous drug use and hemophiliacs [9–12]. In a Spanish cohort of 4709 HIV-infected subjects, the prevalence of HCV coinfection was 95% in intravenous drug users, and 11% in men who had sex with men [13]. In two large United States HIV trials, the overall rate of HIV/HCV-coinfection was 16% [14]. The risk for HCV vertical transmission is higher in infants who are born to HIV coinfected mothers [15]. The prevalence of HIV infection in patients who have chronic HCV was reported among HCV-positive United States veterans in the New York City metropolitan area; the overall rate of HIV infection was 25%, with a higher rate in New York City (29%) than in the suburbs (8.7%) [16].

Screening

Current guidelines recommend that all HIV-infected individuals be screened for HCV antibodies by enzyme-linked immunosorbent assay [9,10]. More than 85% of patients who are positive for anti-HCV antibody show detectable RNA compared with 75% in the HIV-negative setting [17]. HCV antibody–negative patients with repeatedly elevated aminotransferases of unclear cause should be tested for HCV RNA, because this false negative result could be a result of seroreversion [18–20].

Natural History of Hepatitis C Virus in HIV-Infected Individuals

The natural history of HCV varies by HIV status. Levels of HCV RNA are significantly higher in HIV/HCV-coinfected patients than in HCV infection alone, in plasma and liver tissue [4,18,21,22]. HCV also might replicate in lymphoid cells; however, the issue of extrahepatic replication remains controversial [2].

In the pre-HAART era, several studies showed that HIV/HCV coinfection had a negative impact on HCV-induced liver disease [2]. Patients who were coinfected with HIV/HCV had a higher rate of fibrosis progression with more rapid progression to cirrhosis, and a higher prevalence of advanced fibrosis and cirrhosis [23–27]. Additionally, mortality related to liver disease is higher in HIV/HCV-coinfected patients than in HCV-monoinfected patients [28]. The development of decompensation was faster in HIV/HCV coinfection than in HCV monoinfection: 50% versus 13% at 2 years and 70% versus 40% at 5 years ($P = .005$) [29]. Factors that were related to more rapid HCV-related fibrosis progression were HIV coinfection, low $CD4^+$ cell count, alcohol abuse, and older age at initial HCV infection [4]. Liver disease develops after 10 years in HIV/HCV-coinfected patients compared with 15 to 20 years in subjects who are infected by HCV only [23,28,30,31]. In the HAART era, two studies showed slower fibrosis progression in patients who were treated with HAART compared with patients who did not receive HAART [32].

Impact of Hepatitis C Virus Infection on the Course of HIV Disease

The effect of HCV coinfection on HIV disease progression is controversial. Studies show conflicting results, with most data showing no effect; however, some data indicate that HCV may increase the progression of HIV disease [4,33–36]. Two European studies found a more rapid progression of HIV-related disease in HIV/HCV-coinfected subjects [2].

Treatment of Chronic Hepatitis C in HIV/Hepatitis C Virus–Coinfected Patients

The primary goal of HCV treatment in HCV monoinfection is the permanent clearance of the virus or sustained viral response (SVR), defined as undetectable HCV RNA 6 months after the end of therapy. Viral clearance is maintained in greater than 98% of patients after SVR [37,38]. SVR has a lasting impact on HCV-induced liver disease, and prevents clinical complications from liver disease and liver-related death [39,40]. Liver inflammation resolves and HCV-induced liver fibrosis regresses to a mild level or may resolve completely over a 5- to 10-year period [41,42]. Treatment with pegylated (PEG) interferon (IFN) and ribavirin (RBV) is the standard for HCV with response rates of up to 52% for genotype 1 and between 76% and 82% for genotypes 2 and 3 in HCV-monoinfected patients [43–45]. Even in the absence of sustained clearance of HCV in HCV-monoinfected patients, IFN-based therapy can slow the progression of liver fibrosis and may reduce the risk for progression to liver decompensation or HCC [46–49].

Important insights into the effectiveness and toxicity of HCV therapy in HIV/HCV-coinfected patients are provided by two randomized controlled trials that used standard IFN-2b plus RBV and four trials with PEG IFN plus RBV (two with PEG IFN-2a and two with PEG IFN-2b) in 2004.

Interferon-2b Monotherapy

An SVR rate of 23% was seen in an uncontrolled study of monotherapy with standard IFN-2b, 3 million IU (MIU) three times weekly for 12 months, in 80 HIV/HCV-coinfected patients. This was similar to the SVR rate of 26% in 27 HCV-monoinfected patients ($P = .72$) [50].

The AIDS Pegasys Ribavirin International Co-Infection Trial is the largest randomized controlled trial in HIV/HCV-coinfected patients. It assigned 868 patients from 19 countries to receive 48 weeks of 40-kd PEG IFN-2a, 180 μg weekly plus 800 mg/d; PEG IFN-2a plus placebo; or IFN-2a, 3 million IU (MIU) three times weekly, plus RBV, 800 mg/d [51]. The overall SVR was 40% for PEG IFN-2a plus RBV, and was significantly higher than the rate of 20% with PEG IFN-2a monotherapy and 12% with IFN-2a plus RBV (P < .001 for each comparison) [51].

Adult AIDS Clinical Trials Group study A5071 [52] randomly assigned 133 HIV/HCV-coinfected patients to treatment for 48 weeks with PEG IFN-2a, 180 μg weekly, plus RBV, escalating from 600 to 1000 mg/d as tolerated, or standard IFN-2a, 3 MIU three times per week (6 MIU in the first 12 weeks), with the same dosage of RBV. The primary end point was week 24 viral response. Week 24 viral response was better in the group that received PEG IFN (44% versus 15%; P < .001). The SVR of all patients also was superior in this group (27% versus 12%; P = .03), but when stratified by HCV genotype, the differences did not reach significance because of the small sample size (genotype 1, 14% versus 7%; genotype non-1, 73% versus 33%).

RIBAVIC [53], a large French randomized controlled trial of 412 HIV/HCV-coinfected patients, compared 48 weeks of 12-kd PEG IFN-2b, 1.5 μg/kg/wk, with standard IFN-2b, 3 MIU three times weekly, each in combination with RBV, 800 mg/d. The overall SVR rate was significantly better in the group that received PEG IFN-2b plus RBV (27% versus 20%; P = .047); however, PEG IFN-2b therapy was only superior to standard IFN-2b (each with RBV) in genotype 1 or 4 (17% versus 6%; P = .01), but not in genotypes 2 and 3 (44% versus 43%; P = .88).

A randomized controlled trial at the University of Barcelona [54] assigned patients to receive PEG IFN-2b, 100 μg (weight <75 kg) to 150 μg (75 kg) once weekly, or standard IFN-2b, 3 MIU three times per week, each with RBV, 1200 mg/d (patient weight >75 kg), 1000 mg/d (weight 60–74.9 kg), and 800 mg/d (weight <60 kg). The arm that received PEG IFN-2b plus RBV had a significantly higher SVR in genotypes 1 and 4 (38% versus 7%; P = .03), but there was no difference in the SVR rates in genotypes 2 and 3 (53% versus 47%; P = .73).

Although these randomized studies clearly show the superior efficacy of PEG IFN plus RBV over standard IFN plus RBV in coinfected patients, it is unclear whether one PEG IFN product is better than the other in combination with RBV. Similarly, there is a general notion that SVR rates to PEG IFN plus RBV are lower in HIV/HCV-coinfected patients than in HCV-monoinfected individuals; however, it is not certain whether this is really the case. Most HCV monoinfection studies used higher RBV doses of 1000 to 1200 mg/d, compared with 800 mg/d in HIV/HCV-coinfection trials, and the patient profiles are different from the coinfection trials. Until more information is available, HIV/HCV-coinfected patients can be advised that therapy with PEG IFN plus RBV is safe and effective, but that a direct comparison with this treatment and HCV monoinfection has not been performed [2]. The consensus for treatment of HIV/HCV coinfected individuals is to treat when HIV disease is stable, and preferably before HAART treatment.

Hepatocellular Carcinoma

HCC occurs at a younger age in HIV-infected patients compared with HIV-negative persons. In the HIV/HCV-coinfected group, which makes up most HIV patients who are diagnosed with HCC, progression from initial HCV infection to HCC is more rapid than in HIV-negative patients. This accelerated development of HCC is likely to be due to a more rapid progression to cirrhosis in the setting of HIV/HCV coinfection compared with HCV monoinfection. Furthermore, survival of HCC is decreased in HIV-positive patients, at least when they have ongoing HIV viremia [23–26].

HIV AND HEPATITIS B

Hepatitis B virus (HBV) is the world's leading cause of chronic liver disease, including cirrhosis and HCC [55,56]. Coinfection with HBV and HIV-1 is common because of the shared mode of transmission [57]. Data indicate a wide range of coinfection prevalence (7%–70%) in patients who are infected with HIV [58,59]. An increasing incidence of HBV is seen among injection drug users, individuals with multiple sexual partners, and male homosexuals [60]. Individuals who are coinfected with HIV1 and HBV, especially those with low CD4$^+$ nadir counts, are at an increased risk for liver-related mortality [61]. Vaccination rates in high-risk populations remain low, despite an available and effective vaccine for HBV infection [60,62].

Natural History of Hepatitis B Virus/HIV Coinfection

When HBV infection occurs in HIV-negative, immunocompetent adults, up to 95% mount an immune response, which clears hepatitis B surface antigen (HBsAg) and HBV DNA from circulation. Of the 5% of individuals who develop chronic HBV infection, approximately 20% progress to cirrhosis within 1 to 13 years [63]. The effect of HIV on the natural history of HBV in the pre-HAART era demonstrated that individuals who were infected with HIV were more likely to become chronic carriers of HBV than were those who did not have HIV. The ability to clear HBsAg is dependent upon the CD4$^+$ count [64]. The natural history of HIV and HBV has been altered with the advent of HAART. There is evidence to suggest that the reconstituted immune system itself can cause an initial flare of transferase levels, as a result of the onset of a strong cytotoxic T-lymphocyte response [64]. Lamivudine, often administered as a component of HAART for HIV, is highly inhibitory of HBV and can lead to reductions in HBV DNA and HBeAg and normalization of aminotransferase levels in HBV-infected patients [65–68].

Screening and Diagnosis

The Centers for Disease Control and Prevention recommends screening for HBV in all HIV-infected individuals. Current guidelines recommend testing for HBsAg, antibody against core (anti-HBc), and anti hepatitis B antibody (anti-HBs) [69]. These three serologic markers identify most persons with pre-vious exposure to HBV, including those who have chronic infection. Subjects who are negative for all three markers are candidates for vaccination.

HBV DNA in the liver or serum, with the absence of HBsAg, represents oc-cult hepatitis B infection. Anti-HBc alone has been identified as a predictive marker of occult HBV infection. Several studies have shown that the preva-lence of anti-HBc alone is greater in HIV-infected individuals than in HIV-negative persons, although the prevalence and clinical significance of this phenomenon remain controversial [70–74]. The clinical implications of occult HBV infection remain undetermined. This infection pattern has been impli-cated in significant liver pathology that leads to HCC, and it has been identified as the causative agent in HBV transmission by way of liver transplantation and blood donation [75–82].

Treatment

Treatment of HBV in the setting of HIV coinfection is complex, with guide-lines from the major organizations differing in terms of patient selection for ini-tiation of intervention and the role and timing of liver biopsy. The goals of treatment intervention are to prevent disease progression, reduce morbidity and mortality, and reduce the risk for development of HCC. Most experts agree that alanine aminotransferase (ALT) levels that are greater than two times the upper limit of normal require treatment. Some would treat at lower levels based on viral activity and histologic status. Treatment algorithms use a combination of ALT and HBV DNA levels, because HBV DNA levels of greater than 10^5 copies/mL are significantly more likely to be associated with progressive injury than are lower HBV DNA titers. Patients with ALT values of more than two times the upper normal limit and with HBV DNA levels of more than 10^5 copies/mL are candidates for treatment. Liver biopsy before ini-tiation of treatment may not be required in these patients. For individuals with normal ALT levels, values of less than two times the upper limit of normal or lower HBV DNA levels, a liver biopsy to evaluate histologic activity, and the degree of fibrosis may provide useful information before starting therapy.

Vaccination for hepatitis A virus should be done in patients who have chronic HBV infection if antibodies from natural infection are not present. A work-up to determine other liver diseases should be undertaken. Patients should be counseled to avoid alcohol and chronic acetaminophen in high dos-ages (>2–4 g/d). Screening for HCC with α-fetoprotein levels twice yearly and liver imaging once a year should be undertaken.

Four drugs are approved for the treatment of chronic HBV infection: IFN-α, lamivudine, adefovir dipivoxil, and entecavir. Other drugs that are used against HIV (eg, tenofovir and emticitabine) or HCV (PEG IFN-α) have been shown to have anti-HBV activity. Although not approved for use against HBV, these drugs are used often in HIV-infected patients.

HBV response to IFN-α in HBV/HIV-coinfected patients is lower when com-pared with HIV-negative individuals [83,84], with anti-Hbe seroconversion occurring in around 10% of cases, and becoming even lower in the absence of control of HIV replication [85]. The response to treatment with IFN-α is worse when HCV or hepatitis D virus infection is present. HIV-positive individuals with chronic HBV coinfection have substantially lower aminotransferase levels, which is an unfavorable predictor of response to IFN-α [85,86]. Reasons for the lower response to IFN-α that is seen in HBV/HIV-coinfected patients include low CD4 cell counts, low aminotransferase levels, and frequent HCV coinfection [87].

Recent data suggest that PEG IFN products are highly effective against a variety of outcome measures in HBV-monoinfected subjects. No prospective, randomized controlled trials have been conducted in HBV/HIV-coinfected cohorts [88].

Lamivudine is a cytosine analog with anti-HIV and anti-HBV activity, which inhibits HBV replication in up to 86% of HBV/HIV-coinfected patients [24]. It is tolerated well by patients, but exhibits a high degree of mutational emergence that leads to drug resistance [88]. The emergence of lamivudine-resistant virus, in the setting of immune reconstitution, can be associated with the development of an acute hepatitis B flare, significant morbidity, and even death [89,90].

Adefovir dipivoxil, a nucleoside analog, was safe and well tolerated in patients who already had experienced lamivudine resistance breakthrough. It significantly reduced HBV viral load from baseline levels [91]. Subsequent studies did not find evidence of expected or unexpected mutations in HIV reverse transcriptase resistance profiles [92].

Tenofovir disoproxil fumarate is a nucleotide analog that exhibits significant activity against HBV and HIV. Much of the data for use in HBV infection is derived from studies of HIV/HBV-coinfected patients [60]. In a pilot study, patients who received tenofovir for lamivudine-resistant HBV had a more profound suppression of HBV DNA at week 48 than did those who received adefovir [93].

Entecavir is the newest nucleoside analog. It has no activity against HIV [88]. It is tolerated well and is highly effective in promoting rapid multilog decreases in HBV DNA in HBV-monoinfected subjects [94,95].

HEPATOTOXICITY OF ANTIRETROVIRAL DRUGS

Anti-HIV medications that are used to control the reproduction of the virus and to slow the progression of HIV-related disease are implicated in hepatotoxicity. HAART is the recommended treatment for HIV infection. HAART combines three or more anti-HIV medications in a daily regimen. Current HAART medications fall into four classes: nonnucleoside reverse transcriptase inhibitors (NNRTIs), nucleoside reverse transcriptase inhibitors (NRTIs), protease inhibitors (PIs), and fusion inhibitors.

There has been a decline in HIV mortality since the availability of HAART [96]. Studies have shown higher proportions of deaths that are attributable to non–HIV-related conditions (eg, liver failure) [7,97–99].

Patients who have HIV should undergo a complete clinical and laboratory evaluation, including liver enzyme levels and specific testing for chronic HBV and HCV infection before starting antiretroviral therapy. Patients who have hepatitis B and C and unexplained hypertransaminasemia may require further investigation with a liver biopsy. After initiation of HAART, liver enzyme tests should be repeated within 2 to 4 weeks and then measured routinely as part of the quarterly clinical assessment that is recommended for all HIV-infected patients on HAART [100,101]. Drug-related hypersensitivity syndrome should be suspected if liver enzymes are elevated within the first 4 to 6 weeks of therapy along with fever, rash, malaise, and peripheral eosinophilia [100,102,103]. This should prompt the immediate and permanent discontinuation of all antiretroviral agents, because delayed withdrawal and rechallenge after initial clinical improvement has been associated with increased morbidity [100,101,104].

The presence or treatment of viral hepatitis (HBV, HCV), opportunistic infections, alcoholism, or the use of various intravenous or other recreational drugs can affect liver disease adversely [105,106]. Chronic HCV infection is associated with 2.8-fold greater risk for hepatotoxicity with the use of HAART [107]. The mechanism of drug-related toxicity in patients who have chronic viral hepatitis is not known; it may be due to enhanced HCV replication and CD8 cell activity during HAART-associated immune reconstitution [108–112].

Although most cases involve asymptomatic elevation of liver enzymes [105], every class of anti-HIV drug class has been associated with major toxic effects that can compromise quality of life significantly, and, in some cases, jeopardize survival. The risk for hepatotoxicity of antiretroviral drugs is between 3% and 12%, depending on the therapeutic agent [113]. Major long-term liver-related toxic effects that are associated with antiretroviral therapy include hepatitis, hepatic steatosis, liver failure, lactic acidosis, and insulin resistance [114]. Mechanisms of liver toxicity are listed in Box 1 and Table 1.

Nucleoside Analog–Associated Mitochondrial Toxicity

Nucleoside analog–associated mitochondrial toxicity is a major source of concern during HAART in patients who have HIV. Mitochondrial toxicity is induced by the effects of nucleoside analogs on mitochondria through their inhibition of mitochondrial DNA polymerase gamma, the mitochondrial enzyme that is necessary for mitochondrial replication [113]. Inhibition of replication leads to decreased mitochondrial gene transcription that results in reduced respiratory chain enzyme activity [115–118]. This disturbed $NADH^+/NAD^+$ equilibrium results in decreased ATP production, which leads to accumulation

---

Box 1: Mechanisms of liver toxicity

Direct toxicity

Hypersensitivity reactions

Mitochondrial toxicity

Metabolic abnormalities

Immune reconstitution in HCV/HBV-infected patients

Table 1
Liver toxicity of commonly used anti-HIV medications

Drug type	Drug name	Pattern of liver injury	Comments
Protease inhibitors	Indinavir Saquinavir Nelfinavir Ritonavir	Hepatocellular, distinct histologic pattern, including hepatocyte ballooning, Kupffer cell activation, and pericellular zone 3 fibrosis	<10% of patients have transaminases greater than five times the upper limit of normal. Indinavir increases indirect bilirubin in 10% of patients, resembling Gilbert's syndrome. Ritonavir inhibits P450.
NRTIs	ddC d4T ddl AZT	Microvesicular Steatosis	Mitochondrial toxicity (a result of enhanced pyruvate conversion to lactate), manifesting as lactic acidosis (a consequence of impaired fatty acid oxidation). Obese women are at particular risk for AZT hepatotoxicity.
NNRTIs	Nevirapine Efavirenz	Hepatocellular	Nevirapine associated with grade 4 toxicity; FDA issued an alert.

Abbreviations: AZT, zidovudine; d4T, stavudine; ddC, zalcitabine; ddl, didanosine; FDA, U.S. Food and Drug Administration.

of lactate and reactive oxygen species. This can damage mitochondrial DNA further. As a result of this impaired oxidative phosphorylation and compensatory glycolysis, alteration of lactate hemostasis occurs and fatty acids accumulate in hepatocytes [115,119,120]. Severe liver enlargement with microvesicular steatosis occurs when abnormal mitochondrial oxidation of free fatty acids results in accumulation of fat in liver cells [114,121]. Because liver is the main lactate-metabolizing organ, patients who have compromised liver function that is due to HCV infection are more vulnerable to hyperlactatemia and lactic acidosis than are those who do not have compromised liver function. Symptomatic lactic acidosis, although rare, is rapidly progressive and life threatening. Other common causes of lactic acidosis are malignancy, organ failure (particularly liver), cardiovascular disease, and diabetes mellitus. Box 2 describes the assessment of lactic acidosis in patients who have HIV. Risk factors for mitochondrial toxicity include female gender, HCV/HBV co-infection, liver disease, pregnancy, and obesity (Box 3) [105].

Lactic acidosis syndromes vary from asymptomatic mild hyperlactatemia (2.5–5 mmol/L), to chronic symptomatic hyperlactatemia (8–25.6/1000

Box 2: Assessment of lactic acidosis in patients who have HIV

Common causes and risk factors

Drugs

Obesity

Coinfection with hepatitis viruses

Advanced disease

Malignancy

Organ failure (particularly liver failure)

Cardiovascular disease

Diabetes mellitus

Pathophysiology

Mitochondrial toxicity

Riboflavin deficiency

Signs and symptoms

Nausea

Vomiting

Weakness

Abdominal pain

Diarrhea

Malaise

Anorexia

Dyspnea

Cardiac dysrhythmias, followed rapidly by progression to severe, often fatal, acidosis

Management

Discontinue antiretroviral therapy, deliver adequate oxygen to tissues, reduce oxygen demand through sedation and mechanical ventilation

Comments

It is not clear if alternative NRTIs can be given safely to patients with a history of lactic academia; abacavir may be safe.

Asymptomatic hyperlactatemia is common in patients who are receiving NRTIs. Stavudine is associated with a higher prevalence than other nucleosides.

person-years), to the most severe form with fulminant hepatitis (1.3–3.9/1000 person-years). Asymptomatic mild hyperlactatemia is a common finding in patients who take certain NRTIs and is of unknown clinical significance [115]. The fulminant subtype presents with nausea, vomiting, abdominal pain, acidosis, and hepatic and renal dysfunction. Mortality of 40% to 50% has been associated with fulminant hepatitis in this setting [120,122].

Box 3: Risk factors for lactic acidosis that are not associated with nucleoside reverse transcriptase inhibitors

Obesity

Coinfection with hepatitis viruses

Advanced HIV infection

NRTIs have variable impact on lactic acid production. A review suggested that the drugs should be ranked in the following order from the greatest to the least effects on inhibition of mitochondrial DNA polymerase gamma: zalcitabine, didanosine, stavudine, lamivudine, zidovudine, abacavir [123]. Lactic acidosis may occur suddenly, after months, or even years, of NRTI treatment [124,125]. Reports suggest that the incidence of HAART-related lactic acidosis with hepatic steatosis, although still low, is increasing; unfortunately, the exact prevalence cannot be determined because many cases are not reported to the US Food and Drug Administration (FDA) as adverse drug reactions [126].

Antiretroviral Therapy Containing HIV-1 Protease Inhibitors

PIs (see Table 2) are peptidomimetic molecules that target the active site of HIV-1 aspartic protease, the enzyme that is responsible for cleaving the precursor viral polyprotein, gag-pol, into its constituent proteins, which include reverse transcriptase. Inhibition of the cleavage of the viral polyprotein results in the formation of immature noninfectious viral particles [127]. PIs are metabolized in the liver by the cytochrome P450 3A4 enzyme system. It is likely that hepatic impairment may affect the metabolism of these agents by P450 cytochromes, although few studies have evaluated the clinical pharmacology of PIs in patients who have chronic liver disease. Of the currently available HIV-1 protease inhibitors in the United States (Box 4), prescribing information for amprenavir and indinavir provide recommendations for dosage reduction in the setting of significant liver disease [128].

Significant drug–drug interactions may contribute to hepatotoxicity by increasing the plasma concentration of other drugs that are metabolized by the P450 system given that some PIs are potent inhibitors or inducers of cytochrome P450 isoenzymes [129].

The pathogenesis of PI-associated liver injury is not known [101]. Liver injuries that are associated with protease inhibitors have been characterized poorly. The first case of acute liver failure after exposure to the PI ritonavir was reported in 1998 [130]. Several cases of liver toxicity that were associated with the use of indinavir and saquinavir also have been reported [100,127]. None of the studies has been able to prove the higher potential for liver toxicity of this class of drugs [131]. Well-designed studies are needed to characterize better the histopathologic nature of HAART-associated liver injury; however, such studies are difficult to conduct because liver histology would need to be examined before and during HAART-associated hepatotoxicity [100].

Box 4: Currently available HIV-1 protease inhibitors in the United States

Indinavir

Nelfinavir

Amprenavir

Ritonavir

Saquinavir

Lopinavir/ritonavir

Randomized controlled trials that were conducted for the purpose of obtaining FDA approval for PIs reported a prevalence of significant elevations in serum ALT or AST levels of between 1% and 9.5% [128,132–136]. Indinavir is associated with the development of a 2.5-fold increase in total bilirubin level in 11.9% of subjects. This does not reflect drug-induced liver injury, but rather an indinavir-mediated impairment of bilirubin uridine diphosphate–glucuronosyl-transferase activity that leads to the inhibition of bilirubin conjugation and the development of a reversible, asymptomatic hyperbilirubinemia [128,137].

Insulin resistance develops by HIV protease inhibitors and HCV infection [105]. Insulin resistance is associated with increases in visceral abdominal fat and fatty liver in HIV-seronegative persons and HIV-seropositive persons.

Nonnucleoside Reverse Transcriptase Inhibitors

NNRTIs, in general, and nevirapine, in particular, can cause hepatitis in the first 2 or 3 months of therapy, sometimes as part of a hypersensitivity reaction [138,139]. Hepatotoxicity of nevirapine may be seen with late onset, beyond the fourth month, with an increase in cumulative incidence over time. There seems to be a second mechanism through which nevirapine causes liver toxicity, which is much more common than the hypersensitivity syndrome [138,140].

SUMMARY

HIV-infected individuals have myriad causes of hepatotoxicity that range from mild hepatitis to significant liver failure with its associated morbidity and mortality, especially in the setting of chronic viral hepatitis (HCV and HBV). Immune restoration by HAART therapy can contribute liver-related toxicity in HIV-coinfected patients. Clinicians need to be aware of this problem and individualize management in this challenging clinical scenario. Avoidance of potentially hepatotoxic agents or close monitoring during treatment of HIV may prevent liver failure in patients who have HIV. Furthermore, vaccination against hepatitis A virus and HBV in nonimmune HIV individuals may prevent acquisition of hepatitis A virus and HBV infections in patients who have HIV. Finally, treatment of HIV, and, if appropriate, treatment of those who are coinfected with HCV and HBV with close monitoring, may improve the outcome of patients who have HIV and are at risk for significant hepatotoxicity during treatment from immune restoration or hypersensitivity reactions.

References

[1] Lee LM, Karon JM, Selik R, et al. Survival after AIDS diagnosis in adolescents and adults during the treatment era, United States 1984–1997. JAMA 2001;285:1308–15.

[2] Bräu N. Treatment of chronic hepatitis C in human immunodeficiency virus/hepatitis C virus-coinfected patients in the era of pegylated interferon and ribavarin. Semin Liver Dis 2005;25(1):33–51.

[3] Klein MB, Lalonde RG, Suissa S. Hepatitis C (HCV) coinfection is associated with increased morbidity and mortality among HIV-infected patients. Presented at The 8th Conference on Retroviruses and Opportunistic Infections. Chicago, February 4–8, 2001.

[4] Bräu N. Update on chronic hepatitis C in HIV/HCV-coinfected patients: viral interactions and therapy. AIDS 2003;17(16):2279–90.

[5] Cacoub P, Geffray L, Rosenthal E, et al. Mortality among human deficiency virus-infected patients with cirrhosis or hepatocellular carcinoma due to hepatitis C virus in French Departments of Internal Medicine/Infectious Diseases, in 1995 and 1997. Clin Infect Dis 2001;32:1207–14.

[6] Jain MK, Skiest DJ, Cloud JW, et al. Changes in mortality related to human immunodeficiency virus infection: comparative analysis of inpatient deaths in 1995 and in 1999–2000. Clin Infect Dis 2003;36:1030–8.

[7] Bica I, McGovern B, Dhar R, et al. Increasing mortality due to end-stage liver disease in patients with human immunodeficiency virus infection. Clin Infect Dis 2001;32:492–7.

[8] Sulkowski M, Thomas D. Hepatitis C in the HIV-infected person. Ann Intern Med 2003;138:197–207.

[9] Soriano V, Puoti M, Sulkowski M, et al. Care of patients with hepatitis C and HIV co-infection Updated recommendations from the HIV-HCV International Panel. AIDS 2004;18:1–12.

[10] Alberti A, Clumeck N, Collins S, et al. Short statement of the first European Consensus Conference on the treatment of chronic hepatitis B and C in HIV co-infected patients. J Hepatol 2005;42:615–24.

[11] Rockstroh J, Spengler U. HIV/HCV coinfection. Lancet Infect Dis 2004;4:437–44.

[12] Hagan H, Thiede H, Weiss N, et al. Sharing of drug preparation equipment as a risk factor for hepatitis C. Am J Public Health 2001;91:42–6.

[13] Roca B, Suarez I, Gonzalez J, et al. Hepatitis C virus and human immunodeficiency virus coinfection in Spain. J Infect 2003;47:117–24.

[14] Sherman KE, Rouster SD, Chung RT, et al. Hepatitis C virus prevalence among patients infected with human immunodeficiency virus: a cross-sectional analysis of the US adult AIDS Clinical Trials Group. Clin Infect Dis 2002;34:831–7.

[15] Pappalardo B. Influence of maternal human immunodeficiency (HIV) co-infection on vertical transmission of hepatitis C virus (HCV): a meta-analysis. Int J Epidemiol 2003; 32:727–34.

[16] Bräu N, Bini EJ, Shahidi A, et al. Prevalence of hepatitis C and coinfection with HIV among United States veterans in the New York City metropolitan area. Am J Gastroenterol 2002;97:2071–8.

[17] Soriano V, Martin-Carbonero L, Maida I, et al. New paradigms in the management of HIV and hepatitis C virus coinfection. Curr Opin Infect Dis 2005;18(6):550–60.

[18] Cribier B, Rey D, Schmitt C, et al. High hepatitis C viremia and impaired antibody response in patients coinfected with HIV. AIDS 1995;9:1131–6.

[19] Beld M, Penning M, van Putten M, et al. Low levels of HCV RNA in serum, plasma, and PBMCs of IDUs during long antibody-undetectable periods before seroconversion. Blood 1999;94:1183–91.

[20] George S, Gebhardt J, Klinzman D, et al. Hepatitis C viremia in HIV-infected individuals with negative HCV antibody tests. J Acquir Immun Defic Syndr 2002;31:154–62.

[21] Sherman KE, O'Brien J, Gutierrez AG, et al. Quantitative evaluation of hepatitis C virus RNA in patients with concurrent human immunodeficiency virus infections. J Clin Microbiol 1993;31:2679–82.

[22] Bonacini M, Govindarajan S, Blatt LM, et al. Patients co-infected with human immunodeficiency virus and hepatitis C virus demonstrate higher levels of hepatic HCV RNA. J Viral Hepat 1999;6:203–8.

[23] Benhamou Y, Bochet M, Di Martino V, et al. Liver fibrosis progression in human immunodeficiency virus and hepatitis C virus coinfected patients. The Multivaric Group. Hepatology 1999;30:1054–8.

[24] Mohsen AH, Easterbrook PJ, Taylor C, et al. Impact of human immunodeficiency virus (HIV) infection on the progression of liver fibrosis in hepatitis C virus infected patients. Gut 2003;52:1035–40.

[25] Martinez-Sierra C, Arizcorreta A, Diaz F, et al. Progression of chronic hepatitis C to liver fibrosis and cirrhosis in patients coinfected with hepatitis C virus and human immunodeficiency virus. Clin Infect Dis 2003;36:491–8.

[26] Poynard T, Mathurin P, Lai CL, et al. A comparison of fibrosis progression in chronic liver disease. J Hepatol 2003;38:257–65.

[27] Soto B, Sanchez-Quijano A, Rodrigo L, et al. Human immunodeficiency virus infection modifies the natural history of chronic parenterally-acquired hepatitis C with an unusually rapid progression to cirrhosis. J Hepatol 1997;26:1–5.

[28] Darby SC, Ewart DW, Giangrande PL, et al. Mortality from liver cancer and liver disease in haemophilic men and boys in UK given blood products contaminated with hepatitis C. UK Haemophilia Centre Directors' Organization. Lancet 1997;350:1425–31.

[29] Di Martino V, Ezenfis J, Tainturier MH, et al. Impact of HIV coinfection on the long-term outcome of HCV cirrhosis. Presented at The 9th Conference on Retroviruses and Opportunistic Infections. Chicago, February 4–8, 2001.

[30] Thomas DL, Astemborski J, Rai RM, et al. The natural history of hepatitis C virus infection: host, viral, and environmental factors. JAMA 2000;284:450–6.

[31] Seeff LB, Miller RN, Rabkin CS, et al. 45-year follow-up of hepatitis C virus infection in healthy young adults. Ann Intern Med 2000;132:105–11.

[32] Benhamou Y, Di Martino V, Bochet M, et al. Factors affecting liver fibrosis in human immunodeficiency virus- and hepatitis C virus-coinfected patients: impact of protease inhibitor therapy. Hepatology 2001;34:283–7.

[33] Greub G, Ledergerber B, Battegay M, et al. Clinical progression, survival, and immune recovery during antiretroviral therapy in patients with HIV-1 and hepatitis C virus coinfection: the Swiss HIV Cohort Study. Lancet 2000;356:1800–5.

[34] De Luca A, Burgarini R, Lepri AC, et al. Coinfection with hepatitis viruses and outcome of initial antiretroviral regimens in previously naïve HIV-infected subjects. Arch Interm Med 2002;162:2125–32.

[35] Sulkkowski MS, Moore RD, Metha SH, et al. Hepatitis C and progression of HIV disease. JAMA 2002;288:199–206.

[36] Rancinan C, Neau D, Saves M, et al. Is hepatitis C virus coinfection associated with survival in HIV-infected patients treated by combination antiretroviral therapy? AIDS 2002;16:1357–62.

[37] McHutchison JG, Davis GL, Esteban-Mur R, et al. Durability of sustained viral response in patients with chronic hepatitis C after treatment with interferon alfa02b alone or in combination with ribavarin [abstract]. Hepatology 2001;34:244A.

[38] Swain M, Lai MY, Shiffman ML, et al. Durability of sustained virological response (SVR) after treatment with peg interferon alfa-2a (40KD) alone or in combination with ribavarin: result of an ongoing long-term follow-up study [abstract]. Hepatology 2004;40(Suppl 1):400A–1A.

[39] Camma C, Di MV, Lo IO, et al. Long-term course of interferon-treated chronic hepatitis C. J Hepatol 1998;28:531–7.

[40] Shindo M, Ken A, Okuno T. Varying incidence of cirrhosis and hepatocellular carcinoma in patients with chronic hepatitis C responding differently to interferon therapy. Cancer 1999;85:1943–50.

[41] Lau DT, Kleiner DE, Ghany MG, et al. 10-year follow-up after interferon-alpha therapy for chronic hepatitis C. Hepatology 1998;28:1121–7.

[42] Reichard O, Glaumann H, Fryden A, et al. Long-term follow-up of chronic hepatitis C patients with sustained virological response to alpha-interferon. J Hepatol 1999;30:783–7.

[43] Manns MP, McHutchison JG, Gordon SC, et al. Peg interferon alfa-2b plus ribavarin compared with interferon alfa-2b plus ribavarin for initial treatment of chronic hepatitis C: a randomized trial. Lancet 2001;358:958–65.

[44] Fried MW, Shiffman ML, Reddy KR, et al. Peg interferon alfa-2a plus ribavarin for chronic hepatitis C virus infection. N Engl J Med 2002;347:975–82.

[45] Hadziyannis SJ, Sette H Jr, Morgan TR, et al. Peg interferon–alpha 2a and ribavarin combination therapy in chronic hepatitis C: a randomized study of treatment duration and ribavarin dose. Ann Intern Med 2004;140:346–55.

[46] Shiratori Y, Imazeki F, Moriyama M, et al. Histology improvement of fibrosis in patients with hepatitis C who have sustained response to interferon therapy. Ann Interm Med 2000;132:517–24.

[47] Nishiguchi S, Kuroki T, Nakatani S, et al. Randomized trail of effects of interferon-alpha on incidence of hepatocellular carcinoma in chronic active hepatitis C with cirrhosis. Lancet 1995;346:1051–5.

[48] Yoshida H, Shiratori Y, Morimyama M, et al. Interferon therapy reduces the risk for hepatocellular carcinoma: national surveillance program of cirrhotic and noncirrhotic patients with chronic hepatitis C in Japan. IHIT Study Group. Inhibition of Hepatocarcinogenesis by Interferon Therapy. Ann Intern Med 1999;131:174–81.

[49] Nishiguchi S, Shiomi S, Nakatani S, et al. Prevention of hepatocellular carcinoma in patients with chronic active hepatitis C and cirrhosis. Lancet 2001;357:196–7.

[50] Soriano V, Garcia-Samaniego J, Bravo R, et al. Interferon alpha for the treatment of chronic hepatitis C in patients infected with human immunodeficiency virus. Hepatitis-HIV Spanish Study Group. Clin Infect Dis 1996;23:585–91.

[51] Torriani FJ, Rodrigues-Torres M, Rockstroh JK, et al. Peg interferon alfa-2a plus ribavarin for chronic hepatitis C virus infection in HIV-infected patients. N Engl J Med 2004;351:438–50.

[52] Chung RT, Anderson J, Volberding P, et al. Peg interferon alfa-2a plus ribavarin versus interferon alfa-2a plus ribavarin for chronic hepatitis C in HIV-coinfected persons. N Engl J Med 2004;351:451–9.

[53] Carrat F, Bani-Sadr F, Pol S, et al. Pegylated interferon alfa-2a vs. standard interferon afa-2b, plus ribavarin, for chronic hepatitis C in HIV-infected patients: a randomized controlled trial. JAMA 1994;292:2839–48.

[54] Laguno M, Murillas J, Blanco JL, et al. Peg interferon alfa-2b plus ribavarin compared with interferon alfa-2b plus ribavarin for treatment of HIV/HCV co-infected patients. AIDS 2004;18:F27–36.

[55] Tsukuma H, Hiyama T, Tanaka S, et al. Risk factors for hepatocellular carcinoma among patients with chronic liver disease. N Engl J Med 1993;328:1797–801.

[56] Shi J, Zhu L, Lui S, et al. A meta-analysis of case-control studies on the combined effect of hepatitis B and C virus infections in causing hepatocellular carcinoma in China. Br J Cancer 2005;92:607–12.

[57] Thomas DL, Cannon RO, Shapiro CN, et al. Hepatitis C, hepatitis B, and human immunodeficiency virus infections among non-intravenous drug-using patients attending clinics for sexually transmitted diseases. J Infect Dis 1994;169:990–5.

[58] Law WP, Ducombe CJ, Mahanomtharit A, et al. Impact of viral hepatitis co-infection on response to antiretroviral therapy and HIV disease progression in the HIV-NAT cohort. AIDS 2004;18:1169–77.

[59] Konopnicki D, Mocroft A, de Wit S, et al. Hepatitis B and HIV: prevalence, AIDS pro-gression, response to highly active antiretroviral therapy and increased mortality in the EuroSIDA cohort. AIDS 2005;19:593–601.

[60] Scott FK, Anna SFL. Update on viral hepatitis in 2004. Curr Opin Gastroenterol 2005;21:300–7.

[61] Thio CL, Seaberg EC, Skolasky R Jr, et al. HIV-1, hepatitis B virus, and risk of liver-related mortality in the multicenter cohort study (MACS). Lancet 2002;360:1921–6.

[62] Bonacini M, Louie S, Bzowej N, et al. Survival in patients with HIV infection and viral hep-atitis B or C: a cohort study. AIDS 2004;18:2039–45.

[63] Fattovich G, Brollo L, Giustina G, et al. Natural history and prognostic factors for chronic hepatitis type B. Gut 1991;32:294–8.

[64] Bodsworth NJ, Cooper DA, Donovan B. The influence of human immunodeficiency virus type1 infection on the development of the hepatitis B virus carrier state. J Infect Dis 1991;163:1138–40.

[65] Hoff J, Bani-Sadr F, Gassin M, et al. Evaluation of chronic hepatitis B virus (HBV) infection in coinfected patients receiving lamivudine as a component of anti-human immunodeficiency virus regimens. Clin Infect Dis 2001;32:963–9.

[66] Benhamou Y, Bochet M, Thibault V, et al. Long-term incidence of hepatitis B virus re-sistance to lamivudine in human immunodeficiency virus-infected patients. Hepatology 1999;30:1302–6.

[67] Neau D, Schvoerer E, Robert D, et al. Hepatitis B exacerbation with a precore mutant virus following withdrawal of lamivudine in a human immunodeficiency virus infected patient. J Infect 2000;41:192–4.

[68] Piroth L, Grappin M, Buisson M, et al. Hepatitis B virus seroconversion in HIV-HBV coin-fected patients treated. J Acquired Immune Defic Syndr 2000;23(4):356–7.

[69] Benson CA, Kaplan JE, Masur H, et al. Treating opportunistic infections among HIV-infected adults and adolescents. MMWR Morb Mortal Wkly Rep 2004;53:54–8.

[70] Rodriguez-Mendez ML, Gonzalez-Quintela A, Aguilera A, et al. Prevalence, patterns, and course of past hepatitis B virus infection in intravenous drug users with HIV-1 infection. Am J Gastroenterol 2000;95:1316–22.

[71] Hofer M, Joller-Jemelka HI, Grob PJ, et al, for the Swiss HIV Cohort Study. Frequent chronic hepatitis B virus infection in HIV-infected patients positive for antibody to hepatitis B core antigen only. Eur J Clin Microbiol Infect Dis 1998;17:6–13.

[72] Vasquez-Vizoso F, Eiroa P, Ledo L, et al. HIV infection and isolated detection of anti-HBc. Gastroenterology 1994;106:823–4.

[73] Sanchez-Quijano A, Jauregui JI, Leal M, et al. Hepatitis B virus occult infection in subjects with persistent isolated antiHBc reactivity. J Hepatol 1993;17:288–93.

[74] Jilg W, Sieger E, Zachoval R, et al. Individuals with antibodies against hepatitis B core antigen as the only serological marker for hepatitis B infection: high percentage of carriers of hepatitis B and C virus. J Hepatol 1995;23:14–20.

[75] Mezzalani P, Quaglio G, Venturini L, et al, for the Intersert Group of Scientific Collabora-tion. The significance of the isolated anti-HBc carrier. A study of 1797 drug addicts. Recent Prog Med 1994;84:419–24.

[76] Shiota G, Oyama K, Udagawa A, et al. Occult hepatitis B virus infection in HBs antigen-negative hepatocellular carcinoma in a Japanese population: involvement of HBx and p53. J Med Virol 2000;62(2):151–15.

[77] Koyama H, Nishizawa Y, Kinoshita H, et al. Hepatocellular carcinoma with occult chronic hepatitis-hepatitis B virus as a pathogenetic factor of hepatocellular carcinoma. Osaka City Med J 1988;34:51–66.

[78] Uchida T, Shimojima S, Gotoh K, et al. Pathology of livers infected with "silent" hepatitis B virus mutant. Liver 1994;14:251–6.

[79] Takeuchi M, Fujimoto J, Niwamoto H, et al. Frequent detection of hepatitis B virus X-gene DNA in hepatocellular carcinoma and adjacent liver tissue in hepatitis B surface antigen-negative patients. Dig Dis Sci 1997;42:2264–9.

[80] Paterlini P, Poussin K, Kew M, et al. Selective accumulation of the X transcript of hepatitis B virus in patients negative for hepatitis B surface antigen with hepatocellular carcinoma. Hepatology 1995;21:313–21.

[81] Thiers V, Nakajima E, Kremsdorf D, et al. Transmission of hepatitis B from hepatitis–B-sero-negative subjects. Lancet 1988;2:1273–6.

[82] Hoofnagle JH, Seefe LB, Bales ZB, et al. Type B hepatitis after transfusion with blood containing antibody to hepatitis B core antigen. N Engl J Med 1978;298:1379–83.

[83] Puoti M, Airoldi M, Bruno R, et al. Hepatitis B virus co-infection in HIV-infected subjects. AIDS Rev 2002;4:27–35.

[84] Wong D, Cheung A, O'Rourke B, et al. Effect of alpha-interferon treatment in patients with hepatitis Be antigen-positive chronic hepatitis B. A meta-analysis. Ann Intern Med 1993;119:312–23.

[85] Di Martino V, Thevenot T, Colin JF, et al. Influence of HIV infection on the response to interferon therapy and the long-term outcome of chronic hepatitis B. Gastroenterology 2002;123:1812–22.

[86] Di Martino V, Thevenot T, Boyer N, et al. Serum alanine transaminase level is a good predictor of response to interferon therapy for chronic hepatitis B in HIV-infected patients. Hepatology 2000;31:1030.

[87] Nunez M, Soriano V. Management of patients co-infected with hepatitis B virus and HIV. Lancet Infect Dis 2005;5:374–82.

[88] Shire NJ, Sherman KE. Management of HBV/HIV-coinfected patients. Semin Liver Dis 2005;25(1):48–57.

[89] Bessesen M, Ives D, Condreay L, et al. Chronic active hepatitis B exacerbations in human immunodeficiency virus-infected patients following development of resistance to or withdrawal of lamivudine. Clin Infect Dis 1999;28:1032–5.

[90] Bonacini M, Kurz A, Locarnini S, et al. Fulminant hepatitis B due to a lamivudine-resistant mutant of HBV in a patient coinfected with HIV. Gastroenterology 2002;122:244–5.

[91] Benhamou Y, Bochet M, Thibault V, et al. Safety and efficacy of adefovir dipivoxil in patients co-infected with HIV-1 and lamivudine-resistant hepatitis B virus: an open-label pilot study. Lancet 2001;358:718–23.

[92] Delaugerre C, Marcelin AG, Thibault V, et al. Human immunodeficiency (HIV) type 1 reverse transcriptase resistance mutations in hepatitis B virus (HBV)-HIV-coinfected patients treated for HBV chronic infection once daily with 10 milligrams of adefovir dipivoxil combined with lamivudine. Antimicro Agents Chemother 2002;45:1586–8.

[93] van Bommel F, Wunsche T, Mauss S, et al. Comparison of adefovir and tenofovir in the treatment of lamivudine-resistant hepatitis B virus infection. Hepatology 2004;40:1421–5.

[94] de Man RA, Wolters LM, Nevens F, et al. Safety and efficacy of oral entecavir given for 28 days in patients with chronic hepatitis B virus infection. Hepatology 2001;34:578–82.

[95] Lai CL, Rosmawati M, Lao J, et al. Entecavir is superior to lamivudine in reducing hepatitis B virus DNA in patients with chronic hepatitis B infection. Gastroenterology 2002;123: 1831–8.

[96] Crum NF, Riffenburgh RH, Wegner S, et al. Comparisons of causes of death and mortality rates among HIV-infected persons: analysis of the pre-, early, and late HAART eras. J Acquir Defic Syndr 2006;41(2):194–200.

[97] Macias J, Melguizo I, Fernandez-Rivera FJ, et al. Mortality due to liver failure and impact on survival of hepatitis virus infections in HIV-infected patients receiving potent antiretroviral therapy. Eur J Clin Microbiol Infect Dis 2002;21:775–81.

[98] Sansone GR, Ferndale JD. Impact of HAART on causes of death of persons with late-stage AIDS. J Urban Health 2000;77:166–75.

[99] Wolfe MI, Hanson DL, Selik DL, et al. Deaths from non-AIDS-related diseases have increased as a proportion of deaths of HIV-infected persons since the advent of HAART. Presented at The Ninth Conference on Retroviruses and Opportunistic Infections. Seattle, February, 2002.

[100] Sulkowski MS. Hepatotoxicity associated wit antiretroviral therapy containing HIV-1 protease inhibitors. Semin Liver Dis 2003;23(2):183–94.

[101] Splengler U, Licherfeld M, Rockstroh JK. Antiviral drug toxicity-a challenge for hepatologist? J Hepatol 2002;36:283–94.

[102] Fagot JP, Mockenhaupt M, Bouwes-Bavinck JN, et al. Nevirpine and the risk of Stevens-Johnson syndrome or toxic epidermal necrolysis. AIDS 2001;15:1843–8.

[103] Kessler HA, Johnson J, Follansbee, et al. Abacavir expanded access program for adult patients infected with human immunodeficiency virus type1. Clin Infect Dis 2002;34:535–42.

[104] Frissen PH, de Vries J, Weigel HM, et al. Severe anaphylactic shock after rechallenge with abacavir without preceding hypersensitivity. AIDS 2001;15:289.

[105] Dieterich D. Managing antiretroviral-associated liver disease. J Acquir Immune Defic Syndr 2003;34:S34–9.

[106] Aceti A, Pasquazzi C, Zechini B, et al. The LIVERHARRT Group. Hepatotoxicity development during antiretroviral therapy containing protease inhibitors in patients with HIV: the role of hepatitis B and C virus infection. J Acquir Immune Defic Syndr 2002;29(1):41–8.

[107] Rodriguez-Rosado R, Garcia-Samaniego J, Soriano V. Hepatotoxicity after introduction of highly active antiretroviral therapy. AIDS 1998;12:1256.

[108] Rutschmann OT, Negro F, Hirschel B, et al. Impact of treatment with human immunodeficiency virus (HIV) protease inhibitors on hepatitis C viremic patients coinfected with HIV. J Infect Dis 1998;177:783–5.

[109] Vento S, Garofano T, Renzini C, et al. Enhancement of hepatitis C virus replication and liver damage in HIV-coinfected patients on antiretroviral combination therapy. AIDS 1998;12:116–7.

[110] John M, Flexman J, French MA. Hepatitis C virus-associated hepatitis following treatment of HIV-infected patients with HIV protease inhibitors: an immune restoration disease? AIDS 1998;12:2289–93.

[111] Verdon R, Vabret A, Goubin P, et al. HIV-HCV coinfection: is HIV viral load decrease associated with HCV viral load variations. Presented at the 38th Interscience Conference on Antimicrobial Agents and Chemotherapy. San Diego, September 24–27, 1998.

[112] Zylberberg H, Chaix M-L, Rabian C, et al. Tritherapy for human immunodeficiency virus infection does not modify replication of hepatitis C virus in coinfected subjects. Clin Infect Dis 1998;26:1104–6.

[113] Schiff ER, Sorrell MF, Maddrey WC. Schiff's diseases of the Liver. 9th edition. Wilkins (PA): Lippincott Williams; 2003.

[114] Powderly WG. Long-term exposure to lifelong therapies. J Acquir Immune Defic Syndr 2002;29:S28–40.

[115] Ristig M, Drechsler H, Powderly WG. Hepatic steatosis and HIV infection. AIDS Patient Care STDS 2005;19(6):356–65.

[116] Brinkman K, Kakuda TN. Mitochondrial toxicity of nucleoside analogue reverse transcriptase inhibitors: a looming obstacle for long-term antiretroviral therapy? Curr Opin Infect Dis 2000;13:5–11.

[117] Walker UA, Setzer B, Venhoff N. Increased long-term mitochondrial toxicity in combinations of nucleoside analogue reverse-transcriptase inhibitors. AIDS 2002;16:2165–73.

[118] Carr A, Miller J, Law M, et al. A syndrome of lipoatrophy, lactic academia and liver dysfunction associated with HIV nucleoside analogue therapy: contribution to protease inhibitor-related lipodystrophy syndrome. AIDS 2000;14:F25–32.

[119] Tien PC, Grunfeld C. The fatty liver in AIDS. Semin Gastrointest Dis 2002;13:47–54.

[120] Ogedegbe AE, Thomas DL, Diehl AM. Hyperlactatemia syndromes associated with HIV therapy. Lancet Infect Dis 2003;3:329–37.
[121] Johri S, Alkhuja S, Siviglia G, et al. Steatosis-lactic acidosis syndrome associated with stavudine and lamivudine therapy. AIDS 2000;14:1286–7.
[122] Coghlan ME, Sommadossi JP, Jhala NC, et al. Symptomatic lactic acidosis in hospitalized antiretroviral treated patients with human immunodeficiency virus infection: a report of 12 cases. Clin Infect Dis 2001;33:1914–21.
[123] White AJ. Mitochondrial toxicity and HIV therapy. Sex Transm Infect 2001;77:158–73.
[124] John M, Moore CB, James IR, et al. Chronic hyperlactatemia in HIV-infected patients taking antiretroviral therapy. AIDS 2001;15:717–23.
[125] Sundar K. Zidovudine-induced fatal lactic acidosis and hepatic failure in patients with acquired immunodeficiency syndrome: report of two patients and review of the literature. Crit Care Med 1997;8:1425–30.
[126] US Department of Health and Human Services and the Henry J. Kaiser Family Foundation. Guidelines for the use of antiretroviral agents in HIV-infected adults and adolescents. Available at: http://www.hivatis.org/trtdlns.html. Accessed January 2005.
[127] Flexner C. HIV-protease inhibitors. N Engl J Med 1998;338:1281–92.
[128] Crixivan® (indinavir sulfate) package insert. West Point (PA): Merck and Co., Inc; 1999.
[129] Moyle GJ, Back D. Principles and practice of HIV-protease inhibitor pharmacoenhancement. HIV Med 2001;2:105–13.
[130] Picard O, Rosmorduc O, Cabane J. Hepatotoxicity associated with Ritonavir. Ann Intern Med 1998;129(8):670–1.
[131] Nunez M. Hepatotoxicity of antiretrovirals: incidence, mechanisms and management. J Hepatol 2006;44:S132–9.
[132] Viracept® (nelfinavir mesylate) package insert. La Jolla (CA): Agouron Pharmaceuticals, Inc.; 2001.
[133] Agenerase® (amprenavir) package insert. Research Triangle Park (NC): GlaxoSmithKline, Inc.; 2002.
[134] Norvir® (ritonavir capsules) package insert. North Chicago (IL): Abbott Laboratories; 2001.
[135] Fortavase (saquinavir soft gelatin capsule) package insert. Nutley (NJ): Roche Laboratories, Inc; 2002.
[136] Kaletra™ (lopinavir/ritonavir) package insert. North Chicago (IL): Abbott Laboratories; 2002.
[137] Zucker SD, Qin X, Rouster SD, et al. Mechanism of indinavir-induced hyperbilirubinemia. Proc Natl Acad Sci U S A 2001;98:12671–6.
[138] Martinez E, Blanco JL, Arnaiz JA, et al. Hepatotoxicity in HIV-1 infected patients receiving nevirapine-containing antiretroviral therapy. AIDS 2001;15(10):1261–8.
[139] Boehringer-Ingelheim International Viramune product monograph, version 3.0. Ingelheim am Rhein, Germany: Boehringer-Ingelheim International GmbH.
[140] Bonnet F, Lawson-Ayayi S, Thibaut R, et al. A cohort study of nevirapin tolerance in clinical practice: French Aquitaine cohort, 1997–1999. Clin Infect Dis 2002;35:1231–7.

GASTROENTEROLOGY CLINICS
OF NORTH AMERICA

INDEX

Note: Page numbers of article titles are in **boldface** type.

0889-8553/06/$ – see front matter
doi:10.1016/S0889-8553(06)00047-1

Moving?

Make sure your subscription moves with you!

To notify us of your new address, find your **Clinics Account Number** (located on your mailing label above your name), and contact customer service at:

E-mail: elspcs@elsevier.com

800-654-2452 (subscribers in the U.S. & Canada)
407-345-4000 (subscribers outside of the U.S. & Canada)

Fax number: 407-363-9661

Elsevier Periodicals Customer Service
6277 Sea Harbor Drive
Orlando, FL 32887-4800

*To ensure uninterrupted delivery of your subscription, please notify us at least 4 weeks in advance of move.